# Nursing as Therapy

## SECOND EDITION

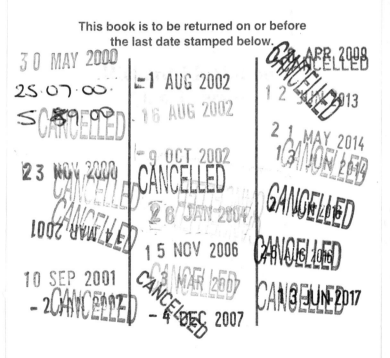

First published by Chapman and Hall in 1991.

Second edition published in 1998 by:
Stanley Thornes (Publishers) Ltd
Ellenborough House
Wellington Street
Cheltenham
GL50 1YW
UK

99  00  01  02  /  10  9  8  7  6  5  4  3  2

A catalogue record for this book is available from The British Library

ISBN 0-7487-3326-4

Typeset by The Florence Group, Stoodleigh, Devon
Printed and bound in Great Britain by
TJ International Ltd., Padstow, Cornwall

# Contents

# Contributors

**Nick Bowles**, Division of Nursing, School of Health Studies, University of Bradford, UK

**Gerald Bowman**, School of Nursing, University of Hull, UK

**Michael Clinton**, Ashford Community Hospital, Adelaide, Australia

**Steven Ersser**, Oxford Centre for Healthcare Research and Development, School of Healthcare, Oxford Brookes University, UK; visiting scholar, St John's College, Cambridge, UK

**John Field**, Department of Health Care Studies, University of New England, New South Wales, Australia

**Mary FitzGerald**, Department of Clinical Nursing, University of Adelaide, Australia

**Jillian MacGuire**, formerly at University of Wales College of Medicine, Cardiff, UK

**Christine McKee**, Division of Nursing, School of Health Studies, University of Bradford, UK

**Richard McMahon**, Northwick Park and St Mark's NHS Trust, Harrow, UK

**Sioban Nelson**, Faculty of Medicine, Melbourne University, Australia

**Nigel Northcott**, Independent Nursing Consultant and Practitioner, Oxford, UK

**Alan Pearson**, Department of Clinical Nursing, University of Adelaide, Australia

**Jean Powell**, Faculty of Health Studies, Buckinghamshire University College, Chalfont St Giles, UK

**Beverley Taylor**, School of Nursing and Health Care Practices, Southern Cross University, Lismore, Australia

**David Thompson**, Department of Health Studies, University of York, UK

**Elizabeth Tutton**, RCN Institute, Oxford, UK

**Barbara Vaughan**, King's Fund, London, UK

**Jean Watson**, Center for Human Caring, School of Nursing, University of Colorado, USA

**Stephen Wright**, European Nursing Development Agency, Mungrisdale, UK

# Preface

The first edition of *Nursing as Therapy* was published at a time of rapid change and increasing creativity in nursing. This growth in the confidence of nurses in their own professional activity coincided with the emergence of unprecedented change in the management of health care. In the UK, Australasia and North America nurses were embracing the concept of primary nursing, considering the implications of moving the preparation of nurses exclusively into higher education and experiencing the introduction of market forces into public health-care systems.

Seeing nursing as a therapeutic activity emerged as an exciting, though somewhat ethereal concept in this period of energetic development. Thus, when we published the first edition of this book, we did not envisage that it would move from being a work on the periphery of nursing literature to one that has become a regularly used text by graduates and undergraduates alike. Moreover, the concept of therapeutic nursing has found acceptance both within nursing and among other health-care professionals. The intermediate care movement in the United Kingdom clearly has the core idea of assisting patients who are out of the acute phase of their illness but in need of intensive nursing. Similarly, the development of subacute units in the United States reflects the growing acceptance of the view that, whilst the increasing sophistication of medicine can treat patients more quickly, many require intensive nursing before they are well again. Similar movements can be identified in Australia where transitional care units have been established under the leadership of nurses. In Canada and Australia, the recognition of nursing as the key to the success of managed care has placed nursing in the forefront of health-care delivery. All these developments embody elements of nursing as therapy and provide real opportunities for nurses to practise therapeutically.

With the second edition, we hope to advance the debate and the opportunities that therapeutic nursing brings. The book contains five new chapters and the original chapters have been extensively revised. We believe that the book has a greater balance between scientific and artistic thought and draws from a wider pool of international authors. It is our view that this enhances the book and provides different perspectives on the concept.

Throughout history, people have sought human caring in times of illness or vulnerability. An intuitive recognition of the therapeutic potential of caring and nursing is evident in the historical record. We hope that this expanded second edition will generate further recognition of and debate on nursing's therapeutic nature and motivate nurses and other health-care professionals to deliver care which promotes healing and celebrates the fundamental therapeutic process of nursing.

Richard McMahon
Alan Pearson

# Foreword

Jean Watson

This second edition of *Nursing as Therapy* comes at a time when the original work stands as a beacon for some of the latest thinking and challenges in current nursing and health-care practices. That is, can nursing be considered a form of therapy in and of its own, distinct from medical cure practices?

As I have increasingly become acquainted with the work and thinking related to nursing as a form of therapy, I have used Pearson, Ersser, McMahon and others, from Australia and the United Kingdom, as exemplars for some of the most modern thinking in nursing. However, in doing so, I have asked large and small audiences and classes around the world to identify and name the 'therapies' of nursing that could be considered primary and distinct forms of treatment, separate from medical treatments and medical therapeutics. What is shocking is that in almost all instances, nurses around the world have to really pause and think about nursing as a form of therapy. In many instances, the audiences cannot come up with tangible nursing practices which could be considered therapeutic in their own right. What that says to me, and to nursing itself, is that nursing is so conditioned into a nursing qua medicine definition that it requires a radical rethinking to entertain nursing itself as valued and valuable therapeutic practices.

While nursing is socialized into considering itself so connected with medical cure practices and treatment regimes, it is often inconceivable for nurses themselves to consider that what they have to offer can and does stand alone as a form of health care and, indeed, exists as a form of therapy in its own right. However, the reality is that the profession and the public alike have to rethink nursing in light of its caring, healing and health-care practices. These practices have to be seen as modalities that stand as distinct as well as complementary practices to conventional medicine.

The pressing question about nursing is posed in relation to the movement to so-called evidence-based practice for all health professionals. The question is posed in relation to the latest developments in mind-body medicine, the developments of 'alternative-complementary' practices occurring around the globe and the emphasis on 'outcome' based practices.

McMahon and Pearson have created the conceptual and pragmatic framework by which to further the work of nursing as a distinctive health profession, while sustaining nursing as complementary to medicine as it has evolved during this century. As such, their first work on *Nursing as Therapy*, and now this second edition of the work, together provide a refreshing new way to reconsider and revalue nursing practice and the arts and artistry of nursing care.

Without rethinking the significance of nursing as a form of therapy, much of its standard human caring practices can, and have been, dismissed as less than medical treatments. As a result, nursing care itself has been marginalized, de-emphasized and demeaned as tasks to be completed by anyone, threatening nursing's very existence. Without reversing the objectification and task orientation, whereby nursing is defined only by 'doing', nursing is in jeopardy of becoming extinct.

Indeed, in the shift to 'buyer's market' health-care systems in the Westernized world, nursing has been placed in an even more vulnerable position. That is, if nursing is allowed to be defined in mechanical-economic terms as a rank ordering of tasks, then of course, others can be trained to do the tasks at the least level of education and experience. However, in redefining nursing as a mature health and human caring profession, in redefining the nurse as a knowledge worker, with direct accountability to the public for its form of therapy, then nursing is not only able to sustain its own purpose for being but demonstrate its significance to society.

Further, when nursing is considered as a form of primary therapy, which balances and complements conventional medicine, then both the profession and the public can see the positive impact nursing makes when present. Moreover, when nursing is considered a form of therapy which facilitates health and healing, then both the profession and the public can witness the negative impact upon the system and society when nursing is absent.

But first, both the nursing profession and the public must redefine nursing in terms beyond the modern, industrial, production line view toward a mature professional practice that indeed makes a significant difference. McMahon and Pearson are masters at helping us both to see the difference and redefine nursing within the most contemporary discourse demanded by systems and society alike.

Within the latest turn in health care related to patient and system 'outcomes', nursing must take its mature place in this arena and demonstrate its effect on patient welfare and outcomes. As this occurs, then we must consider nursing as a form of therapy in its own right. As nursing accomplishes this important transition toward the next century, it will likewise need to be further developed and systematically practised in ways that demonstrate its efficacy and healing outcomes, regardless of the medical treatment and diagnosis demands.

While others may quarrel about definitions and theories of nursing, this work moves beyond theory to pragmatic conceptualizations of the day-to-day world and work of nursing. In doing so, it transforms our definitions and extant theories while simultaneously grounding them in practice and pointing the way to research-based outcomes that demonstrate nursing's essential aspects.

This shift toward revaluing nursing itself and demonstrating nursing as significant in its own right, separate from medicine, is all the more reason for this book. The strength of this second edition is that it not only offers some major revision and updates on the first edition, it also introduces new sections such as Beverley Taylor's work on 'ordinariness', Michael Clinton and Sioban Nelson's chapter on 'quality', Gerald Bowman and Dave Thompson's section on 'practice' and Nigel Northcott's contribution on 'the political dimension'. In addition, John Field and Mary Fitzgerald offer new insights into emerging imperatives for nursing curricula and previous authors from the first edition provide major revisions and new perspectives.

Finally, what I find the most hopeful and helpful of all about this work is the core framework that it offers: first and foremost, by shifting nursing's thinking about nursing itself and second, the timeless, insightful, wise grounding it offers to nursing as a reference for rethinking its most common, yet uncommon, everyday practices which consist of caring-healing relationships; conventional nursing care acts; expanded holistic nursing practices; teaching-learning with increasing emphasis on self-care and self-caring practices for self and others; and lastly, creating a therapeutic healing environment.

While nursing participates in all of these practice activities and processes, McMahon and Pearson are the originators of this seminal, concise, organized framework for reconsidering nursing as a primary therapy. It is through their work that the profession and the public alike can 'see' nursing in all its complexity and wholeness as distinct from, yet complementary to, conventional medicine and other health practices. It is the grasp of the whole that they captured in the original work; it is the grasp of the whole, in relation to the parts and the politics of change and progress, that is captured in the revised edition. This work ushers in new traditions to advance nursing practice and research, while serving as a foundation for transforming old traditions into timeless essentials that must be sustained, if nursing itself is to be.

# Therapeutic nursing: theory, issues and practice

1

Richard McMahon

## INTRODUCTION

Ask a group of nurses or other health workers 'Which occupations are therapists?' and they will often initially respond by mentioning physiotherapists, occupational therapists and maybe another group such as dieticians. Someone will then say doctors (of course!) and then slowly other occupations such as chiropody, psychology and dentistry will be suggested. If the same group is then asked whether pharmacists or radiographers fit into that category, the answer is normally 'no'. The group is then frequently left perplexed by the question 'What about nurses?'

The reason why the association of the concept of therapy with nursing may be baffling to some people is that the listeners compare the idea of nursing as a therapy with their experience of nursing, the stereotypes of nurses and their instinct about the concept. Some people have no hesitation in responding that nursing not only makes you feel better, but that it makes you better. However, all too often groups, including groups of nurses, express considerable doubt that nursing is therapeutic, except when undertaking therapy by proxy through carrying out the doctor's orders.

The purpose of this book is to examine in detail the therapeutic potential of nursing and to explore both the prerequisites for therapeutic practice and the contribution to health care that could be made if nurses recognized themselves to be therapists and made the contribution to care commensurate with that position.

## THE NATURE OF NURSING

It may seem somewhat banal in the late 1990s still to be exploring the question 'What is nursing?' as for 30 years the occupation as a whole seems to have been obsessed with introspection. Indeed, in 1985 Virginia Henderson, who probably provided the most quoted answer to that question, commented that:

> I don't know of any other profession that is beating its breast trying
> to say what it is and what it does. (Campbell 1985)

Yet it would seem that in the minds of many nurses, managers and the public that question is still either unanswered or based on a stereotype that has the potential for constraining nursing. This would seem not to be a new phenomenon; indeed, Nightingale (1859) commented that the word nursing '... has been limited to signify little more than the administration of medicines and the application of poultices' whereas she clearly recognized that by manipulating the environment – the air, the temperature, the food, the quality of the sanitation and so on – nurses could positively influence the outcome for patients.

It is this very idea of how nursing affects the outcome for the patient which holds the key to the nature and contribution of nursing. Nearly all the theorists since Nightingale, in one way or another, seem to have identified nursing as being separate from medicine and having a role in improving the patient's health, whether it be in terms of assisting the patient in those activities that contribute to health or its recovery (Henderson 1966), enabling patients to overcome their self-care deficits (Orem 1985) or by helping patients become independent in the activities of daily living (Roper *et al.* 1985).

Yet nurses have struggled to understand and in particular to articulate and effectively share this conceptualization of nursing with other health care workers and the public. Whilst perhaps there has been some recognition that nurses are not assistants to doctors, this conceptualization has been replaced with an idea of nursing as providing 'care' whilst others provide the 'cure'. This perceived difference between nursing and medicine, with its emphasis on 'caring' as the territory of nurses, was part of the ideological movement away from a biomedical model of nursing and is seductive. However, this in itself was not sufficient to liberate nursing and could be a contributing factor to the functional redundancy of nurses, for if a simplistic conceptualization of caring is made, it is not at all clear why expensively trained nurses are required to provide it (Levi 1980).

Caring has been interpreted by many, including nurses, to mean an activity that is predominantly maintaining the patient's hygiene, dietary and other needs: simply keeping the patient comfortable. In Britain, the concept of care being the domain of the nurse has been widely accepted.

However, the view that caring is an activity that only affects the patient's levels of comfort may have been reinforced by teaching nurses from the outset of their training the writings of Virginia Henderson, who stated:

> The physician is regarded as pre-eminent in diagnosis, prognosis and therapy . . .
>
> . . . The unique function of the nurse is to assist the individual, sick or well, in the performance of those activities contributing to health or its recovery (or a peaceful death) that he would perform unaided if he had the necessary strength, will or knowledge. And to do this in such a way as to help him gain independence as rapidly as possible. (Henderson 1969)

Whilst elements of this definition can be interpreted as identifying aspects of therapy (such as the last line), the part that seems to be most often remembered is 'assisting the individual' with its connotation of helping and doing for. This passive concept of caring suggests the maintaining or supporting of the patient's current health situation. Indeed, patients for whom all active medical intervention for a cure has been withdrawn are sometimes described as being for 'all nursing care', or the comment that a patient is for 'tender loving care' is used where the aim is comfort and little else.

The achieving of comfort is, of course, a fundamental outcome that nurses can attain for their patients (Wilson-Barnett 1984), yet comfort is not an end in itself. Instead, the provision of nursing care is a dynamic process that has the patient's health as the objective, which is demonstrated through such aspects as increased self-care ability, self-determination and coming to terms with a situation. Therapeutic nursing is about that dynamic process, which is not merely supporting the work of others but is potentially a major force for achieving health for the patient.

Whilst attempting to define nursing can be entertaining and a stimulating intellectual exercise, it is not at all clear whether it makes sufficient difference to patients to warrant the investment in effort. There is an old, unattributed definition of nursing that states that 'Nursing is what nurses do'. Whilst this is simplistic and theoretically full of holes, it is a definition to which nurses return (e.g. Castledine 1994) because of its simplicity and pragmatism. It provides no values or ideas which can in any way influence the direction of nursing practice, education or research; indeed, it is the opposite in that it is what nurses *do*, that determines what nursing *is*. As nurses' roles change, so does nursing. Thus debates about whether trained nurses who take roles acting purely as carers or in a different setting as 'mini-doctors' are in fact practising nursing become somewhat academic.

Clearly, such a definition needs to clarify what a nurse is and to identify the 'doing' in terms of health care, but the adoption of such a definition changes the agenda for those, such as the contributors to this book, who wish to influence nursing. It is only by influencing nursing practice that one can really influence nursing and it is this idea which is fundamental to understanding and practising therapeutic nursing.

## TRENDS IN NURSING

A comprehension of nursing's past is fundamental to understanding nursing today and to developing a vision of the future and how this might be achieved (Cushing 1995). For much of its history, nursing has been viewed as an adjunct to medicine in an assisting role. The way nurses thought about their work was dominated by the biomedical model which laid emphasis on the medical diagnosis and the physical tasks required to assist doctors in achieving a cure (Pearson and Vaughan 1986). For example, even 30 years ago one of the central items in the final examination for nurse registration involved the learner setting up a trolley in preparation for a medical procedure.

This division of labour between doctors and nurses arose out of a number of factors. Decisive leadership based on hard science compared to docility, sacrificing behaviour and instinct reflected the traditional stereotypical gender differences in society. This, along with the class division between doctors and nurses, has resulted in medicine being viewed hierarchically above nursing (Salvage 1985) and led Oakley to comment that 'If Florence Nightingale had trained her lady pupils in assertiveness rather than obedience, perhaps nurses would be in a different place now' (Oakley 1984). As a result of these factors, a value system emerged whereby the more experienced nurses undertook the more scientific tasks associated with medicine (giving injections, attending to machines and so on) whilst junior staff gave what was referred to as basic nursing care (helping patients to wash, feed and other activities associated with everyday living).

The biomedical model and the focusing on tasks have been major contributors to passivity in nursing. Similarly, the legacy of the asylums and the workhouses prolonged the concept of nursing as custodial care with Evers describing the care in the wards she observed as 'warehousing' (Evers 1981a,b). Alfano (1971) compared 34 nursing behaviours and attitudes that make up what she called the '"caring", task-oriented kind of practice' which focuses on caretaking, as opposed to those that characterize a professional, healing approach to practice. Unfortunately, much nursing practice up to the present day has displayed aspects of the former, rather than the latter.

The first reference to nursing as a process, as opposed to a series of tasks, has been attributed to Lydia Hall in 1955 (de la Cuesta 1983). Since then the literature on the subject has expanded, with the concepts of viewing the patient as an individual, the planning and prescribing of research-based care given by a nurse 'allocated' to that patient and the evaluation of the effectiveness of the care being explored in detail. Whilst the nursing process has been analysed and criticized (Varcoe 1996), it has embodied a number of varied concepts that have changed the way nurses work and of patients' experiences of nursing. The effectiveness of individualized care in promoting independence among the elderly was demonstrated by Miller (1985) and the key element in implementing individualized care has been shown to be the characteristics of the ward sister (Kitson 1986, Pembrey 1980). Indeed, many of the trends in nursing have affected the organization of care, rather than care itself. Following on from the introduction of the nursing process and individualized care came the introduction of nursing models, primary nursing (Ersser and Tutton 1991, Manthey 1980, Pearson 1988) and the setting up of nursing development units (Pearson 1988, 1992, Salvage and Wright 1995) with the focus on providing holistic care for patients.

At the same time external influences have led to major changes in nursing practice. The reduction in junior doctors' hours in Britain at the same time as a chronic shortage of trained nurses placed greater emphasis on the nurse being able to relieve doctors of some of their tasks, providing both a threat and an opportunity for nursing. In order to accommodate this change and to provide sufficient manpower, health-care assistants are being provided with competency-based training which increasingly leads to their taking on roles and tasks previously performed by nurses.

Finally, it is nearly three decades since Professor Briggs stated that 'Nursing should become a research based profession' (Briggs 1972) but despite the exhortations of educationists and nurse leaders, little progress has been made. However, the recent emergence of the evidence-based medicine movement has led to the government encouraging health authorities to demand clinically effective practice from the health professionals in the units from which they purchase services. The demand is for far more than research-based practice. Evidence-based practice requires that research is scrutinized for its reliability and validity, studies on the same subject to be compared and subject to combined analysis and research to be brought into practice rapidly and consistently. Nursing is having some difficulty in meeting these expectations, not least because of the dearth of research into practice.

These changes make more pressing the need for nursing to identify its therapeutic potential. Nurses have to balance the emphasis on extended roles and the development of evidence-based protocols with a multi-directional development of nursing-based practices for which qualification as a nurse is a prerequisite. Nurses are increasingly recognizing that they too are healers and facilitators who allow and empower patients to heal themselves. This role is not a new one for nurses, but they now have the means through different research methodologies to demonstrate that nursing is a dynamic force in helping patients towards health. As this evidence becomes available, nurses have a moral and professional duty to realign practice along these lines.

## THERAPEUTIC NURSING IN THEORY

### Nursing models

All the principal nursing models view health holistically and see it as the objective of nursing care. However, over time the approach to the therapeutic aspects of nursing has changed. Nightingale believed strongly that good nursing was as responsible for the cure of patients as was the administration of medical preparations. She believed that effective nursing involved the manipulation of environmental variables to put the patient in the best condition to be healed by nature. Whilst much of the emphasis was on influencing the physical environment, Nightingale also recognized the importance of the interpersonal environment; for example, she urged the nurse to keep the patient informed as 'apprehension, uncertainty, waiting, expectation, fear of surprise, do a patient more harm than any exertion' (Nightingale 1859).

Few models use the term 'therapeutic' specifically in their vocabulary, but Myra Levine makes a distinction between supportive and therapeutic nursing interventions. To Levine (1973), supportive interventions prevent further deterioration in the health status of patients who are ill, whilst therapeutic interventions are those which promote adaptation and healing and hence contribute to the restoration of health. Similarly, Hildegard Peplau emphasizes the potential therapeutic value of the nurse–patient relationship, maintaining in particular that 'The nursing process is educative and therapeutic when nurse and patient come to know and respect each other, as persons who are alike, and yet, different, as persons who share in the solution of problems' (Peplau 1952). The themes of the patient knowing the nurse as a person and of the nurse and the patient working in partnership are still receiving considerable emphasis as part of effective nursing practice.

### Therapeutic nursing

In the foreword to the first edition of this book, Lisbeth Hockey analysed the semantics of the term 'therapeutic nursing', and came to the conclusion that it can be explained as '... the practice of those nursing activities which have a healing effect or those which result in a movement towards health or wellness'. It is important to note the importance of the nurse's understanding of the relationship between her care and the effect it has on the patient. Too often, patients have got better despite their nursing care and not because of it. Therefore, therapeutic nursing can be broadly defined as nursing that deliberately leads to beneficial outcomes for the patient.

Four activities that might fall into the category described by Hockey were described by McMahon (1986), including the nurse–patient relationship, the practising of both conventional nursing interventions as well as others – such as complementary therapies – and patient teaching. A number of activities were discussed by Ersser (1988), contributing the concepts of the 'therapeutic environment' and 'providing comfort'. Muetzel (1988) provided a sophisticated model of the nurse–patient relationship as a therapeutic process, identifying the three elements of partnership, intimacy and reciprocity as the key concepts in that process. If these works are combined, a simple description of some of the therapeutic activities of nursing can be listed (Table 1.1). This is not intended to be a 'model' of therapeutic nursing – it has inconsistencies and difficulties which make it incompatible with definitions of a model – rather, it may serve as a framework for analysing some of the key concepts and issues in therapeutic nursing. However, in order to make use of this framework, it is helpful to consider the prerequisites for therapeutic practice.

**Prerequisites of therapeutic nursing**

There are a number of characteristics of the nurse that may affect the individual's ability to practise therapeutically. Many of these are discussed in greater depth in the subsequent chapters of this book, but they all depend to a greater or lesser extent on the values and critical skills such as analysis and decision-making developed by nurses during their training.

**Table 1.1** Therapeutic activities in nursing

- Developing
  - *partnership*
  - *intimacy*
  - *reciprocity*
  in the nurse–patient relationship
- Caring and comforting
- Using evidence-based physical interventions
- Teaching
- Manipulating the environment
- Adopting complementary health practices

*Holism and self-determination*

The concept of therapeutic nursing reflects an underlying belief in the concept of holism (Smuts 1926). Holism assumes that the mind and the body are inextricably linked and that an influence on one will lead to change in the other. The value of holism has been widely discussed and accepted by nurses. Levine (1971) stated that 'Human beings are more than and different from the sum of their parts' and clearly health is about the well-being of both. This is fundamental to therapeutic nursing and provides a wide frame for the assessment of the patient and understanding the causes of the patient's problems. It also clearly implies that nursing interventions should be holistic in their nature and application if they are to be effective in healing the person and their body.

It is important that the relationship between the nurse and the patient should, except under exceptional circumstances, be negotiated, with the nurse empowering the patient to take responsibility for identifying his own goals and using the nurse as a resource in regaining his own health. Hall (1969) suggests that this means helping the patient change his behaviour from that based on being ill to behaviour based on being well.

*The need to be proactive*

The subservience and custodial approach of nursing in the past has already been referred to. If nurses are to be therapeutic, it is critical that they themselves recognize that they have the ability, authority and a moral duty to intervene positively to solve patients' problems. Whilst many nurses may feel instinctively that they do this, research examining nurse-to-nurse communication has demonstrated that, on some wards at least, the nurses being observed seemed to be unaware that they were discussing problems to which nursing may have provided a solution (McMahon 1990). Under such circumstances, it is not surprising that other disciplines take on aspects of patient care in which nurses show no desire to intervene.

However, it would seem that when nurses do take decisions, they are still based primarily on experience as opposed to an explicit reliance on theory or research (Watson 1994). The knowledge base of nurses and their ability to recognize and act effectively on patients' nursing problems is determined by their basic education, the environment and the role models where they work and their ability to be reflective. All these aspects are explored at greater length elsewhere in this book.

*The ability to take risks*

Nurses who practise therapeutic nursing need strength and courage, as prescribing and administering care involves an element of risk taking for which the nurse may be called to account. Gilchrist (1987) illustrated an example of risk taking in the care of the elderly. As 23% of patients who came to his ward did so following a fall, the likelihood of further falls on the wards was high. However, this did not negate the need to rehabilitate those patients by encouraging them to mobilize independently again, even though another fall could in some cases have resulted in the further loss of functional ability or confidence to the extent that the patient could not return home.

Unfortunately, nurses are rarely taught how to take risks; indeed, due to the increasing amount of litigation against health organizations, they are encouraged to do the opposite. However, professional practice is about making decisions and taking risks and so if nurses are to be proactive, to prescribe dynamic nursing care which has an effect on patients and their families, then nurses must accept the risk of occasional failure and any consequent legal action. Carson (1988) distinguishes between a gamble (something that is done voluntarily and which has a high chance of failure), a risk (which involves weighing pros and cons) and facing a dilemma (where a decision has to be made between options which may each have benefits or the possibilities of harm). Clearly nurses should rarely gamble in patient care and when taking a risk, the patient should be included in the making of the decision.

*Professional boundaries*

Patients' problems are frequently expressed in terms that suggest that they are the property of a particular health profession: the patient's walking is the physiotherapist's problem, the patient's depression is the psychologist's problem and his angina is the doctor's problem. This reductionist division of patients' problems into disciplinary areas is a popular but problematic practice. Many health professionals reveal understandable territorial attitudes when they start to feel that nurses may in some way be encroaching into their own area of practice. Conflict can also arise from the differing expectations and theoretical frameworks inherent in different occupations. For example, the medical model may be stereotypically described as being based on the declaration of a diagnosis followed by pharmacological or surgical treatment with the goal of curing or suppressing the pathology identified. In contrast, the nurse may identify and prioritize the patient's problems in partnership with the patient, with a goal of the achievment of self-care.

In order for nurses to work in an environment in which they can maximize the potential to work therapeutically, they must explore the values and expectations of their close working colleagues in other professions.

A recognition that practice boundaries are frequently based on tradition can assist in developing a common understanding of the various contributions to care. Developing an approach that focuses on identifying problems and needs as belonging to the *patient*, as opposed to a profession, can help to overcome disharmony between health workers. These problems can then be addressed through the collaborative application of interventions by nurses, doctors or other health-care workers.

Therapeutic nursing involves achieving beneficial outcomes for the patient's problems, using interventions that acknowledge and complement the work of other therapists and with due regard for the goals and individuality of the patient.

## Therapeutic activities in nursing

Earlier in this chapter, reference was made to therapeutic activities in nursing (Table 1.1). These elements should be considered from a holistic perspective and not viewed as a series of disconnected and isolated parts.

### Developing partnership, intimacy and reciprocity in the nurse–patient relationship

There is much evidence that nurses' interactions with patients are frequently inadequate (Lyall 1990) and fail to be therapeutic. For example, Macleod-Clark (1983) demonstrated how many nurses on surgical wards failed to recognize and take any action about patients' psychological discomforts. There may be many reasons for this, which may relate more to the ward culture and nurses' own attitudes rather than levels of training (Wilkinson 1991). Hall (1969) believed that the way the nurse approached and interacted with the patient is fundamental in moving his behaviour to that which is based on being well. She supported the Rogerian method of being non-directive to allow the patient to explore his own feelings and to find solutions to his own problems (Alfano 1985). This has been succinctly described by Peplau who states that 'Self-insight operates as an essential tool and as a check in all nurse–patient relationships that are meant to be therapeutic' (Peplau 1952).

Muetzel (1988) links the three concepts of partnership, intimacy and reciprocity which she suggests come together in a therapeutic encounter between the nurse and the patient (Figure 1.1). The interaction between each pair of concepts builds three further elements of atmosphere, spirit and dynamics. For each of these, Muetzel identifies qualities that characterize that particular element. The purpose of these subconcepts is to demonstrate that it is valid for both the nurse and the patient to benefit from the relationship and that this self-awareness is a necessity for the achievement and the evaluation of a subjectively therapeutic encounter (Muetzel, personal communication 1989). It is beyond the scope of this chapter to analyse the model in detail, but each of the three primary concepts will be briefly examined.

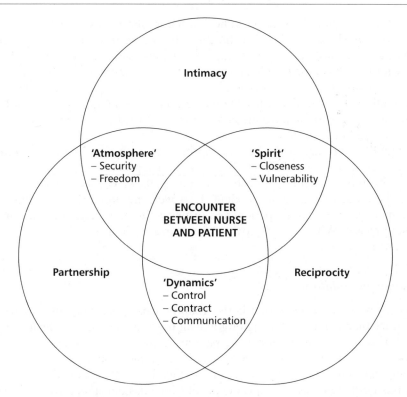

**Figure 1.1** Muetzel's model of activities and factors in the therapeutic nurse–patient relationship (adapted from Muetzel 1988).

Partnership is now well established in British nursing literature as a desirable characteristic of the nurse–patient relationship. In the late 1980s, in its *Position Paper on Nursing*, the Royal College of Nursing stated that:

> Each patient has a right to be a partner in his own care-planning and receive relevant information, support and encouragement from the nurse which will permit him to make informed choices and become involved in his own care. (RCN 1987)

As partners, both the nurse and the patient have responsibilities to and expectations of, each other.

Intimacy, like partnership, is a two-way process (Kadner 1994). In the past, the nurse was expected to maintain a relationship which did not encourage the expression of feelings by the patient or the nurse. This was justified on the grounds that it was not 'professional' to do so and that nurses could not cope with the stress that would ensue. Clearly, the nurse must have insight and security in herself before she can use intimacy safely and effectively (Jourard 1971). Indeed, Muetzel argues that the ability of the nurse to participate in a therapeutic relationship is dependent on her having first developed both as a person and as a member of the nursing team. Whilst intimacy in this context refers to an interpersonal closeness, it should be remembered that the performing of intimate physical care by nurses can provide opportunities and a level of trust that support psychological closeness.

Finally, there are elements of reciprocity in both partnership and intimacy. However, as a distinct characteristic reciprocity reflects the belief that the nurse–patient relationship may be beneficial, and indeed necessary, for the nurse as well as the patient. However, the nurse clearly needs to balance her own and the patient's priorities within the relationship against its purpose. Without reciprocity, the nurse–patient relationship lacks balance and depth.

*Caring and comforting*

As has been discussed earlier in this chapter, caring in therapeutic nursing is more than a general feeling of goodwill towards the patient which leads to no more than maintaining the patient. Campbell (1984) describes the skilled care of a professional nurse as a form of 'moderated love' or skilled companionship. The concept of caring is explored in greater depth later in this book, but it is a complex concept which has developed from caring being a duty in nursing through caring as a therapeutic relationship to caring as an ethical position in nursing (Kitson 1993). This latter development is wholly consistent with Muetzel's elements of the nurse–patient relationship.

Providing comfort may be a part and an expression of caring and has been described as one of nursing's key functions (Wilson-Barnett 1984). However, as a therapeutic activity it can be controversial. For example, it is sometimes necessary to help the patient overcome a level of necessary discomfort in order to elicit a therapeutic effect. A patient who has had hip surgery finds it more comfortable to remain in bed or in a chair than to walk, but the discomfort of the walk needs to be overcome if the patient is to regain independence. Also, it may be argued that comfort is an outcome rather than an intervention and as such is not an activity in itself.

The justification for including comforting as a therapeutic activity lies in the suspicion that activities such as giving a patient a drink, plumping their pillows or getting an extra blanket are therapeutic beyond their physical effect. Rather, it is the psychological comfort and warmth that they express in caring for another human being which epitomizes nursing and which does itself aid recovery.

*Using evidence-based physical interventions*

The body of research evidence into the efficacy of different physical interventions is expanding, yet there is evidence that even where evidence
exists, it does not find its way into practice (Gould 1986), for a variety of
reasons (Hunt 1987). However, as a proportion of nursing research
activity, studies into the effects of nursing on patients form a small
minority – about 8% according to one British study (French 1997).
Whatever the difficulties in transferring theory to practice, if research into
practice is not the main focus of nursing research it is difficult to imagine
how nurses can consistently deliver care which is therapeutic.

It may be that the imperative to provide therapeutic nursing will lead
to a change in current emphasis where nurse researchers beseech practitioners to modify practice as a result of their work. Instead, practitioners
should govern the direction of knowledge development in the future.

*Teaching*

The investigation of the therapeutic effect of nurses giving information to
patients is one of the successes of nursing research. Davis (1985), having
examined much of the research into the subject of preoperative information
giving, concluded that:

> There would seem, therefore, to be a substantial body of evidence
> demonstrating that patient outcomes, related to a model of stress
> reduction involving both physiological and psychological factors, can
> be significantly influenced by nurses giving preoperative information.
> (Davis 1985)

Other studies have demonstrated the benefits of information giving in
other situations, such as prior to investigations (Wilson-Barnett 1978) and
following myocardial infarction (Thompson 1989).

However, patient teaching has a wider range of interventions than
just giving information (Wilson-Barnett 1988). Increasingly nurses are
adopting methods that involve the patient undergoing experiential
learning. For example, newly diagnosed diabetics are from an early
stage taught to test their own blood and to prepare and give their own
insulin.

One area that remains poorly covered by nurses is the health promotion aspect of educating patients, as attention to this aspect remains
extremely variable and the increasing acuity of patients in hospital, along
with poor staffing levels make this aspect of care a difficult one to fulfil
(Macleod-Clark *et al.* 1992).

*Manipulating the environment*

The creation of a therapeutic environment can be interpreted to mean the interpersonal as well as the physical environment. Actions such as the implementation of primary nursing can maximize the contact and continuity between nurse and patient and the values of the nurses will influence the quality of that contact: a ward in which the nurses take their coffee breaks in the day-room with the patients, using the same set of cups, has a different ethos to a ward where nurses find the use of patients' cups distasteful.

However, what constitutes a therapeutic physical environment requires, and is amenable to, further investigation. For example, should the bath on a care of the elderly facility be one that can be tipped and the side raised to allow easy access for a patient in a wheelchair or should it be a traditional one into which the patient has to be hoisted, as he will be at home? Clearly, knowledge of the patient's home, maybe gained by visiting it, can allow the nurse to manipulate the ward environment to simulate problems the patient will face on discharge (McMahon 1988).

*Adopting complementary health practices*

The adoption of some complementary therapies would seem to be a logical extension to traditional nursing practices as they too are founded on the concept of holism. Indeed, some nurses seem to interpret the concept of therapeutic nursing wholly in terms of adopting complementary therapies. However, as Newbeck (1986) pointed out, implementing complementary health practices without fundamental change in other aspects of care is like trying to ice an uncooked cake. Holism may be practised without necessarily adopting such therapies as massage or reflexology, but the converse is not true.

It is also clear that the research base is, for a variety of reasons, particularly weak for many of these activities. Nurses who implement complementary practices need to ensure that they have been trained to the highest level and that they have established their medicolegal position with their employer.

## THERAPEUTIC NURSING IN PRACTICE

It is easy to assume that therapeutic nursing can only take place in an environment in which nurses can practise independently as the lead professional. However, this is erroneous and is an assumption that can lead to therapeutic nursing not being practised in most of the areas where care takes place. Nurses working in almost any area have enormous potential to orchestrate beneficial outcomes for their patients, if they have the necessary skills, knowledge, attitudes, support and facilities.

The preparation of nurses to act therapeutically should be the focus of preregistration training. Luker *et al.* (1996) examined the 'fitness for purpose' of Project 2000-trained nurses and noted that although they were perceived as having a greater research awareness, they seemed to have difficulties applying it. Innovations such as courses which focus heavily on theory being taught in practice through models such as lecturer/ practitioners have not been evaluated, but it is clear that if learners are going to be therapeutic nurses, they must have the ability to find, analyse and make decisions based on evidence available. The majority of nurses in practice were trained in 'traditional' ways and managers have a challenge in empowering these nurses with the skills to identify and implement changes which make genuine and positive improvements in patients' conditions. The relationship between education and nursing as therapy is considered in greater depth later in this book.

In order to start to refocus nursing practice across an organization such as a hospital, it is necessary to have clear leadership with a strategic objective to make clinical effectiveness a reality. This means ensuring that the organization has the right educational facilities and culture, that staff have the necessary skills to access information and that individuals have the authority and ability to create change which directly influences practice to the benefit of the patient.

The organizational aspects of facilitating therapeutic practice are discussed later in this book, but it has been demonstrated that it is necessary to have sufficient trained nurses on the wards if the nursing is to be effective (Carr-Hill *et al.* 1992). However, the opportunities for providing therapeutic nursing through nurse-led services need to be fully explored.

It has taken many years for the concept of nurse-led services to become broadly understood and acceptable to nurses, managers and doctors in Britain. However, such innovations are now widely recognized as providing great opportunities for therapeutic nursing to be practised. Unfortunately, in some situations, the services that have been set up have been a simple replacing of the doctor with a nurse, rather than being nurse led in the sense of nursing being the lead therapy. In many cases, it has been a mixture of the two, with the nursing adding an enhanced quality of care which improves either the process of giving care, the outcome of the care or both.

A number of models of nurse-led care have developed.

## Nurse-led inpatient services

The inception of inpatient hospital services where nursing was seen as the central therapy was in New York at the Loeb Center, under the leadership of Lydia Hall (Hall 1969). The Loeb Center admitted patients whose need for acute medical care had passed but who needed intensive nursing in order to regain their health. The concept of such units was examined in detail by Pearson (1983) who set up the first two units in Britain at Burford and Oxford. Both of these units were subject to research into their effectiveness and both studies demonstrated direct benefits for the patients in terms of their level of independence and consequently the likelihood of them being discharged to their own homes (Pearson 1992, Pearson *et al.* 1992). Whilst the Loeb Center ceased to function as a nurse-led inpatient unit in 1984 (Griffiths 1997) and the Oxford Nursing Development Unit closed in 1989, the British nursing journals have reported the opening of a number of other nurse-led units (Alderman 1996, Gaze 1989, Turner 1989). The unit at the Dulwich site of King's Healthcare NHS Trust has also been the subject of evaluation and has demonstrated similar beneficial outcomes for patients (Griffiths and Evans 1995).

The essence of these units has not simply been that nurses have gained the authority to admit and discharge patients but rather that the nursing has been the main therapy and that the standard of practice has been extremely high. In addition, the patients admitted to such units have been those whom it is surmised would derive the greatest benefit from intensive nursing therapy.

### Nurse-led outpatient services

Clinical nurse specialists in such fields as continence, stoma care and diabetes have been running nurse-led clinics for many years. With the reduction in junior doctors' hours, the number of clinical nurse specialists and nurse practitioners has escalated, with nurses running clinics and services (such as minor injuries) associated with many fields and specialities.

Whilst it may be argued that on the face of it, many of these new roles are substitutions of doctors with nurses and therefore not really nursing roles, it has been suggested earlier in this chapter that nursing is what nurses do. Therefore the test of nursing's contribution is whether nurses undertaking doctors' roles actually provide something additional that enhances the patient's care. This has been demonstrated to be so in a number of studies. For example, Hill (1997) used a randomized, blind trial to examine patient satisfaction with a nurse-led rheumatology clinic compared with a medically led clinic and demonstrated that the patients were significantly more satisfied than those who attended the consultant rheumatologist's clinic. Also, in a four-year trial, Curzio *et al.* (1989) demonstrated that a nurse-led blood pressure clinic could be more effective clinically (in terms of blood pressure control) than consultant-led clinics, even with both doctors and nurses using the same medication protocol. Therefore, the contribution of nursing to patient care through providing nurse-led services has great potential.

## THE FUTURE

It has been suggested that the empowerment of nurses to develop therapeutic nursing provides a challenge to medicine which nurses cannot win
(Salter and Smee 1997). Whilst elements within medicine may view any
interference with their control, even from other doctors, as a challenge,
there are an increasing number of medical staff who take a collaborative
approach and are critical when they see other professionals failing to make
their contribution to care. The rise of managerialism in the health service
has given nurses the opportunity to demonstrate their contribution to
improving care and hence the efficiency of the service.

Kitson (1997) has examined nursing's position with regard to the
evidence-based medicine and clinical effectiveness initiatives. She identifies one of the assumptions underlying these as being that clinicians
directly involved in a patient's care can influence the outcome for the
patient. She suggests that there are three dimensions on which nurses
have been shown to influence patient outcomes: these are through individual nursing interventions, the development of new nursing roles
and the organization of nursing. The challenge to all nurses is to influence each of those dimensions in such a way as to maximize the
therapeutic potential for nursing and hence have the maximum impact
on the patient.

The chapters that follow examine many aspects relating to the preparation and practice of nurses, and the environment in which they work.

Therapeutic nursing is about nurses using their creativity to assist
patients in their quest for health and healing. It relies on nurses being
committed to clinical practice and on managers, educators and researchers
providing the necessary milieu for nursing practice to be effective.
Educators and researchers need to make practice their principal focus.
Nurses have a duty to adopt therapeutic nursing as the focus of their
activity in order to provide best care for their patients.

## REFERENCES

Alderman, C. (1996) Taking the lead. *Nursing Standard*, **10** (33), 22–23.
Alfano, G. (1971) Healing or caretaking – which will it be? *Nursing Clinics of
North America*, **6** (2), 273–280.
Alfano, G. (1985) Whom do you care for? *Nursing Practice*, **1** (1), 28–31.
Briggs, A. (1972) *Report of the Committee on Nursing*, Her Majesty's Stationery
Office, London.
Campbell, A. V. (1984) *Moderated Love: A Theology of Professional Care*, SPCK,
London.
Campbell, C. (1985) Virginia Henderson: the definitive nurse. *Nursing Mirror*, **160**
(26), 12.

Carr-Hill, R., Dixon, P., Gibbs, I. *et al.* (1992) *Skill Mix and the Effectiveness of Nursing Care,* University of York, York.

Carson, D. (1988) Taking risks with patients – your assessment strategy. *Professional Nurse,* **3** (7), 247–250.

Castledine, G. (1994) A definition of nursing based on nurturing. *British Journal of Nursing,* **3** (3), 134–135.

Curzio, J. L., Reid, J. L., Rubin, P. C., Elliott, H. L. and Kennedy, S. S. (1989) *A Comparison of Care of the Hypertensive Patient: Nurse Practitioner Vs Traditional Medical Care,* RCN Research Society Annual Conference, Swansea.

Cushing, A. (1995) An historical note on the relationship between nursing and nursing history. *International History of Nursing Journal,* **1** (1), 57–60.

Davis, B. (1985) The clinical effect of interpersonal skills: the implementation of pre-operative information giving, in *Interpersonal Skills in Nursing,* (ed. C. Kagan), Croom Helm, London.

de la Cuesta, C. (1983) The nursing process: from development to implementation. *Journal of Advanced Nursing,* **8**, 365–371.

Ersser, S. (1988) Nursing beds and nursing therapy, in *Primary Nursing: Nursing in the Burford and Oxford Nursing Development Units,* (ed. A. Pearson), Croom Helm, Beckenham.

Ersser, S. and Tutton, E. (1991) *Primary Nursing in Perspective,* Scutari Press, London.

Evers, H. (1981a) Care or custody? The experience of women patients in long stay geriatric wards, in *Controlling Women: The Normal and the Deviant,* (eds B. Hutter and G. Williams), Croom Helm, London.

Evers, H. (1981b) Tender loving care? Patients and nurses in geriatric wards, in *Recent Advances in Nursing 2: Care of the Aging,* (ed. L. A. Copp), Churchill Livingstone, Edinburgh.

French, B. (1997) British studies which measure patient outcome 1990–1994. *Journal of Advanced Nursing,* **26** (2), 320–328.

Gaze, H. (1989) The shape of things to come? *Nursing Times,* **85** (30), 16–17.

Gilchrist, B. (1987) Taking risks for quality. *Geriatric Nursing and Home Care,* **7** (11), 24–26.

Gould, D. (1986) Pressure sore prevention and treatment: an example of nurses' failure to implement research findings. *Journal of Advanced Nursing,* **11** (4), 389–94.

Griffiths, P. (1997) In search of the pioneers of nurse-led care. *Nursing Times,* **93** (21), 46–48.

Griffiths, P. and Evans, A. (1995) *Evaluation of a Nursing Led In-Patient Service: An Interim Report,* King's Fund, London.

Hall, L. E. (1969) The Loeb Center for Nursing and Rehabilitation, Montefiore Hospital and Medical Center, Bronx, New York. *International Journal of Nursing Studies,* **6**, 81–97.

Henderson, V. (1966) *The Nature of Nursing: A Definition and its Implications for Practice, Research and Education,* Macmillan, New York.

Henderson, V. (1969) *Basic Principles of Nursing Care,* International Council of Nurses, Geneva.

Hill, J. (1997) Patient satisfaction in a nurse-led rheumatology clinic. *Journal of Advanced Nursing,* **25** (2), 347–354.

Hunt, M. (1987) The process of translating research findings into nursing practice. *Journal of Advanced Nursing*, **12**, 101–110.

Jourard, S. (1971) *The Transparent Self*, Van Nostrand, New Jersey.

Kadner, K. (1994) Therapeutic intimacy in nursing. *Journal of Advanced Nursing*, **19** (2), 215–218.

Kitson, A. (1986) Indicators of quality in nursing care – an alternative approach. *Journal of Advanced Nursing*, **11** (2), 133–144.

Kitson, A. (1993) Formalising concepts related to nursing and caring. in *Nursing: Art and Science*, (ed. A. Kitson), Chapman and Hall, London.

Kitson, A. (1997) Using evidence to demonstrate the value of nursing. *Nursing Standard*, **11** (28), 34–39.

Levi, M. (1980) Functional redundancy and the process of professionalisation: the case of registered nurses in the United States. *Journal of Health Politics, Policy and Law*, **5** (2), 333–353.

Levine, M. (1971) Holistic nursing. *Nursing Clinics of North America*, **6**, 253–264.

Levine, M. (1973) *Introduction to Clinical Nursing*, 2nd edn, F. A. Davis, Philadelphia.

Luker, K., Carlisle, C., Riley, E. *et al.* (1996) *Project 2000; Fitness for Purpose. Report to the Department of Health.* University of Warwick Centre for Health Services Studies and Institute for Employment Research/University of Liverpool Department of Nursing.

Lyall, J. (1990) Cycles of evasion. *Nursing Times*, **86** (34), 16–17.

Macleod-Clark, J. (1983) Nurse–patient communication – an analysis, in *Ten Studies in Patient Care*, (ed. J. Wilson-Barnett), John Wiley, Chichester.

Macleod-Clark, J., Wilson-Barnett, J., Latter, S. and Maben, J. (1992) *Health Education and Health Promotion in Nursing: A Study of Practice in Acute Areas*, Nursing Studies Department, King's College, London.

Manthey, M. (1980) *The Practice of Primary Nursing*, Blackwell Scientific Press, Oxford.

McMahon, R. (1986) Nursing as a therapy. *Professional Nurse*, **1** (10), 270–272.

McMahon, R. (1988) Discharge planning: home truths. *Geriatric Nursing and Home Care*, **8** (9), 16–17.

McMahon, R. (1990) Power and collegial relations among nurses on wards adopting primary nursing and hierarchical ward management structures. *Journal of Advanced Nursing*, **15** (2), 232–239.

Miller, A. (1985) Nurse/patient dependency – is it iatrogenic? *Journal of Advanced Nursing*, **10** (1), 63–70.

Muetzel, P.-A. (1988) Therapeutic nursing, in *Primary Nursing: Nursing in the Burford and Oxford Nursing Development Units*, (ed. A. Pearson), Croom Helm, Beckenham.

Newbeck, I. (1986) *How Holistic Therapies Can Be Used In Nursing.* Second Holistic Nursing Conference, City University, London.

Nightingale, F. (1859) *Notes on Nursing* (republished 1980), Churchill Livingstone, Edinburgh.

Oakley, A. (1984) The importance of being a nurse. *Nursing Times*, **80** (50), 24–27.

Orem, D. (1985) *Nursing: Concepts of Practice*, 3rd edn, McGraw Hill, New York.

Pearson, A. (1983) *The Clinical Nursing Unit*, Heinemann, London.

Pearson, A. (1988) *Primary Nursing: Nursing in the Burford and Oxford Nursing Development Units*, Croom Helm, Beckenham.

Pearson, A. (1992) *Nursing at Burford: A Story of Change*, Scutari Press, London.

Pearson, A. and Vaughan, B. (1986) *Nursing Models for Practice*, Heinemann, London.

Pearson, A., Punton, S. and Durand, I. (1992) *Nursing Beds: An Evaluation of the Effects of Therapeutic Nursing*, Scutari Press, London.

Pembrey, S. M. (1980) *The Ward Sister – Key to Nursing*, Royal College of Nursing, London.

Peplau, H. (1952) *Interpersonal Relations in Nursing*, Macmillan Education, London.

RCN (1987) *A Position Paper on Nursing*, Royal College of Nursing, London.

Roper, N., Logan, W. W. and Tierney, A. J. (1985) *The Elements of Nursing*, 2nd edn, Churchill Livingstone, Edinburgh.

Salter, B. and Smee, N. (1997) Power dressing. *Health Service Journal*, 17th February, 30–31.

Salvage, J. (1985) *The Politics of Nursing*, Heinemann, London.

Salvage, J. and Wright, S. G. (1995) *Nursing Development Units: A Force for Change*, Scutari Press, London.

Smuts, J. C. (1926) *Holism and Evolution*, Macmillan, New York.

Thompson, D. R. (1989) A randomised controlled trial of in-hospital nursing support for first-time myocardial infarction patients and their partners: effects on anxiety and depression. *Journal of Advanced Nursing*, **14** (4), 291–297.

Turner, T. (1989) Taking the lead. *Nursing Times*, **85** (43), 16–17.

Varcoe, C. (1996) Disparagement of the nursing process: the new dogma? *Journal of Advanced Nursing*, **23** (1), 120–125.

Watson, S. (1994) An exploratory study into a methodology for the examination of decision making by nurses in the clinical area. *Journal of Advanced Nursing*, **20** (2), 351–360.

Wilkinson, S. (1991) Factors which influence how nurses communicate with cancer patients. *Journal of Advanced Nursing*, **16** (6), 677–688.

Wilson-Barnett, J. (1978) Patients' emotional response to barium X-rays. *Journal of Advanced Nursing*, **3** (1), 37–45.

Wilson-Barnett, J. (1984) *Key Functions in Nursing*, Royal College of Nursing, London.

Wilson-Barnett, J. (1988) Patient teaching or patient counselling? *Journal of Advanced Nursing*, **13** (2), 215–222.

<table>
| Reflection and the evaluation of experience: prerequisites for therapeutic practice? | 2 |
</table>

# Reflection and the evaluation of experience: prerequisites for therapeutic practice? | 2

Jean Powell

## INTRODUCTION

Since the first edition of this book, the title of the chapter has acquired a question mark. This is designed to highlight the criticisms levelled at reflective practice in the past few years and the uncritical way it has been introduced into nursing.

Reflective practice was discussed in the first edition as something which might promote a deeper and more critical approach to practice, using this together with research-based knowledge to promote therapeutic practice. It has largely been introduced to nursing educational programmes, rather than actual practice, and in a generally uncritical way, with perhaps an overemphasis on its usefulness in therapeutic practice and little thought given to the practicalities of its introduction. It is therefore doubtful whether therapeutic practice has been developed or enhanced by its use.

This chapter will discuss the concept of reflection and the criticisms made of reflective practice, give an overview of reflective practice in nursing and some issues for the future.

## EXPERIENTIAL LEARNING AND REFLECTION

Much of the interest in experiential learning developed from both education, through Dewey, and the social sciences, with Lewin's work in the United States and Habermas' in Germany. Dewey produced a problem-solving design, which was an early model of the actual experience of learning. He reasoned that all thinking had its origins in problematic situations and that this thinking is an enabling device for interaction between the individual and his environment. He defined problematic situations as being unable to be resolved by the use of prior solutions. This is very similar to Schön's view of the problems faced by professionals and the development of strategies for solving these (Schön 1983).

Dewey also emphasized the active nature of learning, where an experience is in two parts: first, the undergoing of the experience and second, the thought and consideration of what this experience meant. He wrote that we do not 'learn by doing' . . . 'we learn by doing and realising what came of what we did' (Dewey 1929:367). This type of learning offers developmental and growth potential which exceed the requirements of the immediate situation and which can not only be transferred to other situations but, because of this growth potential, may enable this further experience to be of greater significance.

Other writers have produced problem-solving models (Garrison 1964, Garry and Kingsley 1970, Urban and Ford 1971, among others). Some have highlighted the creative aspects of this, such as Osborne (1953) who developed a seven-stage model on the same lines as Dewey but who added the concept of 'incubation', the stage where the halting of active reasoning appears to allow a spontaneous generation of a solution to the problem.

If Dewey was undoubtedly a major influence on experiential learning, producing new insights from the field of education, particularly with his books published in 1916, 1929 and 1938, an equally important influence came from Lewin's work in the field of social science. This work was mainly carried out in the 1940s and provided further insights into experiential learning. Lewin (1935) refers to the 'life space' of the individual, the interaction of the complexity of factors influencing the context in which learning takes place. This individual interaction affects the development of a learning style that will enable the individual to know, explain and cope with his world and the experiences it provides.

At around the same time, Habermas, one of the Frankfurt school of social philosophers, proposed that knowledge was generated in three separate ways: through the area of work which he saw as comprising the aspects where control and manipulation of the environment were occurring; through the practical area where interaction would assist in interpreting the situations and identifying conditions for furtherance of this; through the emancipatory area which is concerned with self-exploration, leading to self-knowledge and reflection (Habermas, cited in Mezirow 1981:6). This important foundation was further advanced by the work of Kolb and Fry (1975) in their exposition of an experiential learning model with concrete experience followed by observations and reflections, leading to the formation of abstract concepts and generalizations which would then be used to test implications of the concepts in new situations. This work has since been developed more fully by Kolb (1984). The emergence of the model was a rigorous attempt to understand the dynamics of the learning process in experiential learning.

Kolb and Fry (1975) sought to clarify four aspects of experiential learning:

1  The integration of the cognitive and socioeconomic perspectives on learning
2  The role of individual differences in learning style
3  The concept of growth and development inherent in the experiential learning model
4  A model of learning environments that is commensurate with the experiential learning process.

The model is a cyclical one which is designed to be consistent with both the structure of cognition and also with growth and development. One of its major features was the emphasis on learning styles and their individuality. Kolb and Fry defined four main styles: convergent, divergent, assimilating and accommodating. While they recognized that these styles are overlapping and that within each is a great diversity and complexity, they do stress the opposition of reflection and action, claiming that each inhibits the other.

This separation of reflection and action has led to general acceptance of the view of reflection and action as not only very different but as inhibitors of each other. Schön's work on reflective practice (1983) was the first to dispute this and to promote the idea of reflection-in-action, assisting both the action and learning from it. This will be discussed more thoroughly later in this chapter.

The Kolb and Fry learning cycle is, however, extremely important in that it represents a method of separating the learning occurring from experience into various elements which can then be studied. The cycle itself is simplistic and it can be seen that, for example, reflection must also occur at the third stage of formulating concepts (Jarvis and Gibson 1985), but this is possibly more of an aid to examination of the various aspects than a defect.

Reflection in its relation to experiential learning and hence to therapeutic practice is the main concern of this chapter and therefore it is important to examine more directly the whole concept of reflection. Reflection in learning is not a new idea, indeed it is akin to Aristotle's concept of deliberation (Elliot 1983). Dewey also discussed the problems in 'forming habits of reflective thought' (Dewey 1933) and he later defined reflective thought as:

> Active, persistent and careful consideration of any belief or supposed form of knowledge in the light of the grounds that support it, and further conclusions to which it leads . . . it concludes a conscious

and voluntary effort to establish belief upon a firm basis of evidence and rationality.

Dewey undoubtedly has provided a great deal of the foundation for current thinking on reflection and learning, although the present emphasis appears more on the creativity and affective elements of reflection rather than the rationality of it as a process. This can be seen, for example, in the work of Boyd and Fales (1983) who see reflective learning as emphasizing 'the self as the source of learning and ... therefore inherently an individual and ipsative process'. They define reflection: '... as the process of creating and clarifying the meaning of experience (present or past) in terms of self (self in relation to self and self in relation to the world)', and further state that the 'outcome of the process is a changed conceptual perspective'.

They feel that reflection is a natural process used spontaneously by many people and as such is not a new concept, but that its present significance lies in reflection as a 'paradigm shift in professional learning from experience, personal growth ... both in professionals' own continuing learning and in facilitating the learning and growth of their clients'. A further aspect of their work is the emphasis on consciousness raising and their description of beginning reflection as a sense of 'inner discomfort'.

Consciousness raising echoes Freire's (1972) work and his concept of conscientization with its links to reflection. Similar ideas are promoted by Goldstein (1985) in his discussion of discrimination learning which he conceives as being 'primarily focused on the perceptual functions of consciousness and attention to enable the individual to become more sensitive and responsive to these aspects of his experience that, for some reason, remain obscure'.

Boud, working with Keogh and Walker, has produced a model for promoting reflection in learning where they define reflection as:

> a generic term for those intellectual and affective activities in which
> individuals engage to explore their experiences in order to lead to
> new understandings and appreciations. (Boud *et al.* 1985)

This model emphasizes the affective aspects of learning and how these may facilitate or hinder reflection. Feelings throughout the experience are of fundamental importance here and Boud also highlights the relationship of these to past experiences.

This importance given to the affective nature of learning also emphasizes its individuality and therefore the control must always be with the learner, with the teacher acting as facilitator, with access only to such information as the learner wishes him to have (Boud *et al.* 1985). This is similarly emphasized in Knowles' (1985) work, where he places great stress on the building up of trust between learner and teacher.

Knowles acknowledges the control vested in the learner further in his discussions on andragogy, with the involvement of the learner in diagnosing his own needs and planning of learning contracts to meet those needs.

Experiential learning is a key component of andragogy and Knowles highlights the vast range of adult learners' experiences and therefore the complexity of the effects of this on learning experiences and the essential individuality of these (Knowles 1985). While andragogy is not a theory of experiential learning *per se*, it has undoubtedly added much to present-day thinking on and practice of this and also to the thinking on and practice of reflection. His use of learning contracts means they cannot be effective without this reflection and careful consideration at all stages (Knowles 1985).

Further ideas on reflection have been put forward by Kemmis (1985) to suggest that reflection is a social rather than an individual process. This is based on the interesting premise that:

> The fruits of reflection-action have their meaning and significance in a social world, in which others understand us through our actions (including our utterances) and, as Wittgenstein (1974) showed, in which we can invest meaning in our actions only by reference to the forms of life we share with others.

Kemmis separated reflection into three different but parallel forms: problem solving, practical deliberation and speculative thought. The last is closely linked to the Habermas (1971) concept of initial reflection. Each of the three forms is action orienting and therefore Kemmis strongly promotes the concept of reflection as both political and ideological. Although Kemmis does not refer to Freire's writings in his work, there would appear to be strong links between them.

Other writers have related reflection purely to postaction thinking (Clarke 1986, Shotter 1974). While this is valuable, it is only part of the complex process of reflection and more critical studies, such as those of Habermas, whose contribution to experiential learning was discussed earlier in this chapter, and Mezirow, are therefore more relevant to the discussion here.

Habermas (1971) proposed that reflection is always intentional and talked of 'critical intent'. Mezirow has largely built on the work of Habermas but analysed reflection in greater detail and used it to clarify his concept of learning as 'perspective transformation'. Mezirow (1981) classifies reflection as having seven forms which act as a type of hierarchy of reflective activity. This begins with reflectivity, where there is awareness of specific perception, meaning or behaviour or of limits regarding these. Affective reflectivity is becoming aware of feelings with regard to reflectivity, while discriminant reflectivity assesses the effectiveness of perceptions, thoughts, actions and habits. Judgemental reflectivity is closely related to this in that it is concerned with awareness of value judgements regarding perception, thoughts, actions and habits.

These four forms can be seen to be on a different level from the last three which are particularly concerned with perspective transformation. They are all concerned with critical thought rather than simple awareness. The first is conceptual reflectivity, which is a kind of bridge between the first four forms and the last three and where consciousness of awareness, and questioning of the perception that allows this awareness, are present. Psychic reflectivity is the recognition that judgements are made on perceived evidence which may be limited and is certainly influenced by the experiences and awareness of the perceiver. The highest of these three, and therefore of the seven, is what Mezirow describes as the theoretical reflectivity, which is the addition to psychic reflectivity of the capacity to see that although judgements made are limited by personal experience and culture, this is not unchanging and more useful and satisfying judgements might be made using altered perspectives. This perspective transformation relies on conscious and critical awareness and leads to growth and development of the individual. While it is necessary to separate these seven forms for the purpose of understanding Mezirow's concept, it is perhaps more useful to see them as points on a continuum, with reflectivity as the starting point leading to an infinity of perspective transformation.

This concept is vastly different from Kolb's where action and reflection are antagonists. Mezirow, with his awareness of action at all levels and his juxtaposition of thoughts, perceptions, actions and habits, appears to view them as aspects of the whole rather than as separate in themselves. His use of habit is also interesting in the context of reflectivity. It might also be considered that habit opposes reflection, since it leads to routine actions and unthinking behaviour. By incorporating habit into his levels of reflectivity, the seeker after reflection is forced to consider habits, possibly of long standing, and this consideration may in itself lead to perspective transformation. This linking of action and reflection and the incorporation of habits are also important in Schön's work on reflection-in-action.

## REFLECTION-IN-ACTION

Reflection-in-action develops the concept of reflection further, adding the idea of reflecting while acting, rather than postaction. Reflection-in-action is more than this, however, and the philosophy underlying is important here. This is based on both Schön's own work and that done in conjunction with Argyris on theory in practice (Argyris and Schön 1974, 1978). Note that this is not theory related to practice nor theory applied to practice, but theory which is an integral part of practice and which has grown through the experience of varying practice.

Reflection-in-action is also concerned with the professional relationship, where the professional is seen not as the expert offering solutions to problems but as someone with particular skills and knowledge who may be able to help a client. The relationship is one of equals, with the client deciding whether or not the professional may be helpful. Within reflection-in-action, Schön has discussed several concepts of use to professionals, including nurses.

The first of these is the idea of theories-in-use. Schön suggests that the theories-in-use underlying a professional's actions are different from what he refers to as the espoused theories, that is, the ones professed to be used. This has been rigorously researched by Schön, both alone (1983) and with Argyris (1974, 1978). The reasons for this difference are complex, but one of them has to do with the difficulty of relating conventional academic knowledge to actual practice. Schön refers to this conventional academic knowledge as technical rationality, with the basis of this being the formal scientific approach. He is not, however, saying that this technical rational basis is not useful, rather that it needs to be used in conjunction with knowledge developed from practice and that this latter type of knowledge may be the more influential.

Reflection-in-action implies awareness of the individual's own theories-in-use. These theories-in-use, once developed, can be tested in practice and Schön sees reflective practitioners as researchers, although not in the sense of large, conventional research studies but rather as individual action researchers, trying out solutions and using the knowledge gained to assist in future practice.

This view is akin to Kelly's (1963) view of humans as scientists, experimenting on their environment. Kelly is careful to insist that experience in itself does not necessarily make for valid knowledge, that this depends on the validity of the constructs of the person and that only the reconstruing of events leads to development or learning. Schön does not refer to Kelly in his writings but many of his views reflect similar ideas to those inherent in personal construct theory, developed by Kelly.

A further important concept is the recognition that professional practitioners do not generally deal with the type of problems solvable by reference to technical rational means; rather, they encounter very individual, complex, messy and indeterminate situations, demanding an individual and innovative approach. Professionals are taught how to solve problems but the real problem is how to define the problem from the real-life situation. Problem framing or problem setting is the skill professional practitioners acquire with experience . . . sometimes.

Schön (1987) states that:

These indeterminate zones of practice . . . uncertainty, uniqueness and value conflict . . . escape the canons of technical rationality.

> When a problematic solution is uncertain, technical problem solving depends on the prior construction of a well formed problem ... which is not itself a technical task.

Tacit knowledge (Polanyi 1966) is also seen by Schön as a key component in reflection-in-action. 'We know more than we can say' (*ibid*) is seen as contributing to unique solutions for problems, described by Schön as knowing-in-action. This is linked to Freire's (1972) concept of conscientization and certainly awareness raising is essential if past experience is to be used to assist present and future practice. The routinization of practice is called overlearning by Schön and implies unthinking, unhelpful care giving, with little possibility of learning from experience.

The other side of this is the use of disjuncture, where learning may occur because something is out of place and does not fit into the common pattern. This disjuncture will cause a fresh view to be taken of the situation and a reframing of the problem. This is similar to Mezirow's (1981) perspective transformation where disjuncture plays a key part. Mezirow's work also stresses the rigour of 'critical reflection which addresses the validity of taken-for-granted presuppositions' (Mezirow 1988). This examination of assumptions again echoes Schön.

Value conflict is also seen as a major area of concern. Schön discusses the indeterminate areas of practice, where there is no clearcut solution and where value conflict often exists, unrecognized or unresponded to by the professional practitioner. He relates this to the crisis of confidence in professions generally and states 'that the most important areas of professional practice now lie beyond the conventional boundaries of professional competence' (Schön 1987). Certainly, in nursing this is increasingly true and it may be that a move towards professional learning based on the practice exemplar is the way to resolve this. Knowledge developed from practice is relativist and takes account of value conflict, unlike conventional, technical rational knowledge which is positivist and claims to be value free.

Schön's work has been criticized by several writers, Furlong (1995), Day (1993) and Eraut (1995) among others. The basis of these criticisms seems to relate mainly to the concept of reflection-in-action which is felt to lack clarity, particularly in relation to the processes, cognitive and psychological, which lead to reflective practice.

Eraut made a comprehensive critique of Schön's work and feels that parts of this are unclear and almost contradictory at times, although he suggests that:

> Schön's notion of rapid reflection-in-action provides an original and useful theory of metacognition during skilled behaviour. His ideas about referencing and reflective conversations with the situation might be construed as contributing to a theory of metacognition

during deliberative processes. This makes a clear distinction between deliberation and reflective metacognition of that deliberation. (Eraut 1994)

Eraut also raises the question of the time variable in professional practice and feels Schön has ignored this in his discussions of reflection-in-action. Eraut not only raises the question of lack of time whilst making rapid decisions, he states that in those circumstances 'Reflection is best seen as a metacognitive process in which the practitioner is alerted to a problem, rapidly reads the situation, decides what to do and proceeds in a state of continuing alertness' (Eraut 1995). This may appear to be a matter of semantics, particularly since Mezirow (1991) writes that:

> Several psychologists have made reflection, or something closely allied to it, a significant part of their theories. Terms used in those theories that are more or less synonymous with what transformation theory calls reflection include metacognition, reflection-in-action and mindfulness.

A more worrying criticism is that Eraut, and others, have raised the question that Schön's view of technical rationality is strongly argued and this is most easily construed as needing to be replaced by his alternative based on professional practice. Fenstermacher (1988) supports the view that Schön offers rather not an alternative but a complement to existing research-based professional practice and this seems much more realistic for nursing, given that so much of nursing knowledge is founded on other disciplines.

There are also some important criticisms general to reflective practice, such as Day (1993) pointing out that how reflection changes practice is unknown and Ecclestone's (1995) view that reflective practice has become little more than a mantra. Furlong (1995) argues that reflective practice has legitimized the removal of theory from teacher education and its replacement with personal reflection. This echoes fears among some nurse educators. Many professional education programmes now claim to be based on Schön's theory but many of these have great variations. Whilst the quote here from Mumby and Russell (1993) refers to teacher education, it probably applies equally well to nurse education.

> Each of the seven programs has unique assumptions and organising principles, some working with little more than a common sense definition of reflection that seems to come naturally to all teacher educators. The six critiques similarly convey unique senses of reflection.

Most critical approaches to reflective practice are found in teacher education and very few are seen in nursing, although Newell (1992) is an exception here. This is perhaps to be expected since teacher education is likely to take a view on new learning developments. However, a critical approach is useful and it is to be hoped that nurse educators will take note of the many issues raised by teacher educators. It is appropriate now to take a look at what has happened to nursing and nurse education since the first edition.

## NURSING PRACTICE AND EDUCATION

Nurses are doers and this doing is highly valued in the culture of the nursing world. In the past, socialization into this world was assured by the requirement that learner nurses were also a major part of the workforce. This system has now been phased out across the country, having been completed over a few years. The system that replaced this is known as Project 2000, essentially a university-based system whereby students study for a diploma qualification, achieving nurse registration at the same time. This system is intended to prepare students for a future role as nurses through enabling a greater focus on learning in both classroom and clinical areas and through allowing these students the time and space to both apply theory to practice and to try out, in a limited, supervised way, different ways of carrying out practice. This should ensure that nurses are 'thinking doers', able to make informed choices of care within the increasing technological and social complexities of health care. However, given the value placed on doing, the development of a higher education route has inevitably raised the suspicion that the doing aspect of nursing may not continue to receive the emphasis it has in the past.

At the same time, the system is designed to ensure a more stable workforce for individual clinical areas, where students would come and go but as supernumerary members of the team, not as part of the establishment. This should therefore make possible the 'utilization of nursing knowledge by qualified nurses to resolve the dilemma and ambiguities inherent in patient care' which Proctor (1989) felt was not possible within the organizational system heavily reliant on transient staff, as with the past educational system, where much of the workload was carried by learner nurses, spending only a short time in each area.

Until very recently, postregistration courses were either academic diploma/degree courses, often based on either social science or biological science and in some cases not particularly relevant to nursing practice, or very skills-based, content-heavy ENB clinical courses. The latter were certainly relevant to practice but frequently did not encourage critical thinking or the ability to continue to learn on completion of the course. With the UKCC PostRegistration Education and Practice (PREP) guidelines in effect from September 1995, all postregistration courses leading to specialist practitioner status will be at degree level and will build on

Project 2000 and in effect combine the best of the old-style degree programmes with a critical approach to clinical skills. Clearly many nurses, because of their present educational level, are not ready for such a programme, so in the short term, access courses will be developed to enable them to benefit from PREP.

It can be seen, therefore, that over the past few years nurses have had to cope with major changes in education which have affected their day-to-day practice. Concurrently, most nurses have acted as mentors and/or assessors to both learner nurses following the old curriculum and those following Project 2000 programmes. In addition, some of the latter will have been full university students with a very different culture from those earlier learners, with a culture derived from the NHS and, in particular, the hospital where they were undertaking training.

Mentors themselves felt largely unprepared for the new breed of students; they were not often qualified in academic terms to the level for which students were being prepared and although they were clearly experienced and very competent, they often felt insecure in teaching these new students. Many courses were embarked on in a hurry, with insufficient thought given to the role of the mentor; indeed, many of the nurse educators were non-graduates, with little knowledge of university culture and no experience in teaching at diploma level, making them a poor support for the mentors. In addition, many mentors (and some nurse educators) felt that Project 2000 programmes would not produce a nurse who could practise effectively. This was based on the smaller amount of practice time and the supernumerary status of students, often ill understood.

At the same time, the changes in both pre- and postregistration education made it appear as if mentors and nurse educators were continually playing catch-up with qualifications to enhance their own areas.

Educationally, therefore, the picture was somewhat chaotic. Add to this the effects of the NHS reforms and requirements for annual efficiency gains and staff are further stressed. Many of the reforms have beneficial effects, e.g. emphasizing accountability, and certainly have created new opportunities for nurses. However, against this, insecurity of nursing posts and requirements to change established ways of working have led to loss of morale and stressed staff in many areas. The use of health-care assistants in place of the learner nurses and the need for these to be trained through NVQ achievement further added to the workload. It is remarkable that good nurses have been prepared under Project 2000 and that many examples of innovation and practice developments can be cited across the country from qualified, experienced nurses, given these difficult circumstances.

## REFLECTION AND NURSING PRACTICE

It was against the above background that reflective practice was introduced. Like many changes in the last few years, it was introduced without clear direction or even, in some cases, understanding. However, reflective practice was widely accepted by nurse educators and, indeed, expected to be part of nursing curricula. This led to the use of reflective diaries and learning logs in vast quantities. Many of these were not confidential to the student and some were formally assessed. Anecdotal evidence suggests that some students, not particularly effective in actual nursing practice, became very good indeed at writing reflective diaries. In many cases these logs or diaries only added to the workload of the student and teacher and were of dubious benefit.

Clearly, reflective techniques are beneficial to students when used to reflect on what they actually did in real situations and how this could be done differently or more effectively. A key part of this is the identification of the knowledge used to make decisions and of the source of this, whether this be research paper, textbook or from discussion with lecturer or mentor. Equally clearly, it is ludicrous to suggest that students are or can be reflective practitioners. A key part of this is the use of experience of which, by definition, students have a minimal amount. The use of disjuncture to raise awareness and induce learning is also irrelevant here, since to a student most situations appear unusual, again because of lack of experience.

It is with qualified nurses that reflection can be developed more strongly and, indeed, Schön's work is directed at professionals and, moreover, at professionals with substantial experience. Many experienced nurses feel that they have gained a great deal from reflective techniques, although whether some of this benefit from undertaking a course of study and discussing issues with peers, rather than reflection, is open to question. Clearly, reflection is used in courses and possibly this is artificial, even if the usage is real. The really interesting question is whether nurses are using reflection in day-to-day practice. A problem this writer has with the use of reflective techniques in both pre- and postregistration programmes is that they seem to be used almost as the only way to learn, rather than as part of a range of learning tools. Most students have an individual learning style, a combination of some of the four learning styles identified by Honey and Mumford (1986) as:

1  *Activist*:     'I'll try anything once'
2  *Reflector*:    'I'd like time to think about this'
3  *Theorist*:     'How does this fit with that?'
4  *Pragmatist*:   'How can I apply this in practice?'

Using reflection as the major learning method may be disadvantageous to students who are primarily non-reflectors and whilst it may be beneficial to explore each style, it is surely not sound educational practice to place one above the others.

A worry, reflected also in teacher education, is the use of personal reflection and possible overemphasis on the affective areas, so that nurses can describe and analyse their feelings well but are not so able when it comes to cognitive areas, particularly those relating to the hard sciences – physics, chemistry and biology. This is important because it imbalances the nurse–patient relationship. The patient has a right to expect that the nurse will consider the quality of life of the patient suffering, for example, stiff painful knee and hip joints from arthritis and to explore the patient's feelings to determine the most appropriate care. However, this consideration and empathy is of little use if the nurse does not have an up-to-date and critical approach to the drugs and treatments available to the patient. This is what Schön means when he states '... we will also respect the professionals' claim to extraordinary knowledge in the areas susceptible to technical expertise' (Schön 1983).

Aside from this, there are two major problems with reflective practice in nursing. Firstly, for reflective practice to work, it needs support from at least the nursing team, if not the entire organization. Clearly, given the hierarchical organization of the NHS, this may cause a problem in that there will be a degree of resistance to the introduction of such an unhierarchical concept. It would appear at present that reflection is mainly used within education programmes and that reflective practice is not a reality in any meaningful way at present.

A much greater problem is that of time. Increasingly time is at a premium in all areas of practice, nurses have greater responsibilities than in the even fairly recent past and the demands made in a busy and ever-changing environment leave little time for reflection. Reflection-in-action, the focusing on individual situations and using both knowledge and experience to provide a thoughtful decision on action to be taken, is unlikely to occur with any frequency, given the myriad events which make up the working day. In this, Eraut (1994) is probably correct in saying that it is impossible to do as part of everyday practice with any real success and the NHS is possibly one of the worst examples around to demonstrate this. Staff who have worked hard during a shift, remembering that nursing is demanding physically as well as mentally and contains many stressful situations, are unlikely to be able to or wish to reflect on the decisions they made. This also clearly contributes to reflective practice being generally ignored in reality.

## THE WAY FORWARD

Clearly, as nurse education begins to settle down and meet the challenges of Project 2000 and PREP, unencumbered by the many old-style curricula and with one or two intakes a year giving further stability, nurse educators will have more time to evaluate reflective practice and think through strategies for its use. Again, the move of all nurse education into higher education will be helpful in removing the uncertainty of the past few years, enabling this more critical approach to emerge.

The trusts are also beginning to move forward, now that the initial major changes have been carried out. This should mean that more time is spent on determining what education is needed for the staff and how best to ensure this is effective. For reflective practice, further clarity in the terms used and the concept behind these is a priority along with research into how (or if) reflection changes practice and into the relationship between reflection and practice.

This writer believes that reflective practice can add to professional knowledge and complement, not replace, the research-based knowledge of nursing. It would seem a mistake, as the NHS embraces evidenced-based practice, not to include verified experience with individual patients as some, albeit small part of this.

The extensive usage of reflection in education needs to become more rigorous and to be seen as part of education rather than the whole. The balance between affective and cognitive has perhaps swung too far towards affective, possibly because of the total lack of emphasis on this in the past. Perhaps now this can be redressed. A key part of this is not increasing the use of education but determining strategies to help grassroots nurses use it in their practice. There is some anecdotal evidence that this is happening, with a few pockets of reflective practice being developed. However, the future is unlikely to consist of all or even a majority of nurses using reflective practice at all times. Rather, the future may be that nurses are educated in reflective techniques and use these from time to time, both for their normal practice and for unusual occurrences, when their experience tells them there is disjuncture.

Therapeutic practice is an excellent aim and it may be that this is not an absolute but that there are degrees of this, in the same way that Mezirow's concept of reflection may be seen as a continuum. The higher levels of this practice will include using experience and reflection to assist in determining the actions taken and the underlying premises. Whether a new epistemology of practice will eventually result is debatable, but growth and development of professional nurses are certain.

## REFERENCES

Argyris, C. and Schön, D. (1974) *Theory in Practice: Increasing Professional Effectiveness*, Addison-Wesley, Massachusetts.
Argyris, C. and Schön, D. (1978) *Organisational Learning: A Theory of Action Perspective*, Addison-Wesley, Massachusetts.

Boud, D., Keogh, R. and Walker, D. (eds) (1985) *Reflection: Turning Experience into Learning*, Kogan Page, London.

Boyd, E. M. and Fales, A. W. (1983) Reflective learning: key to learning from experience. *Journal of Humanistic Psychology*, **23**(2), 99–117.

Clarke, M. (1986) Action and reflection: practice and theory in nursing. *Journal of Advanced Nursing*, **11**(1), 3–11.

Day, C. (1993) Reflection: A necessary but not sufficient condition for professional development. *British Educational Research Journal*, **19**(1), 83–93.

Dewey, J. (1929) *Experience and Nature*. Grove Press, New York.

Dewey, J. (1933) *How We Think*. D.C. Heath, Boston.

Ecclestone, K. (1995) The reflective practitioner: mantra or a model for emancipation? Conference paper, University of Central Lancashire.

Elliot, J. (1983) Self-evaluation, professional development & accountability, in *Changing Schools, Changing Curriculum*, (eds M. Galton and R. Moon), Kogan Page, London, pp. 183–201.

Eraut, M. (1994) *Developing Professional Knowledge and Competence*. Falmer Press, London.

Eraut, M. (1995) Schön shock: a case for reframing reflection-in-action? *Teachers and Teaching*, **1**, 9–21.

Fenstermacher, G. D. (1988) The place of science and epistemology in Schön's conception of reflective practice, in *Reflection in Teacher Education*, (eds P. P. Grimmett and G. L. Erikson), Teachers College Press, New York.

Freire, P. (1972) *Pedagogy of the Oppressed*, Penguin, London.

Furlong, J. (1995) *Mentoring Student Teachers*, Routledge, London.

Garrison, K. (1964) *Educational Psychology*, Appleton-Century-Crofts, New York.

Garry, R. and Kingsley, H. (1970) *The Nature and Conditions of Learning*, Prentice-Hall, New Jersey.

Goldstein, H. (1985) *Social Learning and Change*, Tavistock, London.

Habermas, J. (1971) *Knowledge and Human Interests*, Beacon Press, Boston.

Honey, P. and Mumford, A. (1986) *The Manual of Learning Styles*, available from Dr P. Honey, Maidenhead.

Jarvis, P. and Gibson, S. (1985) *The Teacher Practitioner in Nursing, Midwifery and Health Visiting*, Croom Helm, Beckenham.

Kelly, G. A. (1963) *Theory of Personality: The Psychology of Personal Constructs*, W.W. Norton, New York.

Kemmis, S. (1985) Action research and the politics of reflection, in *Reflection: Turning Experience into Learning*, (eds D. Bond, R. Keogh and D. Walker), Kogan Page, London.

Knowles, M. S. (1985) *Andragogy in Action*, Jossey-Bass, San Francisco.

Kolb, D. A. (1984) *Experiential Learning*, Prentice-Hall, London.

Kolb, D. A. and Fry, R. (1975) Towards an applied theory of experiential learning, in *Theories of Group Processes*, (ed. C. L. Cooper), John Wiley, London.

Lewin, K. (1935) *A Dynamic Theory of Personality*, McGraw-Hill, New York.

Mezirow, J. (1981) A critical theory of adult learning and education. *Adult Education*, **32**(1), 3–24.

Mezirow, J. (1988) Transformation theory. Adult Educators' Conference paper.

Mezirow, J. (1991) *Transformation Dimensions of Adult Learning*, Jossey-Bass, San Francisco.

Mumby, H. and Russell, L. T. (1993) Reflective teacher education – technique or epistemology? *Teaching Teacher Education*, **9**(4), 431–438.

Newell, R. (1992) Anxiety, accuracy and reflection – the limits of professional development. *Journal of Nursing*, **17**, 1326–1333.

Osborne, A. F. (1953) *Applied Imagination*, Scribners, New York.

Polanyi, N. (1967) *The Tacit Dimension*, Doubleday, New York.

Proctor, S. (1989) The functioning of nursing routines in the management of a transient workforce. *Journal of Advanced Nursing*, **14**(3), 177–185.

Schön, D. (1983) *The Reflective Practitioner*, Temple Smith, London.

Schön, D. (1987) *Educating the Reflective Practitioner*, Jossey-Bass, San Francisco.

Shotter, J. (1974) What it is to be human, *Reconstructing Social Psychology*, (ed. R. Armistead), Penguin, Harmondsworth.

Urban, H. and Ford, D. (1971) Some historical and conceptual perspectives on psychotherapy and behaviour change, in *Handbook of Psychotherapy and Behavior Change*, (eds A. Bergin and S. Garfield), John Wiley, New York.

Wittgenstein, L. (1974) *Philosophical Investigations*, (trans. G. Anscombe), Basil Blackwell, Oxford.

# The presentation of the nurse: a neglected dimension of therapeutic nurse–patient interaction?

3

Steven J. Ersser

The experience of patients and nurses as to the therapeutic effect of nursing has received little attention in the literature. This chapter focuses on one aspect of the findings of a study examining the therapeutic nature of nursing from the perspective of nurses and patients. The complexity of this field makes it necessary to focus this analysis on the area given most emphasis by nurses and patients, namely, the concept of the *presentation of the nurse*. This concept reflects beliefs about the therapeutic significance of the expressive, non-verbal aspects of nursing action. The chapter includes an outline of the two primary features of the nurse's presentation: the importance of the nurse's personal qualities during interaction (*nurse as person*) and the *presence of the nurse*. The chapter begins with an outline of the rationale for adopting an interpretive approach to the study of nursing as a therapeutic activity. The concept of the presentation of the nurse and its therapeutic significance is then examined.

Deepening our understanding of the ways in which nursing may contribute effectively to patient welfare constitutes one of the most important areas of investigation for nursing research. However, few have examined this issue using a qualitative research approach. The interpretive approach taken involved exploring any beliefs patients and nurses may have held about the consequences of nurses' actions for the patient . The study was conducted in several hospital settings. A qualitative research approach was used (ethnography) based on nurses' and patients' accounts given through diaries, interviews and, for nurses, group discussions. Each type of data is used as an illustration within the chapter. The aim of the study was to discover if nurses and patients held views on the therapeutic (beneficial) effect of nursing and, if so, to determine the nature of those actions and compare the views of nurses and patients. Some brief details on the study design are given at the end in the methodological appendix. Full details of the completed study are given in Ersser (1995, 1997).

This chapter builds on and revises work for the earlier edition of this book (Ersser 1991). The latter presented the interim findings of the first stage of fieldwork (data collection) of three months. This chapter incorporates data from a further six months of fieldwork, to the completion of the study. Further extensive analysis has revealed three major categories of nursing action believed to have therapeutic potential.

Throughout the chapter some key findings will be illustrated using data excerpts relevant to the study aims. These excerpts draw from the meaningful building blocks of the data (codes). The codes encompass only those references made by the participating patients and nurses to three areas:

1   The actions of the nurse
2   The corresponding effect those actions were thought to have on the patient
3   Reference to the context of the situation.

The excerpts used here are labelled according to the nurse's action only. First, a case is made for the need to study nursing as a therapeutic activity using an interpretive research approach.


## THE NEED FOR AN INTERPRETIVE STUDY OF THE THERAPEUTIC EFFECT OF NURSING

There is a fundamental need to understand the relationship between nursing activities (process factors) and any corresponding effect these may have on the patient (outcome factors). This need is directly relevant to contemporary issues, such as understanding those factors that influence the effectiveness of health care and wider debates seeking to re-examine the evidential basis of health-care practices.

The literature on nursing as a therapeutic activity is at an early stage of development. Much of the literature consists of either theoretical assertions, for example Peplau's (1952) work on interpersonal relations, or speculative and controversial items, such as Muetzel's (1988) views about therapeutic interaction. There is little empirical research work to be found, although exceptions include, for example, Kitson's (1991) study of therapeutic nursing and the hospitalized elderly. Some studies build on theoretical assumptions about the nature of therapeutic care in nursing, such as Kitson's (1991) study drawing on Orem's (1980) theory of self-care. The limited research literature reflects attempts to examine the therapeutic effect of specific nursing interventions. For example, giving systematic information or massage to patients has been evaluated using the experimental design (e.g. Fortin and Kirouac 1976, Stevenson 1994, Wilson-Barnett 1978). Few have attempted a global evaluation of the therapeutic effect of nursing. An exception is Pearson *et al.*'s (1992) experimental work, based on Hall *et al.*'s (1975) study.

Experimental designs are best for evaluative research, although they have important limitations. For example, experimental designs involve an attempt to minimize variability in the actions of the person delivering the intervention. Crow (1981) highlighted the importance of the variability of nursing actions affecting the quality of care. She was referring to the different ways in which nursing care is delivered and how this may influence the quality of care received. This issue also directly applies to those actions of the nurse that could be defined as therapeutic, where beneficial patient outcome can be attributed to a complex range of nursing actions. From this follows the question of whether there are factors within nurse–patient interaction, beyond any specific procedural-type intervention of the nurse, which are significant in influencing patient outcome. Different explanatory models exist which attempt to depict the ways in which process and outcome factors are related in nursing situations. However, it is argued that these may be too simplistic (Jennings 1991).

An interpretive research approach is a neglected line of analysis in the study of nursing as a therapeutic activity. The study presented here involves an analysis of patients' and nurses' views on the effect of nursing on the patient. The accounts of nurses and patients, the providers and receivers of nursing care, may give insight to those more elusive and subtle but significant features of the nurse's actions. Nursing action has meaning for patients and the sense made of this interaction may have real consequences for the patient. The therapeutic significance of the symbolic nature of nursing action for the patient is discussed later.

Ethnographers recognize the importance of the link between social action and meaning; this view has direct relevance to the study of therapeutic action. Many features of patient experience are defined subjectively to an important degree. This includes aspects such as the patient's feelings of well-being, their comfort or sense of their ability to cope in certain situations. The study presented here only examined those instances in which the nurse's actions were seen as being related to specific patient outcomes. Given that beliefs on these issues were identified early on in the ethnographic study, work could continue with trying to build up a conceptual map. The 'map' encompasses sets of patient- and nurse-defined concepts and hypotheses on nursing as a therapeutic activity. It is apparent from the literature that there are major gaps in this fundamental descriptive work. Descriptive work is needed to provide a basis for studying the subtleties of therapeutic nursing action through labelling the factors (variables) involved and their interrelationship. The call for greater use of interpretive research to examine the interrelationship of process and outcome in nursing has been highlighted by others (Bond and Thomas 1991, 1992, Colledge 1979, Jennings 1991, McGuire 1991).

## INVESTIGATING VIEWS ON THE THERAPEUTIC EFFECT OF NURSING

From the first-stage fieldwork it was evident that nurse and patient participants held views on the therapeutic and adverse effects of nursing on patients. They were able to attribute specific patient outcomes to nurses' actions (Ersser 1991). Patients differentiated nurses from other health-care professionals in giving their accounts. Only occasionally were other staff mentioned by patients, such as doctors or the person delivering newspapers to the ward.

The informants (nurses and patients) described the consequences of nursing care for the patient in a wide range of ways, including reference to the nurse's impact on patient welfare and satisfaction. Particular emphasis was given to various ways in which the nurses helped the patient feel able to cope and adjust to their situation, whether illness, disability or being in hospital. Less prominent reference was made to the effect of nursing on health, well-being, satisfaction, recovery and promoting comfort. The outcome of care was described with varying degrees of specificity in detailing the resultant benefit or adverse effect; this is illustrated below.

*1. Nurse Angela: 'I spent as much time as possible today helping her to drink'*
Diane, who has a stroke, is having great difficulty drinking. I spent as much time as possible today helping her to drink so that hopefully she will not have to go back on IVI (*intravenous infusion*) hydration which is both uncomfortable and an infection risk.

Excerpt 1 can be seen to refer to the impact of nursing on patient outcome which is specifically focused, compared with the rather non-specific and vague recognition of benefit arising from nursing care remarked on in excerpt 2.

*2. Nurse Fay: 'A listening ear'*
There were several people who may have had bad news after investigations, like cancer – a cancerous growth or something, and they,

I think, were thinking about that in their head, although you never can tell ... so to listen to them would do them quite a lot of good, I think, well, in general it does anyway.

## NURSE AND PATIENT VIEWS ON NURSING AS A THERAPEUTIC ACTIVITY

From the detailed study of 17 cases, ten nurses and seven patients, 54 data sets were produced. From these, three core categories were identified, reflecting the broad categories of nurse actions believed to have therapeutic potential. Each core category describes a facet of the nurse's (or group of nurses) action believed by the informants to influence patient outcome beneficially or otherwise. It is interesting that the same three core categories have been identified in both the nurses' and patients' accounts. These categories encompassed the full range of codes reflecting views about nurses' therapeutic actions. They also encompassed codes identifying actions which could have an adverse effect, due to the specific form or absence of particular nursing actions.

The core categories are depicted in Figure 3.1. Specifically, they represent patients' and nurses' beliefs in the therapeutic importance of both the nurses' specific technical or procedural-type actions and their personal-expressive actions. The nurses' personal-expressive actions are embraced by two categories of nurses' actions, the *presentation of the nurse* and the nurse *relating to the patient*. Figure 3.1 also represents the interrelationship of these factors in a nursing situation. Central to the findings of this study is the belief in the therapeutic importance of not only *what nurses do* during their interaction with patients but *how nurses act* during their interaction.

The rest of the chapter will focus on the category of nurses' action, the presentation of the nurse and beliefs about its therapeutic significance. Presentation of the nurse reflects a range of largely expressive non-verbal actions which have received limited attention in the literature, relative to the other core categories of nursing action, namely, *the specifications of the nurse* and *relating to patients*.

### Building concepts on nursing actions believed to have therapeutic potential

The myriad of patterns within the data attributing nursing action to patient outcome were observed in the data. Codes were clustered together into categories identified by patients and nurses. Each code on nursing action or patient outcome, of which there were almost 2000, was organized into an extensive taxonomy or classification system. This is

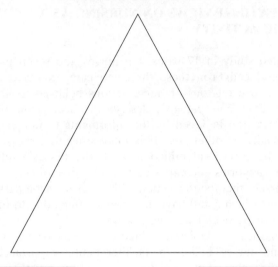

**Presentation of the nurse**

How the nurse appears before the patient;
largely non-verbal, expressive actions
(e.g. giving the patient time)

**Relating to patients**

References to the nurse
and patient having or forming
a relationship or developing rapport;
interaction in which the emotional
quality is emphasised
(e.g. developing rapport with the
nurse)

**Specific actions of the nurse**

The specific procedural-type
activities of the nurse, largely
instrumental in nature
(e.g. washing the patient)

**Figure 3.1** Core categories of nurses' actions believed to have therapeutic potential.

illustrated in Figure 3.2 as it relates to nursing action. The patterns in the codes reflect the variation in the nurses' actions and patient outcomes; these may be seen as characteristics or properties of the core categories. The excerpt labels used in this chapter reflect the terms used by the informant to describe the nurse's action wherever possible.

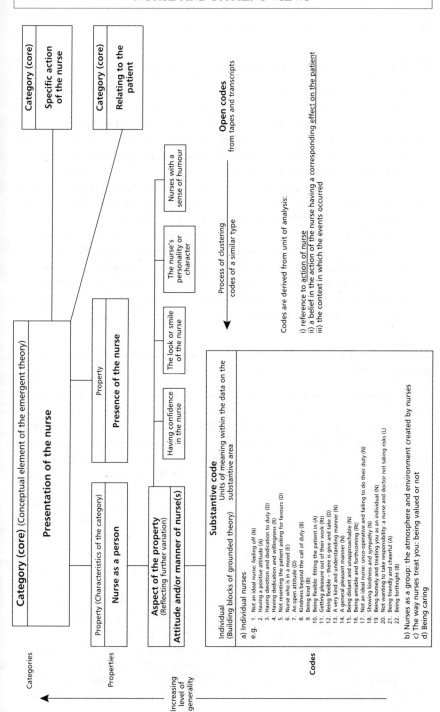

**Figure 3.2** The construction of a core category and taxonomic organization.

## THE PRESENTATION OF THE NURSE

### The therapeutic significance of nurses' expressive actions

Nurses and patients placed greatest emphasis on the way in which nurses present themselves to patients, how this is communicated non-verbally and their belief in its bearing on patient welfare and satisfaction with care. Such 'presentational action' highlights the importance of *how* nurses behave during interaction and the consequences for the patient; it may be viewed as different from what the nurse does in a procedural or task sense.

There are two main characteristics or properties of the nurse's presentation: the importance of the nurse's personal qualities (*nurse as a person*) and the ability of the nurse to communicate their physical or psychological presence with the patient (*presence of the nurse*). These features are now used to illustrate the 'Presentation' category. Due to the 'rich' nature of the data and the large range of views expressed, only a very limited number of illustrative data excerpts is described here. The excerpts are also truncated accounts of the full code. The main features of the nurse's presentational actions are now outlined in turn.

### The nurse as a person: the influence and significance of the nurse's personal qualities

Most emphasis was given by nurses and patients to the belief in the therapeutic potential of the nurse's personal qualities, in terms of the range and frequency of views expressed. 'Nurse as person' accounts referred to the variations in nursing action; for example, the nurse's attitude and manner, whether they appeared to be tired or in a mood, their appearance and whether their actions conveyed to the patient that they were valued by the nurse.

Ann, an adolescent with a chronic skin condition, had not been in hospital before and had impending school exams. She was finding the prolonged hospital stay and the treatment regime arduous. However, the nurse's 'presentation' helped her to cope.

*3. Patient Ann: 'Nurses with a positive attitude'*
If you say 'I've been here for three weeks and it doesn't seem any better' then they say, 'Well I haven't seen it (*her skin*) for four days'. They (nurses) are very positive and keep my spirits up a lot. They're just very positive and easy going. I mean, never having any treatment at all I was feeling a little, you know. I didn't want to go into hospital and have all these people doing things to me, but, you don't feel like that because it's so much a part of their routine that you don't feel at all uncomfortable.

Both nurse and patient referred to the significance of non-verbal aspects of the nurses' actions, such as facial expression or nervous demeanour, and its emotional influence on the patient, however transient. The following excerpt is from a patient who had just been admitted to a ward. She describes in her diary the significant impact of the nurse's presentation in helping her to adjust to being in hospital.

*4. Patient Joan: 'The nurse introducing herself to the patient'*
... the most influential nursing care is that received on direct entry to the ward. Liz met me, introduced herself as 'Liz', the nurse who would look after me that night. She showed me to my room, left me to gather up my thoughts and unpack before coming for a friendly chat. This meeting set the whole of my stay. If Liz had been unfriendly I would have had a hostile feeling and apprehension.

Nurses also show awareness of the importance of their presentation in putting the patient at ease and creating opportunities to help, such as listening or giving them information, whether as individuals or in groups.

*5. Nurse Sarah: 'The nurse's manner'*
I think you can put people at ease with the manner with which you talk to them.

*6. Nurse Fay: 'A happy ward atmosphere'*
It's no good being miserable. I mean, your overall disposition affects the way your patient feels – it doesn't matter where you work, though. It's no good coming into hospital and seeing a bunch of miserable nurses. It's going to make you feel miserable, isn't it? If the ward atmosphere is happy then you have happy patients and happy patients get better quicker.

Further support for the therapeutic effect of the group presentation of nurses (exemplified in 6 above) is also found in patient accounts. Another illustration is given from a dermatology ward, where patients gave emphasis to the therapeutic influence of the nurse's humour and their creation of a light ward atmosphere.

*7. Patient Betty: 'Nurses making treatment a fun time'*
There's three cubicles in the treatment room ... (laughs) there's another (nurse) she's telling outrageous stories about her mother ... It's always a fun time, it's not an ordeal going in for treatment and it could be, couldn't it? That again creates laughter and atmosphere. I think a friendly atmosphere makes such a difference.

This patient goes on to reinforce ('Coming on bright and breezy') the important influence of 'the way the staff are feeling' on the ward atmosphere and how the patient feels.

The differences between nurse and patient accounts were relatively insignificant, compared with the strong similarities in the core categories of nursing actions thought to be of therapeutic importance. One area of difference in the accounts of 'nurse as person' were those features referred to by patients but infrequently by nurses, including the importance of the nurse's humour and those expressive actions which gave patients confidence in the nurse. For example, patient Laura remarked on the distress created by not receiving consistent information on how to manage her new tracheostomy tube (excerpt 8, below). However, nurses repeatedly reported that they were benefiting the patient by giving them information, whilst unknowingly disrupting the patient's ability to gain independence by giving conflicting advice on self-care.

*8. Patient Laura: 'Conflicting advice'*
People constantly have different ideas about care . . . This has caused me a lot of distress – it's unnerving to be told different things.

This highlights the way in which ethnographic data may reveal significant differences between nurses' and patients' views.

## A sociological analysis of presentation of the nurse

Information about the individual helps to define the situation, enabling others to know how best to act in order to call forth a desired response from him. (Goffman 1971:13)

*The social meaning of the nurse's presentation*

A sociological analysis will be used to illuminate further the significance of the nurse's presentation. Recognition that the actions of people in a situation are related to the meaning or sense that the situation has for them is an important theoretical consideration in ethnographic research. Social actions have a symbolic significance for those involved; this applies to the actions of nurses that can communicate information to the patient. An illustration is provided by Chapman's (1983) study which revealed the symbolic importance of social rituals observed in hospitals. An understanding of nursing action therefore requires an interpretation of the meanings which patients and nurses give to nursing actions. The manner in which the nurse and patient define their situation will shape the way they will interact subsequently. Their actions will depend on the interpretation of the action of each party by the other. This process of 'making sense' takes place during interaction and involves negotiation. Each party will attempt to acquire information about the other. Mutual expectations will be held about how the other party will act. Viewed in this way, the presentation of the nurse may influence the outcome of nursing care for the patient. The relationship of the presentation of the nurse to patient outcome is depicted simply in Figure 3.3.

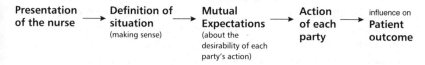

**Figure 3.3** A sociological analysis of the presentation of the nurse and its relationship to patient outcome.

### The nurse's emotional display

A major feature of the data on the nurse's presentation includes the variety of emotional expressions displayed by nurses and the various meanings these conveyed to the patient. The outward appearance of a nurse's emotional display to the patient was often said to affect the outcome of care since the symbolic nature of the encounter was thought to influence the course of interaction. For example, frequent accounts are given of the nurse's ability to convey to the patient that they are valued. This may be conveyed through their manner, attitude and the giving of time. Under these conditions the patient has been found to be more willing to ask the nurse important questions about their welfare. Other examples include the wide range of presentational strategies used by nurses, whether purposeful or not. This includes the nurse being 'professional and friendly' or displaying 'more experience of life'. In this way, the nurse may increase the patient's confidence in their own abilities, during their recovery period.

The findings of this study raise interesting questions about the extent to which the nurse's presentational actions are purposefully intended. The sociologist Weber (1979) studied the meaning and intention underlying social behaviour. He saw 'affectual (emotional) action' as unintentional and not purposefully directed in a rational way and viewed this as distinct from 'rational action'. However, the findings of the study here indicate that the nurse's actions may be construed or experienced as both intentional or deliberative; such emotions have been 'worked on' by the nurse. Such emotional display is in contrast to the more spontaneous expressions of affect which are truly felt by the nurse.

*Emotional labour and intentional emotional display*

> ... I assume that when an individual appears before others he will
> have many motives for trying to control the impression they receive
> of the situation. (Goffman 1971:26)

The deliberate management of emotional display for instrumental
purposes in the work environment has also been examined by the sociologist Hochschild (1983). In a study of air hostesses, she introduces the
concept of 'emotional labour' (p. 7) as '... the management of feeling to
create a publicly observable facial or bodily display: emotional labour is
sold for a wage and therefore has exchange value'.

  Hochschild viewed emotional labour as a form of social engineering within
public service work. She argues that emotional work by women may be used
to affirm, enhance and celebrate the well-being and status of others. Her
work draws on empirical examples using observation and interview from a
range of sources. Smith (1988) identified that nurses were engaging in emotional labour, although limited attention was given to examining its impact
on the patient. Jourard (1971:177) referred to the problems of the nurse's
'bedside manner', '... a peculiar kind of inauthentic behaviour adopted by
nurses', and pointed to the implications this may have for communication
between nurse and patient. The study presented here reveals the capacity of
nurses to use their emotional display in a deliberate way to influence
patients' welfare or satisfaction. This is illustrated in excerpt 3. It is difficult
to identify whether the emotional display of the nurse is deliberate in
the sense of being 'managed' or not. In making sense of each interaction,
however, the patient may make judgements about the sincerity of the nurses'
actions.

*9. Nurse Angela: 'Not being in the mood'*
I mean, whatever your mood is, it's going to have some bearing on
patients ... as a nurse you can't sort of totally throw off your mood
and be all smiles and chit chat to the patient always. I think, most
of the time you can – I'm amazed at myself – how lousy I can feel
and yet how, you know, sort of bubbly I can appear sometimes.

Different forms of emotional display have been described in the literature. Hochschild draws on Goffman's work in viewing social action as
drama, with the use of the terms 'surface acting' and 'deep acting'. 'Surface
acting' describes behaviour in which there is a change in the outward
appearance of a person with the action being in the body language. It is
a way of deliberately disguising what is really being felt, although there
is no self-deception. 'Deep acting' involves a display that results naturally
from working on feeling. The person tries to feel what they believe they
ought or want to feel through the production of real self-induced feelings
in a way often used by actors.

In the study presented here, nurse and patient data appear to depict instances of surface acting by nurses. This may be the case in excerpt 6. Also, excerpt 9 reveals a student's growing awareness of her ability to surface act. It is difficult to define these accounts as referring to one type or another, due largely to the covert nature of such activity. The cases of emotional display described could involve either surface acting or more spontaneous unintentional displays. The patient does not readily refer to the nurse's intent or does not necessarily assume that it is anything other than genuinely felt emotion.

*10. Patient Ella: 'A kind genuine smile'*
... as a patient one perhaps tends to be perhaps oversensitive to what seems unkind treatment, whereas a kind genuine smile from anyone does wonders for the patient.

Hochschild selected the extreme case of the airline hostess to highlight emotion work in public life. She examined the extent to which people may be trained to engage in emotional labour, to a degree which perhaps has not been attempted in nursing. Nurses' accounts from the study presented here suggest that emotional display of therapeutic significance does not necessarily involve emotion management. Furthermore, the pattern of emotional labour displayed by nurses is different from that adopted by flight attendants. The latter may attempt to use a higher degree of surface and deep acting, relative to the level of natural emotional display. The context of health-care services as opposed to the commercial field may largely account for this pattern. The deeper expression of interest and concern for another would of course be more likely to arise in the care context. Also, the high level of stress that often pervades clinical situations may lead to nurses controlling their own true feelings. They may fear (although often perhaps mythically) that such disclosures would threaten their ability to interact successfully with patients.

*Natural and spontaneous emotional display*

The emotional display of the nurse would often appear to involve spontaneous and natural expressions as well as emotional labour. Evidence of the genuine expression of emotions was provided in excerpts 5 and 8. It is also implicit in excerpt 11, from a discussion with the patient expressing feelings of loneliness due her separation from her loved ones:

*11. Patient Laura: 'Being friendly in a kind of ordinary friendly way'*
... hospital can be a very lonely place – you know, I think if you sort of find one or two nurses who are friendly – in a kind of ordinary friendly way – you know what I mean, not just a nurse being

friendly but, but just another person being friendly to you – I think that sort of makes me feel less isolated.

Several accounts describe the failure of emotional management, which may have therapeutic implications for the patient. In excerpt 12, the nurse describes her concern about disclosing her emotions to the patient (see also excerpt 6).

*12. Nurse Angela: 'Avoiding contact'*
The thing about standing at the end of the bed hiding behind the charts, that's more to do with how I'm feeling myself. If I do that then it's probably cos I'm not feeling confident. But, just sometimes you don't feel like it, you're just not in the mood to sort of say who you are and what you're there to do ... I always feel later when I go back to the person, I'm aware that we haven't yet been introduced and it, it would've been easier to have broken the ice earlier.

*The consequences of nurses' emotional display for the patient*

Some of the foregoing accounts reflect a belief in the capacity of emotional display to influence interaction with the patient. This effect, beneficial or not, may be viewed as direct or indirect through influencing the conditions whereby the patient's needs may or may not be met.

*13. Patient Roger: 'Nurses keep smiling'*
Everything is done with a smile and a cheery word. (When) the nurses are changing they wish you 'goodnight: sleep well: we'll see you in the morning.' One has to be in hospital to know what comfort you get.

*14. Nurse Fran: 'Being miserable and sullen and relaying it to the patient'*
They (*patients*) pick up the vibes if you are going onto the ward. They know when two of you have a run in and aren't getting on pretty well. They notice all these things and it prejudices them towards you or if you come across being sullen or if they think you haven't got enough time, they're not going to ask you again because they feel they're being a nuisance and that's not what you're aiming at. I mean, I know you all have your off days. You can't be one hundred percent happy.

The sincerity of the nurses' act does not seem in question here. The 'bedside manner' does not appear to be in evidence. Concern has been expressed that the nurse's bedside manner may lead to a neglect of the nurse's own personal needs. It may be an obstacle to communication with the patient, acting specifically as a barrier to a self-disclosure (Jourard 1971). However, Jourard recognizes the 'armoury function' of the bedside manner, which allows the nurse to work unaffected by excess emotion and insecurity.

The findings also reveal instances of a nurse's conscious awareness of her actions: it is a purposefully directed act *with a belief in the instrumental nature of her expressive actions*. This is an important finding because it highlights that the expressive and instrumental actions of nurses may not be discrete given that they may both be used for instrumental effect. This issue has received little focused attention in the nursing literature.

*15. Nurse Will: 'I try and be friendly and open'*
Obviously, my attitude when giving out drugs can alter, affect the patient's attitude to myself and nurses in general. If I try to be friendly, open and converse, this naturally puts people more at ease, more relaxed.

Strauss *et al.*'s (1982) empirical work is comparable with the findings presented here. They identified the 'sentimental' work that accompanied instrumental work in hospitals. A typology of sentimental work was described which compares with the findings from the study presented here. For example, 'composure work', which may involve an empathic display by the nurse, was found to be the most usual and visible type of sentimental work. It is believed to help patients to remain composed during a frightening or painful procedure. 'Trust work' depicts the display of many subtle gestures which reflect concern and competence; this may help staff to carry out other work such as an unavoidably painful procedure. The significance of sentimental work is captured by Strauss *et al.* (1982:274).

... when the sentimental work is not done, or is done badly in someone's judgement, then not only the main line of medical work may be affected but so may interactions, moods, composures, identities. Patients' feelings of humiliation, insult, invaded privacy, physical and mental discomfort, and resentment at being treated like an object are related to failures of sentimental work.

Gow's (1982) study on how the nurse's emotions may affect patient care examined the accounts of 275 graduate nurses in situations which they believed were 'helpful' and 'unhelpful' to patients. Nurses believed they could be unhelpful to patients when their self-image was being threatened, purposefully disregarding significant cues in patients' behaviour because they themselves had not resolved the issue. Organizational constraints, such as having too little time to devote to patients, were highlighted. Three main helping responses of the nurse were identified. First, 'gave moral support', which was characterized by the nurse as providing verbal reassurance. Second, nurses were seen to act as 'a sounding board' and involved the nurse listening to the patient, and thirdly, 'took time to explain'. An obvious weakness of method in Gow's work was the *a priori* assumptions made about the capacity of the nurse herself to affect the patient, in what was said to be an open-ended enquiry. However, these findings are comparable with those of the study presented here since they embrace both the personal and presence features of the nurse's presentation. Gow (1982:229) concluded:

> In situations where the nurses saw themselves as helpful, it was not because they perceived that they had neutralized their affect but rather because they had directed their affect in a particular way.

### The presence of the nurse: the influence and significance of being with the patient

The importance of the quality of 'presence' during nurse–patient interaction is evident from the accounts of both parties. The presence of the nurse is one of the two major characteristics of the core category 'presentation'. It reflects a belief in the value of the nurse 'being with' or having proximity to the patient, expressed in either physical or psychological (existential) terms. This feature has a range of properties, for example, the giving of time to patients, being with the patient and trying to understand the patient's experience. These extend across the data from patients and nurses. The nurse's presence was often employed when the patient was seen to be under stress to help the patient cope with their situation. This range of action and effect is now briefly illustrated.

Nurses describe the difficulty created when it is not possible to give a patient adequate time, particularly in meeting their needs for information and physical assistance. The patients' accounts of the nurse not being available correspond with the nurses' reports of their intent to 'give' or 'spend' time with the patient.

*16. Nurse Fay: 'Having time for patients'*
I think that quite an important way of affecting someone is letting them have a few minutes of your time, cos they all say 'You're too busy, nurse'. I've had people say 'Can I have a commode – no, you're too busy' or 'Can I have a word? No, you're too busy now, I'll ask you later' or 'I'll wait' or 'Don't bother, don't worry'. I think quite a lot of people miss out on care they could've got by kind of not taking the opportunity to, kind of, talk with a nurse or doctor, whoever they find useful.

The following shows the difficulty the nurse may find in being available for the patient and the risks of reinforcing feelings of dependency in the patient.

*17. Patient Laura: 'Not enough nurses/being very busy'*
Only five nurses to look after the ward this morning. Usually about 11. Felt really annoyed and frustrated because I wanted a shower and a hair wash but it wasn't possible as they were very busy. The student told me the whole week was going to be like this which didn't make me feel any better. She said she could understand how I felt but I'm sure she couldn't possibly understand the frustration of being dependent and there not being enough people to help.

Both nurses and patients convey the importance of the nurse trying to understand the patient's experience and having an awareness of the patient's situation. This is expressed in terms such as the 'sensitivity-insensitivity shown to the patient' (patient data) and 'determining what the problem is from the patient's viewpoint' (nurse data).

*18. Nurse Will: 'Determining what the problem is from their (patients') viewpoint and responding to it'*
. . . the patients often actually know the problems themselves more than, obviously better than, anybody else. So, if you can determine what the problem is from their point of view, then you can actually treat it in a more effective way.

*19. Nurse Angela: 'Helping a patient to accept that their need is under-stood and that they are not a nuisance'*
B was extremely worried about the possibility of her needing to keep calling the night staff to fetch her a commode. I sat and listened to her worries and tried to discover fully if it was such a big worry, I then tried to make her accept that we understood her need and that to us she was in no way being a nuisance as she felt herself to be.

While accepting that suffering is personal and beyond the full comprehension of other individuals, sufferers may seek a more complete understanding of their suffering from others (McGilloway and Myco 1985).

The therapeutic importance of being physically present with a patient was described in various situations. This feature is illustrated below where the potentially therapeutic factor is absent. When circumstances prevent the nurse being with the patient in a time of need, the patient may be affected adversely within circumstances which may seem rather ordinary. For example, the following account has to be seen in the context of the patient having undergone a tracheotomy for a respiratory arrest and being fearful of another.

*20. Patient Laura: 'Not being there'*
I mean, sometimes I'm just sort of on the loo and my chest's a bit rough. I know somebody might not come for a while, you know, it

takes a lot of confidence to sit there, particularly bearing in mind
that I, I did have a, I did stop breathing. I did have a bout in the
ITU and it was bound to have some effect on me. You know, I need
to build up my confidence – that does take (ermm) quite an effort
on my part, just to, you know relax and realize that nothing is going
to happen.

In excerpts 20 and 21, the nurse's presence is seen as a means of helping
to alleviate some of the patient's distress.

*21. Nurse Fay: 'Just by being with him'*
Bill had his treatment applied this morning. He appears to have
become breathless again on exertion. I had to ask for him to be
given oxygen after lunch, as he found no relief from his inhalers. I
think just being with him helped to reassure him that he would soon
be better.

The literature relevant to the value of the nurse's presence spans a wide
field and includes psychology, theology and existential philosophy. An
important nursing example is evident in Paterson and Zderad's (1976)
theoretical work. This compares with the features of the nurse's presence
found in the study data, such as 'being there' and the nurse's 'availability'.
They view 'presence' as a therapeutic dimension of interaction. It allows
the nurse to be in a situation in which they may relate to the patient
and thereby help to increase their capacity to make choices. Similarly,
Muetzal's (1988) analysis of the therapeutic nurse–patient relationship
includes recognition of the element of the nurse 'being there' for the
patient, although this appears to be speculative.

The importance of the nurse being available to understand and be with
another, physically present and not preoccupied with other thoughts, is
evident in empirically based nursing literature (Benner and Wrubel 1989).
Empathy is recognized both as an essential basis for helping (Carkhuff
1969) and 'as integral to therapeutic nursing' (Gagan 1982). The problem
of nurses giving patients adequate time is evident in research exploring
the pattern of verbal interaction between nurse and patient. It reveals
that interaction is often infrequent, of short duration and typically accompanied by nursing activity, in various clinical settings (Cormack 1976,
Macleod-Clarke 1982). Such patterns may have adverse therapeutic implications. Macleod-Clarke warned that patients appear consciously to adopt
a passive role, perceiving the nurse as too busy to be worried; as such,
patients may then be reluctant to express their concerns.

The significance of the nurse 'being with' the patient is evident from a
range of literature. However, little has been derived from interpretive
studies involving patients and nurses. Campbell's (1984) exploratory
account provides a comparable image of the nurse as a companion to the

patient. This is seen in the form of the nurse's physical presence; it involves 'being with' and not just 'doing to' the patient. Companionship is believed to help the person move onward and to provide encouragement in the face of apparent hopelessness. Such accounts do not necessarily differentiate nursing from the activities of other carers or helpers. Descriptions of the care of dying people often describe the value of the 'presence' of another. The fear of death may be experienced as the fear of being alone. Dyck and Benner (1989) describe the care of a person with progressive tracheal stenosis. Listening, checking on the patient and being with them as they confront death were viewed as therapeutic features of nursing.

The protective value of 'presence' can be compared to the specific psychological concept of 'attachment behaviour', which refers to forms of behaviour used to attain and maintain a desired proximity to another. Attachment may help to alleviate anxiety and provide an increased sense of security (Bowlby 1984). However, its place in nature to help protect the vulnerable is not confined to infants. It has a vital role to play in adult life, especially in situations of sudden danger, sickness or calamity (Bowlby 1984, Weiss 1982).

Analysis of the issues highlighted by the nurse's presentation throws into relief an important issue discussed in the literature on therapeutic nursing action, namely, the concept of 'therapeutic use of self'. This concept is now revisited in the light of the study findings discussed.

## THE CONCEPT OF THERAPEUTIC USE OF SELF

The concept of the 'therapeutic use of self' is widespread throughout the nursing literature. It has its origins in the psychotherapy field. The influence of psychotherapy on the theoretical thinking in nursing is evident in the work of, for example, Hall (1969), Peplau (1952) and Travelbee (1971). Emphasis is given to the necessity for the nurse to act with intention when acting in a therapeutic way.

Peplau (1952:5) made no direct reference to the term 'therapeutic use of self' but referred to nursing as '. . . an interpersonal process and often a therapeutic one'. Peplau's interest lay in 'psychodynamic nursing' which she described as understanding one's own behaviour in order to help others. Like Travelbee, Peplau was concerned with the nurse–patient relationship and its implications for patient welfare. Uys's (1980) descriptive paper attempted to formulate an operational definition of the therapeutic use of self concept. However, Uys indicates that the therapeutic effect that may arise from such nursing interaction may result from either natural inclination, luck or developed social skill. This point is implicit in the accounts of the study presented here and is one infrequently expressed in the nursing literature. It is also interesting to view this point in the context of foregoing discussions of emotional display being deliberative or not. In a similar vein to the nursing literature, Balint (1964) studied psychotherapeutic activity in GP clinics and found that by far the most frequently used 'drug' was the doctor himself. Balint's accounts gave little specific reference to doctors' expressive actions but rather focused on activities such as the use of understanding and listening.

### The concept of therapeutic use of self re-examined

An important finding of the study presented here is the recognition by nurses and patients of the therapeutic potential of the nurse's presentational actions. Such actions may be communicated to the patient with or without intention. This is in contrast to the picture created in the theoretical nursing literature which gives emphasis to the deliberate actions of nurses when engaged in the therapeutic use of self (e.g. Orlando 1961). For example, Travelbee (1971:19) defined therapeutic use of self thus:

> When a nurse uses self therapeutically she consciously makes use of her personality and knowledge in order to effect a change in the ill person. This change is considered therapeutic when it alleviates the individual's stress.

Similarly, in the sociological literature, Goffman's (1971) concept of the 'presentation of self' places emphasis on the deliberate management of appearances. Although this is a useful concept from which to examine the symbolic significance of nurses' actions, it does not adequately account for the variation observed in the findings on the nurse's emotional display, some of which is not managed.

The prevailing view of the concept of therapeutic use of self, as found in the literature, would only account for those features of nurses' emotional display which involve deliberate or intentional actions. Such is the case when the nurse engages in emotional labour. In contrast, the study findings convey a belief in the potential value of nurses' natural, spontaneous emotional display for patients, which is not intentionally purposeful. As such, there is a need for re-examination of the received concept of therapeutic use of self which is confined to considerations of deliberate action. The current use of this concept underplays the significance of nurses' ordinary social conduct which may be evident in other areas of their social lives. The emphasis reflected in the 'nurse as person' feature of nurses' presentation is consistent with Taylor's (1994) thesis. Here, the humanity and effectiveness of the nurse's ordinariness during their interaction with patients are given recognition (epitomized here by excerpt 12). Taylor concludes: 'Aspects of ordinariness such as facilitation, fair play, familiarity, family, favouring, feelings, fun and friendship can have advantageous effects', (p. 241). Taylor's analysis is also congruent with accounts about the value of nurses 'relating to patients'; this core category of nurses' action has been mentioned but is not explored further here.

### The therapeutic encounter: the place of the symbolic-expressive actions of the nurse

The qualitative research design adopted in this study has generated concepts and propositions on features of nurse–patient interaction believed to have therapeutic potential. The therapeutic significance of the nurse's symbolic expressive actions has been highlighted; these aspects of nursing action require closer attention in the study of therapeutic nursing activity. Work has begun which highlights the need to examine further the conceptual framework encompassing the interrelationship between the nurse's expressive-personal type actions (presentation and relating) and technical, procedural-type actions (specific actions). The importance of this conceptual framework for the study of patients' evaluation of therapeutic effect, the effectiveness of nursing and patient satisfaction is discussed further elsewhere (Ersser 1995, 1997) but more empirical work is needed in this complex area. It is advocated that a wider theoretical view of the concept of therapeutic use of self in nursing be adopted. Recognition is needed of the therapeutic significance of nurses' deliberative actions and those natural, spontaneous and ordinary features of the nurse's social action, including emotional display.

## METHODOLOGICAL APPENDIX

This study aimed to identify whether hospital nurses and adult patients on medical units hold views about the therapeutic (beneficial) and adverse effects of nursing. If this was found to be so, the aim was to identify the nature of such views and to compare the views of patients and nurses. An attempt has also been made to develop a conceptual framework from the data (depicted at its simplest in Figure 3.1).

### An ethnographic approach

'Ethnography' refers to the description and analysis of aspects of the way of life of a particular culture or subculture (Germain 1986). Ethnography involves the description of culture, the acquired knowledge of what people use to interpret experience and generate social behaviour (Spradley 1979). People learn their culture by observing other people, listening to them and making inferences from this information. The ethnographer employs the same approach to infer what people know. Culture is a shared system of meanings; a significant part of any culture consists of tacit knowledge.

An attempt was made to identify the knowledge or shared meanings related to the study aims among nurses and patients in hospital settings. Participant observation was not employed in this study. It was thought that it would often be impossible to define the consequences of nurses' actions for the patient as beneficial or adverse in effect, simply on the basis of what could be observed. This was an important consideration given the subjective nature of outcomes that are not readily observable, such as the patient's feelings of well-being, coping and comfort.

The theoretical orientation of the study was sociological in nature and of the social action or micro-interpretive type. Interpretive sociology was founded principally by Weber (1979) and is influenced by symbolic interaction theory (Blumer 1969). Interactionism is based on the premise that people act on the basis of the meaning a situation has for them and these meanings arise out of a person's interaction with others (Blumer 1969).

Ethnography may be used to identify discrepancies in patient and professional perceptions (Ragucci 1972), to uncover the complexities of nursing practice and to develop nursing theory (Aamodt 1982) as grounded theory (Spradley 1979). Each of these opportunities was taken during this study. The elements of grounded theory were discovered from the data during the concurrent process of data collection and analysis. The aim was to identify the logical unity of the informants' concepts and their relationships on the therapeutic features of nursing emerging from the data.

## Organization of the study

Fieldwork took place over a nine-month period. Three methods were used to collect the data: diaries (document); in-depth ethnographic interviews and group discussions (nurses only). Data collection began with patients completing diaries. These were analysed and used as a basis for drawing up an interview schedule.

The study was organized with the aim that nurses on the same ward would remain unaware of the content of the diary and interview process for the patient participants. Data collection commenced with patients and proceeded to nurses once complete. This helped to minimize the nurses' awareness that their actions were being reflected upon while the patients were completing diaries. However, it was also not possible to make detailed comparisons of pairs of nurses and patients. Nurses commenced with the same pattern of participation as the patients except that they engaged in a group discussion prior to completing their diary. Details of the ethical aspects of conducting ethnography in clinical situations are given elsewhere (Ersser 1996).

**The setting and sampling methods**

The study was set in general and speciality (neurology and dermatology) medical wards across three different hospitals within the same health authority. Ten nurses and seven patient participants were selected from these settings. A small number of cases are studied in ethnography (Hammersley and Atkinson 1983). There was also a practical requirement to select accessible informants and so to employ opportunistic sampling (Burgess 1984).

The development of grounded theory involves the selection of cases that would generate as many categories from the data as possible following analysis (Glaser and Strauss 1967). Purposive sampling was employed; this refers to a theoretically directed approach in which informants were selected who would facilitate the development of the emerging theory (Field and Morse 1985). As such, the sample included those with knowledge about the experience of receiving nursing care (patients) or experience of providing it (nurses), irrespective of their staff grade. A form of purposive sampling, termed 'theoretical sampling', was also used whereby the direction of data collection was guided by the product of ongoing data analysis.

**Data collection**

The diaries consisted of unstructured notebooks with an accompanying instruction sheet. They provided a form of personal documentary data solely for research purposes. The diaries were designed to enable the informants to provide spontaneous, personalized accounts, freely structured by them on events significant to them. Patients were asked to consider the following.

> I am interested in your experiences of receiving nursing care. In particular, I want you to try and describe how you believe the nursing you receive affects you.

Nurses were asked to consider the comparable question:

> I am interested in your experiences of giving nursing care. In particular, I want you to try and describe how you believe the nursing you give affects your patients.

Informants were requested to reflect on this issue and complete the diary as they felt appropriate over a period of up to five days.

The ethnographic interviews served as a basis for exploring informants' diary entries while allowing the opportunity to request elaboration and clarification. The interview schedules served as flexible *aides-mémoire* in providing a list of topics and questions. 'Ethnographic elements' were introduced during the interview, including explanations about its purpose and the use of ethnographic questions (Spradley 1979).

The group discussions involved nurse informants only for several reasons: the commitment of completing a diary; the potential difficulty nurses may have in recording the adverse effects of their action and the need to provide a basis to explore the use of reconstructed ('public' and 'private') accounts. The group discussions included those nurses or students participating in the study together with other nursing staff who were free to leave the ward. Group discussions have been used in other studies, such as those of Stimpson and Webb (1975).

## Data analysis

The process of data analysis was informed by the work of Chenitz and Swanson (1986), Glaser (1978), Lofland (1971) and Wiseman (1974). Diaries and interviews were transcribed verbatim to provide accurate and detailed records. The diary transcripts and tape recordings of interviews and group discussions were treated as the primary data source. Data analysis took place during the fieldwork period, allowing further data collection to be guided using theoretical sampling. Grounded theory method was adhered to closely and involved several processes. The first was content analysis, in which the contents of the informants' communication were fractured into meaningful units related to the study aims (codes). The identification and labelling of units of meaning within the data are described as coding (Corbin 1986). The nature of codes has been described. Groups of similar codes were clustered in ways faithful to the informants' beliefs. An attempt was made to achieve theoretical saturation of the data, although this was difficult in some areas due to the wide variation in the description of action and effect. Each item of data was compared to other items to identify similarities and differences and thereby to reveal uniformity and variation in the data (constant comparative method). The process of building the categories, identifying their characteristics and variation and generating hypotheses (ideas about how the categories were related) was driven by the writing of memos (Glaser 1978).

## Acknowledgements

The author would like to acknowledge the support and comments of the late Dr Morva Fordham, my first academic supervisor, and Professor Wilson-Barnett. Financial assistance was received from the Nightingale Fund Council, the Tregaski's Bequest, King's College (London) and the National Institute for Nursing, Oxford. The comments of Sue Atkins, Oxford Brookes University, are also valued.

# REFERENCES

Aamodt, A. M. (1982) Examining ethnography for nurse researchers. *Western Journal of Nursing Research*, **4**(2), 209–221.

Balint, M. (1964) *The Doctor, His Patient and the Illness*, London, Pitman.

Benner, P. and Wrubel, J. (1989) *The Primacy of Caring: Stress and Coping in Health and Illness*, Addison-Wesley, California.

Blumer, H. (1969) *Symbolic Interactionist Perspective and Method*, Prentice-Hall, New Jersey.

Bond, S. and Thomas, L. (1991) Issues in measuring outcomes in nursing. *Journal of Advanced Nursing*, **16**, 1492–1502.

Bond, S. and Thomas, L. (1992) Input on outcomes: findings from the *Nursing Times* Readers Survey (Annex 4), in *Outcomes of Nursing: Proceedings of an International Developmental Workshop*, (ed. S. Bond), Centre for Health Services Research Direct Patients Services Programme, University of Newcastle upon Tyne.

Bowlby, J. (1984) *Attachment and Loss. Volume 1, Attachment*, Penguin Books, Harmondsworth.

Burgess, R. G. (1984) *In the Field: an Introduction to Field Research*, Allen and Unwin, London.

Campbell, A. V. (1984) *Moderated Love: a Theory of Professional Care*, SPCK, London.

Carkhuff, R. R. ( 1969) *Helping and Human Relations: a Primer for Lay and Professional Helpers. Volume 1, Practice and Research*, Holt Rinehart and Winston, New York.

Chapman, G. (1983) Ritual and rational action in hospitals, *Journal of Advanced Nursing*, **81**, 13–20.

Chenitz, W. C. and Swanson, I. M. (1986) *From Practice to Grounded Theory: Qualitative Research in Nursing*, Addison-Wesley, California.

Colledge M. M. (1979) Observing nursing: exploration of the familiar, towards the construction of nursing knowledge, in *Readings in Nursing*, (eds M. Colledge and D. Jones), Churchill Livingstone, Edinburgh.

Corbin, J. (1986) Coding writing memos, and diagramming, in *From Practice to Grounded Theory*, (eds W. C. Chenitz and J. M. Swanson), Addison-Wesley, California.

Cormack, D. (1976) *Psychiatric Nursing Observed*, Royal College of Nursing, London.

Crow, R. A. (1981) Research and the standards of nursing care: what is the relationship? *Journal of Advanced Nursing*, **6**, 491–496.

Dyck, B. and Benner, P. (1989) Dialogues with excellence: the paper crane. *American Journal of Nursing*, **89**(8), 824–825.

Ersser, S. (1991) A search for the therapeutic dimensions of nurse-patient interaction, in *Nursing as Therapy*, (eds R. McMahon and A. Pearson), Chapman Hall, London.

Ersser, S. (1995) An ethnographic study of the therapeutic effect of nursing. Unpublished PhD thesis, King's College, University of London.

Ersser, S. (1996) Ethnography in clinical situations: an ethical appraisal, in *Nursing Research: An Ethical and Legal Appraisal*, (ed. L. De Raeve), Baillière Tindall, London.

Ersser, S. (1997) *Nursing as a Therapeutic Activity: An Ethnography*, Avebury, Aldershot.

Field, P. A. and Morse, J. M. (1985) *Nursing Research: The Application of Qualitative Approaches*, Croom Helm, London.

Fortin, F. and Kirouac, S. (1976) A randomised controlled trial of preoperative patient education. *International Journal of Nursing Studies*, **13**, 11–24.

Gagan, J. M. (1982) Methodological notes on empathy.' *Advances in Nursing Science*, **5**(2), 65–72.

Germain, C. (1986) Ethnography: the Method, in *Nursing Research: A Qualitative Perspective*, (eds P. L. Munhall and C. J. Oiler), Appleton-Century-Crofts, Norwalk.

Glaser, B. (1978) *Theoretical Sensitivity*, Sociology Press, California.

Glaser, B. and Strauss, A. (1967) *The Discovery of Grounded Theory*, Aldine, Chicago.

Goffman, E. (1971) *The Presentation of Self in Everyday Life*, Pelican Books, Harmondsworth.

Gow, K. M. (1982) *How Nurses' Emotions Affect Patient Care: Self Studies by Nurses*, Springer, New York.

Hall, L. (1969) The Loeb Center for Nursing and Rehabilitation, Montefiore Hospital and Medical Center, Bronx, New York. *International Journal of Nursing Studies*, **6**, 81–95.

Hall, L., Alfano, G., Rifkin, E. and Levine, E. (1975) Final report: longitudinal effects of an experimental nursing process. Unpublished report, Loeb Center for Nursing and Rehabilitation, New York.

Hammersley M. and Atkinson, P. (1983) *Ethnography: Principles and Practice*, Tavistock, London.

Hochschild, A. R. (1983) *The Managed Heart: Commercialisation of Human Feeling*, University of California Press, Berkeley.

Jennings. B. M. (1991) Patient outcomes research: seizing the opportunity. *Advances in Nursing Science*, **14**(2), 59–72.

Jourard, S. (1971 ) *The Transparent Self*, Van Nostrand Reinhold, New York.

Kitson, A. (1991) *Therapeutic Nursing and the Hospitalised Elderly*, Royal College of Nursing Research Series, RCN, London.

Lofland, J. (1971) *Analysing Social Situations: A Guide to Qualitative Observation and Analysis*, Wadsworth, Belmont, California.

MacGuire, J. (1991) Tailoring research for advanced nursing practice, in *Nursing as Therapy*, (eds R. McMahon and A. Pearson), Chapman and Hall, London.

Macleod-Clarke, J. (1982) Nurse-patient interaction. An analysis of conversations on surgical wards. Unpublished PhD thesis, University of London.

McGilloway, O. and Myco, F. (1985) *Nursing and Spiritual Care*, Harper and Row. London.

Muetzel, P. A. (1988) Therapeutic nursing, in *Primary Nursing: Nursing in the Burford and Oxford Nursing Development Unit*, (ed. A. Pearson), Croom Helm, Beckenham.

Orem, D. (1980) *Nursing: Concepts of Practice*, McGraw-Hill, New York.

Orlando, I. J. (1961) *The Dynamic Nurse–Patient Relationship: Function, Process and Principles*, Putnam, New York.

Paterson, J. G. and Zderad, L. T. (1976) *Humanistic Nursing*, John Wiley, New York.

Pearson, A., Punton, S. and Durand, I. (1992) *Nursing Beds: an Evaluation of the Effects of Therapeutic Nursing*, Scutari Press, London.

Peplau, H. (1952) *Interpersonal Relations in Nursing*, Putnam, New York.

Ragucci, A. T. (1972) The ethnographic approach to nursing research. *Nursing Research*, **21**(6), 485–490.

Smith, P. (1988) The emotional labour of nursing. *Nursing Times*, **84**(44), 50–51.

Spradley, J. (1979) *The Ethnographic Interview*, Holt, Rinehart and Winston, Chicago .

Stevenson, C. J. (1994) The psychophysiological effects of aromatherapy massage following cardiac surgery. *Complimentary Therapies in Medicine*, **2**(1), 27–35.

Stimpson, G. and Webb, B. (1975) *Going to See the Doctor: The Consultation Process in General Practice*, Routledge and Kegan Paul, London.

Strauss, A., Fagerhaugh, S., Suezek, B. and Wiener, C. (1982) Sentimental work in technological hospitals. *Sociology of Health and Illness*, **4**(3), 254–278.

Taylor, B. J. (1994) *Being Human: Ordinariness in Nursing*. Churchill Livingstone, Melbourne.

Travelbee, J. (1971) *Interpersonal Aspects of Nursing*, 2nd edn, F.A. Davis, Philadephia.

Uys, L. R. (1980) Towards the development of an operational definition of the concept 'therapeutic use of self'. *International Journal of Nursing Studies*, **17**(3), 175–180.

Weber, M. (1979) *Economy and Society: an Outline of Interpretative Sociology*, (eds G. Roth and C. Wittich translated from the German by Fischoff, E.), University of California Press, Berkeley.

Weiss, R. S. (1982) Attachment in adult life, in *The Place of Attachment in Human Behaviour*, (eds C. M. Parkes and J. Stevenson-Hinde), Basic Books, New York.

Wilson-Barnett, J. (1978) Patients' emotional response to barium x-rays. *Journal of Advanced Nursing*, **3**, 37–45.

Wiseman, J. P. (1974) The research web. *Urban Life and Culture*, **3**, 317–328.

<table>
<tbody>
<tr><td>**4**</td><td># Ordinariness in nursing as therapy</td></tr>
</tbody>
</table>

Beverley Taylor

Some things in life are so commonplace that they are virtually unnoticed on a daily basis. Arguably, two of the most obvious enduring characteristics of human life are the sky and the earth. Every day, the sky stays above our heads and the earth stays beneath our feet, but they may remain silent and unacknowledged givens for the people who do not stop to ponder the awesomeness of their presence. Nursing is a bit like that. Nursing is about nurses and patients in contexts of care, yet it seems the awesomeness of this goes relatively unnoticed in the daily run of practice.

## THE MEANING OF CERTAIN WORDS

Words carry meaning and at times these meanings can be multiple, so at this point it seems a good idea to arrive at some common understanding for key words for this chapter, specifically ordinariness, patients, illness and nursing.

Malone and Malone (1987) used the word 'ordinariness' in relation to interpersonal relationships. They perceived that people who accepted and nurtured their ordinariness were reacting naturally to life events. They explained that in the attempt to do what people think they should do, rather than what they would like to do, they think that they have to be special. People then attempt to attain specialness by striving to please others, thereby risking the effects of high stress rates, rather than simply being ordinary, which is what they are and how they are meant to be as humans.

Through a research process (Taylor 1991), I defined ordinariness as the common bond of humanity that ties people together. In relation to nursing, ordinariness emerged as a phenomenon of shared sense of humanity between nurses and patients that makes illness experiences manageable somehow. Thus, nursing is what happens between nurses and patients in contexts of care and it is facilitated by the humanity of both parties, as they negotiate the illness experience together.

I make no apologies for the use in this chapter of the words 'patient' and 'illness', even though they have fallen into a certain amount of disrepute in contemporary nursing and health rhetoric. The word 'patient' is derived from *sufferre*, which means to suffer, and I think patients suffer, from the finest degrees of anguish to the thickest layers of misery, from disturbances to their lives, because of their illness circumstances.

Illness is still a useful word for nursing and health because the people experiencing illness do not feel well and that is what matters to them. Perceptions and manifestations of illness are apparent in varying degrees in patients who suffer from disturbances to their life patterns through not feeling well. Nursing finds itself in the context of patients and illness and even as roses by other names, clients, customers and consumers still suffer to some extent and a health focus will always be understood in terms of its opposite, illness.

Nursing practice reflects the ways in which nurses and patients experience the nurse–patient relationship and as this is essentially a person-to-person encounter, it is inextricably bound to the humanness of nurses and patients as people. Therefore, it is the simple claim of this chapter that some basic essentials for therapeutic encounters in nursing lie within the nature of being human. Human qualities are ordinary in that they are commonplace, but this is not the same as saying that they are inconsequential. It was said most eloquently that 'The foundation of genuine helping lies in being ordinary. Nothing special' (Pearson 1988a). In these words lie some clues to the therapeutic nature of ordinariness in nursing.

In order to situate ordinariness in nursing as therapy, it is important at this point to overview briefly the research which explicated the phenomenon, before describing specific insights for nurses of ordinariness. This chapter is based on the original research (Taylor 1991) but components of the following have subsequently been published as the book *Being Human: Ordinariness in Nursing* and in other papers related to the research (Taylor 1992a,b, 1993a,b,c). The purpose of this chapter is to emphasize those elements of the research that relate directly to ordinariness in nursing as therapy.

## OVERVIEW OF THE RESEARCH INTO ORDINARINESS

The idea of researching the phenomenon of ordinariness in nursing originated from discussions with Professor Alan Pearson and through my own previous research into midwifery practice (Taylor 1988). In both cases, it became apparent that when nurses and patients were 'just themselves' in clinical settings, they were happier with each other generally. Based on these casual observations, the research wanted to explore nurse–patient relationships to see whether or not nurses and patients being 'just themselves' enhanced nursing encounters.

A phenomenological approach was used for exploring the phenomenon of ordinariness, because it had the potential to describe everyday human qualities and activities in nursing. A fuller explanation of phenomenology and the reasons for its selection as a guide for undertaking this research can be found in other publications (Taylor 1991, 1993a, 1994). The health-care context for the research was a professorial nursing unit (PNU) in a large acute-care hospital in Victoria, Australia, which was based on the Burford and Oxford Nursing Development Units (Pearson 1988b,c, 1992), in which primary nursing was the system of nursing care.

I was present as a participant observer at 24 nurse–patient interactions, including washes in bed, bowel evacuation, showers, dressings and other specific nurse–patient activities. The interactions included any nurse–patient communications that were part of the negotiated plan of care for each patient. After informed consent was secured from all the research participants, the nurses involved informed me when nursing care interactions were due to happen. After each interaction, I recorded my impressions in my journal, including preinterview and postinterview notes, some demographical information and a full account of the interaction.

After each interaction, I audiotaped a conversation with each patient, after saying to them: 'I was with you when you interacted with (the nurse) this morning. What did you like about being with (the nurse) this morning? What didn't you like about being with (the nurse) this morning?'. When audiotaping a conversation with each nurse after the respective nurse–patient interactions, I said: 'I was with you when you were with (the patient) this morning. Tell me your impressions of being with (the patient) this morning'.

The transcribed audiotapes and the journal notes became text for a hermeneutical interpretation of the respective nurse–patient interactions. The text was analysed to find the main aspects illuminating the phenomenon. Initially, this was done by using a computerized qualitative data analysis package, to search for frequently recurring words and phrases. Following the initial search, the data were read and re-read to immerse myself fully in the contextual features of each interaction. A large set of qualities and activities emerged from the initial searches of the impressions, which were then grouped into aspects, which will be explained in detail later in this chapter. Having arrived at the aspects of the phenomenon, I tried to explain the nature of the aspects themselves and the resultant actualities that emerged from this process will also be explained in detail later in this chapter.

The interpretation of the meaning of each interaction was shared and checked at the time of conversation with the patients and nurses. A draft of each set of interactions was given to respective nurses for them to check the validity of my impressions against their own impressions of the interactions and to offer feedback on their perceptions.

## THE ESSENTIAL FINDINGS OF THE RESEARCH

### Aspects of ordinariness

The eight major aspects were facilitation, fair play, familiarity, family, favouring, feelings, fun and friendship.

*Facilitation* refers to the enabling qualities and activities of both nurses and patients, whereby certain challenges being experienced by one person are made easier to face by the other person. In relation to learning about diabetes management, Jean (a patient) said this about Peter (a nurse):

> I feel that Peter explains things very plain to you ... He puts it in English that I can understand ... It was special, because I thought that he was doing it for me ... I thought he was doing it especially for me ... I hope he can keep on getting through to people like he got through to me.

*Fair play* refers to the sense of reasonableness that we possess as humans, through which we are forthright in saying what we feel we have to say, knowing that the least we can do, even partially, is to tolerate frustrating elements in others that we recognize in ourselves. Tolerating one another's humanness was best described by Andrew (a nurse), who said:

> We're (nurses are) only human, that's right. It's probably one of the hardest jobs I know, because you've got to put it aside, you're supposed to. One of the things I've always found in nursing is honesty with the patient. You have some days when you come to work and you really don't want to be there and (that was) one of the things Donald (a patient) and me understood with each other. I could be really tired and I could just say to Donald: 'I'm not in the mood today, Donald' and those days he didn't make as many demands ... Like, he always got bread but it was toast that he wanted, not that you minded, but you know some days you'd say you don't feel like it and you'd notice that Donald would sort of give you sort of a breather. But that was through being able to be honest with Donald.

*Familiarity* refers to that sense we have of someone else, through the sense we have of ourselves, as individuals with a lifetime of experiences. Naomi (a patient) expressed relating to the nurse as person, when she said this about Sue:

> Well, she seems to be such a normal sort of, she's a nurse, but as well as being a nurse, she's a friendly sort of person, who gives you confidence, I think. That makes a big difference, doesn't it, you don't look at her as a clinical sort of figure altogether, she's a friend as well. It's hard to explain. Well, when I say normal, to me normal is to be friendly and helpful, as well as being that trained person, who knows what it's all about anyway, but you feel that you can talk to her as a friend. Not to be afraid to ask questions, whether it be foolish or not. Because she treats you very sensibly and in a friendly manner. I just can't explain it ... I don't have to be afraid of her training and because she knows so much about this and that, that I'm scared of asking her something. I don't feel like that at all. I feel I can ask her anything, sensible or not.

*Family* refers to the sense of home we have within ourselves, which binds us to people with whom we have blood ties or special affinities. Expressing 'family-like' ties was exemplified by Donald (a patient), who said of Andrew (a nurse):

> Yeah, yeah. Andrew and I get on really well together. I'd say he was more or less like a brother.

*Favouring* refers to the approval we give to other people and ourselves for commendable qualities, which remind us of our essential nature as human beings. Elizabeth (a nurse) explained her pleasure when Mary (a patient) requested that Elizabeth become her primary nurse:

> I was quite pleased that she chose me (to take over her care). She said she'd seen me interact with the patient across the room and she felt quite comfortable with me. That was nice to think that she felt that way ... (It made me feel) good, naturally. Everybody likes a compliment.

*Feelings* refers to the way we sense ourselves in relation to our worlds of people and things; sometimes as feeling high, sometimes as feeling low, sometimes as feeling somewhere in between. Sue (a nurse) expressed her feelings about massaging Ralph (a patient) thus:

> It seems weird, when we talk about giving enemas and shaving people and that, but massage is probably one of the most intimate things we do with patients, because it creates the most intimate responses ... He just seemed very relaxed ... When you think of it, it is so intimate to have someone laying hands on you.

*Fun* refers to a sense of merriment, which lightens our day-to-day lives and reacquaints us with the child within us all. Gus (a patient) said this in relation to Sophie and Sally (night nurses):

> As I say, I have a lot of fun with them. I know I'm a bit cheeky sometimes, but I have a lot of fun with them.

*Friendship* refers to knowing people well enough to regard them with affection. The importance of company and talking in developing friendship was shown in an interaction between Sally, Sophie and Gus. Gus explained it in this way:

> Well, myself, I found it (the conversation with Sally) good. I mean to say, she's a busy girl and I could talk to her all day and all night. Do you know what I mean? Well, they'll (the nurses will) do anything for you, to help you. Anytime. I could sit here all night and I'd still get my cups of tea or coffee and all that. They'd come in at night time, cos I'd be in trouble at night time. I used to prop that (the amputated leg) and make a noise some nights. They'd hear me and they'd come in and say: 'I don't think that this (the phantom pain) can be fixed. It's gotta just take its own course, I think.' So they stop and talk with me and that would help.

The eight aspects illuminated something of the nature of ordinariness in nursing. The ontological nature (of existence) of ordinariness in nursing was the nature within the aspects illuminating the phenomenon, that is, it was at the level of what I termed its actualities. The research process found that within facilitation there was 'allowingness'; within fair play there was 'straightforwardness'; within familiarity there was 'self-likeness'; within family there was 'homeliness'; within favouring there was 'favourableness'; within feelings there was 'intuneness'; within fun there was 'lightheartedness' and within friendship there was 'connectedness'. The methodological reasoning for this phenomenological process is described fully in the thesis (Taylor 1991), but what this basically means is that a deeper interpretation of the phenomenon allowed for more to be said and known about its nature.

## The actualities of deeper meaning

Allowingness is when people try to make things easier for other people. In nursing, allowingness creates the potential for patients and nurses to help themselves, by providing some guidance and support until such a time, if at all, that people feel able to take over their own daily life business. Allowingness is considerate of the other person's needs to be independent and dignified; it helps quietly and carefully, always attentive to the cues within the other person that suggest a preparedness to resume increasingly autonomous thoughts and actions. Allowingness is the essential quality of facilitation that relates to the other person through sensitive helping.

Straightforwardness is when people express their thoughts in relation to others. In nursing, straightforwardness creates the potential for patients and nurses to speak to each other as frankly as possible, saying whatever is in need of being said, while tolerating each other's humanness. Straightforwardness is clear and concise in its delivery and generous in its intent; it speaks to the other to unblock impasses and puts the perceived focus of contention plainly on view, to trigger discussion. straightforwardness is the essential quality of fair play that relates to people through sensitive straight talking.

Self-likeness is when people see themselves mirrored, to some degree, in other people. In nursing, self-likeness creates the potential for patients and nurses to understand the humanness of themselves in others, sharing an affinity as humans together bonded by the commonality of their ordinary human existence. Self-likeness is the glue of oneness, wherein people share a sense of togetherness, regardless of a variety of differences. It is a source of recognition of being within human beings, a sense of the ultimate sameness of all people and things in the universe. Self-likeness is the essential nature of familiarity.

Homeliness is the regard people have for others as family, either through blood ties or special affinities. In nursing, homeliness creates the potential for patients and nurses to develop close interpersonal relationships that encompass perspectives of people as family. Homeliness is sharing common understandings with people and in so doing, accepting a share of their joys and pains, which are integral to closer human relationships. Homeliness is the essential nature of family that relates to people through sensitive family bonding.

Favourableness is being reminded of our own commendable qualities by seeing them in other people, as a mirror of our essential nature as human beings. In nursing, favourableness creates the potential for patients and nurses to give approval to other people and themselves and in so doing, to magnify the attractive aspects of themselves. Favourableness is seeing beauty in people at the inside level; it recognizes everyday human qualities that defy adequate description and realizes that only through sensing them within itself is it possible to know that these qualities exist and how they are. Favourableness is the inner nature of favouring that relates to people through sensitive recognition and acceptance.

Intuneness is when humans are sensitive to their feelings and find licence to express them as a legitimate part of themselves and the polarity of things within our worlds. In nursing, intuneness creates the potential for patients and nurses to acknowledge and express the polarity of their feelings. Intuneness is clearing away the debris of rationality to face up to and embrace the rawness of emotions which, when expressed, unblock the streams of human reactivity and cause our life energies to flow a little more easily. Intunencss is the inner nature of feelings that relates to people through sensitive expressions of emotion.

Lightheartedness is about sharing a sense of fun. In nursing, light-heartedness creates the potential for patients and nurses to express themselves through humour. Lightheartedness is levity above the everyday circumstances that cloud our minds and weigh our bodies down. Lightheartedness seeks to aerate the lead ball of life and turn it into a bright balloon. Lightheartedness is the essential nature of fun that relates to people through sensitive exchanges of humour and levity.

Connectedness is when people sense themselves as friends. In nursing, connectedness creates the potential for patients and nurses to know one another well enough to regard each other with affection. Connectedness is recognizing friendly aspects in other people and coming in closer to get to know them. Connectedness takes time to get to know the other person, through keeping company and talking. Connectedness is the essential nature of friendship that relates to people through sensitive affection and liking.

The actualities were expressed as potentiating energies within the aspects of ordinariness. In the end, though, I realized that I had found no words to express the inexpressible, that clusive thing called existence. I knew that I was in good company, though, because Heidegger (1962) knew the frustration of a lifelong search for explicating being (the nature of existence), resorting as he did finally, after many years of ontological enquiry, to naming being 'Es' (itself).

## THE THERAPEUTIC NATURE OF ORDINARINESS

Nursing involves people being thrown together in complex human rela-tionships, that are exacerbated by the effects of illness and changed life circumstances. This and other contingencies make nursing complex work. When nurses understand the centrality of their role with people, they can begin to appreciate their potential for understanding the people in their care. Nursing happens whenever nurses and patients are together in contexts of care; it is about how nurses and patients relate to one another and work through the circumstances that have brought them together. The therapeutic ingredient of nursing is the humanness of inter-personal encounters.

Patients recognize and respect nurses' knowledge and skills and they trust in these professional prerequisites, but they receive a bonus when they find that nurses are humans, similar to themselves. It is this affinity as humans, this thing that I have called 'ordinariness', that allows nurses and patients to acknowledge each other as humans and to share in the transitory imposition of illness. Ordinariness in nursing makes the nurse–patient relationship therapeutic, so that healing occurs and patients feel that their time spent in the health-care facility has been made manageable by its familiarity as a human place.

Healing in this sense is not about cure. Cure may be possible in healing as it is applied to nursing, but it is not the main intention. In a therapeutic sense, healing means a personal movement towards integrity, as sensed and defined by individuals, even if it is to their death. This view of healing turns the cure perspective on its head by allowing a good death (Taylor 1993d) to be an appropriate nursing care outcome.

The therapeutic nature of ordinariness nursing is related to the healing effects that accrue for both parties when nurses and patients interact as humans together. There is something about the humanness of both parties and the ways in which they combine together in the relatively strange contexts of health-care facilities that hold some reasons for therapeutic effects in nursing. The phenomenon of ordinariness in nursing is about some qualities of being human that are shared by nurses and patients alike and it is through the recognition of the affinity of being human that a bond is formed, which transcends apparent differences nurses and patients may have in terms of knowledge, skills and other specific differentiating features.

Ordinariness in nursing is therapeutic through the effects of genuine human relationships. There is reciprocity in allowingness, although the flow of facilitation is determined by who has the need and how much need there is, as well as who is in the best position to make the other's challenge easier to face. In nursing encounters, patients often have the greatest need for help because of their illness circumstances but patients can facilitate nurses' needs through their allowingness.

Straightforwardness frees nurses and patients to speak their minds clearly and plainly, having taken into account the relative strengths and weaknesses of their own human condition, before dispensing their straight talking to the other person. The enhancement of nursing encounters is through the frankness and forthrightness of the speaking and the reactive freedom of the listening. When nurses and patients know each other well enough to share straight talking, they know each other well enough to risk a friendship worth keeping, so nursing encounters are enhanced through nurses and patients being at that level of rapport that allows straightforwardness to express itself.

Self-likeness raises the possibilities of nurses and patients relating, acknowledging, equating, recognizing, and being part of their respective worlds, through a shared sense of being human. Whilst recognizing and respecting the different talents each person brings to nursing encounters, patients and nurses are connected more by their similarities as humans than they are disconnected by their differences as clients and professionals respectively.

Homeliness affords the possibilities of acknowledging, valuing, expressing, appreciating and preparing for treasured qualities and activities in relation to family and home. Homeliness centres nurses and patients inwardly with a sense of home and belonging, through blood ties or special affinities, because it creates strong bonds between them, allowing the potential for greater self-growth, from a personal base made stronger through feelings of inner security and family-like relationships. Even in the face of the strangeness of hospitals and other inhospitable health-care settings, nurses and patients can manage to feel 'at home'.

Favourableness is the recognition and endorsement of human qualities as an expression of human nature. When human qualities are recognized and approved by nurses and patients, they have the potential to bring out a stronger alignment with these positive human qualities, thus creating a firmer affinity for each other and a stronger sense of purpose in planning care collaboratively.

Intuneness acknowledges and expresses feelings, thus reaffirming the shared sense of reactivity to the polar extremes and places in between of feelings. Enhancement of nursing encounters comes about through nurses and patients sensing that life is about highs and lows and in-betweens and realizing that it is reasonable to acknowledge and express these feelings to themselves and to others.

There is mutual enjoyment in lightheartedness, as nurses and patients invite one another to take a brief respite from the heaviness of their circumstances, to be lifted momentarily by some light relief. Nursing encounters are enhanced through sharing the surprise of humour and revisiting the child within, by virtue of its transitory liberating and lightening effects. The therapy is within the fun and lightheartedness, even when tragedies are imminent. There is a special brand of humour in nursing that sends up the rawness of human illness experiences and dares to laugh at them.

There is mutual acknowledgement and expression in connectedness, with the potential for ever-increasing bonds of friendship, through knowing one another over time. Enhancement of nursing encounters occurs through connectedness, when nurses and patients step outside their patient–nurse roles that favour distancing and detachment to risk the vulnerability of closeness, for the therapeutic effects of friendship that it brings. The masks come off when people connect at deep levels. Nursing has a way of opening up possibilities for connectedness, because the everyday dramas of caring for ill and unhappy people encourage nurses to 'get over' feeling important and superior, to relate genuinely as an 'in-the-moment' person actively attentive to people in their care.

**CONCLUSION**

Ordinariness in nursing refers to the sense of shared affinity that nurses and patients have for one another as humans which gives them a common bond in the face of their singular existence as a nurse or a patient. Although ordinariness may seem to be a commonplace thing, it may be its very familiarity that renders it relatively invisible in daily nursing practice. If ordinariness in nursing is named and described, it may become more visible and actually very important to nurses and patients in the development of their relationships and their therapeutic value.

Self-knowing is implicit in being oneself, because it might be easier to mimic someone else or act out a role that may be more consistent with what may be expected in a situation. For instance, some nurses may choose to hide behind their professional masks and talk in high falsetto pitch to mimic the 'soapie' representations of a 'real' nurse. Acting out the role of a nurse may also serve to protect the hapless practitioner from the everyday battlefront of clinical work, where emotional knocks and bruises may be the norm. In this uncertain context a professional facade may act as armour to protect nurses from the daily drama of human suffering. In this sense, nurses are patients of sorts, in that they also suffer because of the illness experiences of the people for whom they care.

Clinical settings throw nurses and patients together in 'on-the-spot' scenarios with a host of potential possible outcomes. The challenge is for nurses to be themselves as human beings, to be attentive in the moment and have genuine loving and knowledgeable concern for patients, relatives, friends and colleagues. This is no small challenge but it may be possible if nurses are willing to allow themselves to be themselves, in spite of their knowledge and skills and in spite of temptations to hide themselves away from patients and other people.

Nursing is what happens between nurses and patients in contexts of care and it is facilitated by the humanity of both parties, as they negotiate the illness experience together. This does not mean that nursing is a simple practice and that any person can do it without prior knowledge or skills. Nurses are selected and educated carefully, to ensure that they are able to manage the demands of the work. I have argued elsewhere (Taylor 1992b) that the absolute need for high standards of professional education and continuing practice is beyond doubt. What is being claimed here is that nurses are able to transcend the limitations of their professional roles and responsibilities to show their human qualities and to be at ease with them. In this way, ordinariness in nursing is therapeutic through the dynamic potential of genuine human simplicity. The therapeutic potential is housed in people and activities in nursing and it is as simple and exquisitely commonplace as facilitation, fair play, familiarity, family, favouring, feelings, fun and friendship.

# REFERENCES

Heidegger, M. (1962) *Being and Time*, (trans. J. Macquarrie and E. Robinson) Harper and Row, New York.

Malone, T. P. and Malone, P. T. (1987) *The Art of Intimacy*, Prentice-Hall, New York.

Pearson, A. (1988a) Just an ordinary nurse. Lakeside graduation address (unpublished).

Pearson, A. (1988b) *Primary Nursing: Nursing in the Oxford and Burford Nursing Development Units*, Croom Helm, Beckenham.

Pearson, A. (1988c) *Therapeutic Nursing: The Effects of Admission to a Nursing Unit*, Oxfordshire Health Authority, Oxford.

Pearson, A. (1992) *Nursing at Burford: A Story of Change*, Scutari Press, London.

Taylor, B. J. (1988) What are the patients' perceptions of the usefulness of information given to them by nurses and what are the nurses' perceptions of their roles and constraints as teachers in giving effective patient education in a postnatal ward? A research paper submitted in partial fulfilment of the requirements for the degree of Master of Education, Deakin University, Geelong.

Taylor, B. J. (1991) The phenomenon of ordinariness in nursing. Unpublished PhD thesis, Faculty of Nursing, Deakin University, Geelong.

Taylor, B. J. (1992a) Relieving pain through ordinariness in nursing: a phenomenological account of a comforting nurse–patient encounter. *Advances in Nursing Science*, **15** (1), 33–43.

Taylor, B. J. (1992b) From helper to human: a reconceptualisation of the nurse as person. *Journal of Advanced Nursing*, **17**, 1042–1049.

Taylor, B. J. (1993a) Phenomenology: one way to understand nursing practice. *International Journal of Nursing Studies*, **30**, (2), 171–179.

Taylor, B. J. (1993b) Ordinariness in nursing: a study, part 1. *Nursing Standard*, **7** (39), 35–38.

Taylor, B. J. (1993c) Ordinariness in nursing: a study, part 2. *Nursing Standard*, **7** (40), 37–40.

Taylor, B. J. (1993d) What does a good death of people in their care mean to hospice nurses? Unpublished research report. School of Nursing, Deakin University, Geelong.

Taylor, B. J. (1994) *Being Human: Ordinariness in Nursing*, Churchill Livingstone, Melbourne.

# 5

# Patient education in therapeutic nursing

Barbara Vaughan and Alan Pearson

*No man can reveal to you aught but that which lies half asleep in the dawning of your knowledge.*

Gibran (1926) *The Prophet* on speaking of teaching.

As is stated elsewhere in this book, therapeutic nursing which promotes wellness is grounded in a partnership between nurse and patient and thus patient independence in decision making and goal setting is fundamental to being therapeutic. To be independent is to be 'not subject to the control of others' (*King's English Dictionary* 1938) and wellness is the subjective experience of well-being – of being at peace with, in harmony with and happy with one's world. Independence and wellness are inextricably linked with being powerful, rather than powerless. Of course, all of us are, to a greater or lesser extent, controlled by other forces in the world, be it natural forces, governments or those with whom we live in interdependent relationships. So, to some extent, none of us is in fact *not* subject to the control of others and all of us are sometimes out of tune with or unhappy in our world. Total independence is, therefore, out of reach to most of us. *Relative* independence and wellness are, however, within the reach of most of us who exist in modern society.

Promoting independence and wellness through therapeutic nursing in the community, residential settings such as nursing homes and hostels and in hospitals is becoming an increasingly popular goal. However, in Western countries, where economic rationalism has become the guiding principle, independence is less and less possible for those who are disabled, who suffer from any form of ill health or who are economically or culturally disadvantaged. Furthermore, the attitudes and values of many health and welfare workers, such as nurses, more often create dependence rather than enable independence.

Well-established structures and roles in health and welfare systems in Western countries serve to limit independence and to avoid broad concepts such as wellness and to concentrate on narrow perspectives, frequently related to specific outcome measures.

Nurses who seriously wish to promote independence in clients and who view wellness as their goal, no matter how worthy, moral or logical this may seem, simply have to confront the powerfulness of the few and the powerlessness of the many. In other words, promoting independence is a political business, because it involves power sharing. Sharing power can only occur if there is a serious attempt to share knowledge and well-planned patient education is a central component of therapeutic nursing.

This central importance of patient education in therapeutic nursing is now widely acknowledged and is implicit, if not explicit, in the majority of conceptual or theoretical frameworks of nursing which are found in the literature. For example, nurses cannot help patients to maximize their ability to self-care, as advocated by Orem (1980), unless they share information with them. Orem describes teaching as one of the essential nursing acts. Similarly, there is a fundamental need to become involved in patient education in Roy's (1976) notion of helping patients to adapt to stressors, King's (1981) theory of goal attainment or Roper *et al.*'s (1985) ideas about independence. Neuman (1982) argues that care planning should be divided into primary, secondary and tertiary components, the first being concerned with preventive factors, the second with dealing with an acute phase of ill health and the third with helping patients to prevent recurrence. The implications for teaching are self-evident in such an approach but particularly conspicuous in the primary and tertiary phases of care.

Health education has also attracted many nurses working both clinically and in research as they recognize this need which has been so widely neglected to date. While this fundamental area of health care may not be the sole province of nurses, there is certainly a major contribution which they can make. Yet again, there is a suggestion that the teaching function of the nurse must be acknowledged and developed if he or she is to be able to work effectively as a health educator.

According to Watson (1985), nurses have always maintained that teaching about health is one of the main functions of nursing. She suggests that this is one of the criteria which may differentiate professional nursing from 'technical nursing', commenting that:

> The amount and level of teaching done by a nurse who has a baccalaureate or masters degree is expected to be greater than the amount done by a nurse who has a diploma or associate degree. Patients/clients as well as health professionals expect that.

It is interesting to speculate how easily such a comment transfers from the expectations of American society to other cultures such as the UK, Australia or Africa. Nurses with degrees or higher degrees are still in the minority in many countries. Furthermore, there is as yet little evidence to suggest that the general public acknowledge nurses as credible sources of information.

Furthermore, the sharing of knowledge which is implicit in such a statement does not comply with the traditional view of professions who, it can be suggested, maintain part of their status by retaining a 'mystical body of knowledge' (Friedson 1975). Such a stance would be antithetical to therapeutic nursing where partnership with patients and sharing of knowledge are crucial. Alternatively, however, Watson's words imply that there is a depth of knowledge in nursing which is commensurate with studying to higher degree levels and, more importantly, that studying to this level should enhance the practising skills of the nurse.

Such thoughts go some way to offering a sound rationale for the current transfer of nursing education to the higher education sector since if patient teaching is a core part of practice, it cannot be achieved effectively without advanced knowledge of health and nursing, which includes knowledge of learning and teaching theories. Furthermore, Watson's words could be taken as a guide to some of the criteria which could be used in evaluating nursing in terms of both the skills required and the service which nurses offer.

## SHARING KNOWLEDGE THROUGH PATIENT TEACHING

Although patient teaching is now widely accepted as an important part of health care, education that enables the patient to engage in the self-care they themselves desire and design is fundamentally different from current approaches to client teaching, which emphasize the nurse's role of encouraging patients to do what they and their medical colleagues think is right. In a study which described an attempt to introduce self-medication in a professorial nursing unit, Pearson and Baker (1992) found a high level of allegiance to patient teaching which focuses on compliance and little understanding of the difference between this kind of approach and an approach which maximizes the patient's abilities to engage in self-care. Levin (1978) points out that the aim of both processes is to teach patients skills and ideas which will help them to deal with the problems of their present state and also, if possible, to avoid disease in the future, thus maintaining a level of health which is optimal for the particular person. A non-therapeutic approach to patient teaching pursues this aim by passing on relevant information (as determined by the health worker) in an appropriate way, whereas education for self-care focuses on the patient's own lifestyle, aspirations and abilities.

A focus on self-care and independence demands that professionals set aside the values they hold about what the patient needs to know and consider what is important for the attainment of specific goals generated from the perspective of the patient. According to Levin (1978), contemporary patient teaching often has an inherent view of the patient as a sick person. Self-care education, however, does not assume sickness but views the role of the patient from a perspective of wellness. Levin (1978) suggests that health-care skills which do not compete with professional services (for any reason) are frequently offered, but when caregivers perceive disadvantage to their group, only patient teaching which maintains the dependence of the client is countenanced. When this is the case, patient teaching is carried out only to safeguard the professional from blame, should unexpected occurrences reflect adversely upon their practice.

When patient teaching is offered within a framework of therapeutic nursing, it is based on patients' perception of their needs. The patient determines the desired outcomes, content, method and evaluation. It is directed toward the reduction of dependence and thus the control over the situation moves from the health professional to the patient.

The existing personal resources of any individual are taken into account and the lay practices which are already part of their lives are used as the foundation for further education. The inherent capabilities of the patient in diagnosing, monitoring and healing themselves are recognized and encouraged.

In many health-care settings, real obstacles to patient teaching aimed at self-care exist. These obstacles are many and varied in style, but often relate to the confusion between self-care and compliance; the increase in 'defensive practice' designed to minimize litigation; the continuing dominance of the biomedical model in health care; and interprofessional rivalry in health care.

**Patient teaching and 'compliance'**

The term 'compliance' is used frequently in health-care circles and is closely associated with the biomedical model of health care. Compliance with therapeutic regimens is defined in different ways, depending upon the world view of the occupational group framing the definition. Bergen (1987) cites two definitions from the biomedical model, which vary only in degree. They are from Norton (1982) who says that compliance consists of client behaviour which is controlled by the physician, while Haynes *et al.* (1979) write of a coincidence of client behaviour with medical advice. Kent and Dalgleish (1973, cited by Bergen 1987) define non-compliance as any error in dosage or timing and O'Hanrahan and O'Malley (1981, cited by Bergen 1987) write of non-compliance as deviation from a regimen which is sufficient to interfere with the therapeutic goal.

### Patient teaching and defensive practice

In a society which is becoming increasingly litigious, resulting in a health-care environment in which quality of care is emphasized, the risks involved in self-care may be unacceptable to the organization. For example, in Pearson and Baker's (1992) self-medication study, pharmacy, nursing and medical staff were legally responsible for the ordering, dispensing and administration of drugs within institutions. While all these groups were quick to agree that self-care is desirable, few were prepared to take the risk of litigation involved if a client should suffer severe health outcomes as a result of missed medications, overdosage of self-administered medication or accidental self-administration of drugs prescribed for another person in the hospital.

### The biomedical model and patient teaching

Most of the nurses practising in health-care institutions at present are products of hospital-based training programmes and a socialization process which enhanced the hegemonic status of the biomedical model of nursing. The traditional role of nurses in this model is to carry out the orders of the medical practitioner in a distant and uninvolved way. This puts nurses into a position of superiority over the patient, militates against the development of individualized strategies for self-care and focuses on compliance with the medically prescribed regimen.

### Patient teaching and interprofessional rivalry

The giving of information has become a matter of controversy within the health-care team, with some occupations claiming ownership of knowledge and suggesting that only they are competent to determine the content and amount of information 'suitable' for patients. Pearson and Baker (1992) report that the giving of information on medications to patients in their study was eventually stopped when the claims of medical practitioners and pharmacists that nurses were inadequately qualified to assess patients' information needs, or to give information, were accepted by hospital authorities.

## TEACHING AND LEARNING – THE STATE OF THE ART

If it is accepted that teaching is part of nursing then the fundamental questions which have to be addressed relate to how both nurses and patients perceive teaching and learning. It is not the intention of this chapter to give detailed explanations of theories of teaching and learning since they are widely available elsewhere. It is, however, useful to clarify these terms.

## Teaching

Wilson-Barnett (1989) describes patient teaching as the process of increasing patients' or clients' understanding about their state of health, disease, treatment and rehabilitation by giving information in a planned and structured way. However, in nursing much of the teaching which occurs is aimed at helping people to manage their own lives more independently. Thus it can be argued that helping patients/clients to increase their theoretical understanding of what is happening to them is only the beginning of the process. What is even more vital is that the teaching occurs in such a way that it is meaningful to the recipients in making decisions about any changes in their way of life which may be beneficial to their health and which they wish to make. It is, of course, much more difficult to interpret knowledge in this way so that it can be of practical use to the learner and requires much more skilful teaching.

Such difficulties are widely understood by nurses themselves as evidence grows of the well-known theory–practice gap. As far back as the mid-1970s, Bendall (1975) presented evidence of the lack of correlation between what nurses said they did and what they actually did. In the same way, while patients may learn new facts about different things which could affect their health status, this does not mean that those facts can be easily transferred into a change of behaviour. Thus, teaching undertaken by nurses must go well beyond the simple imparting of new knowledge to an assurance that the patients/clients have not only absorbed that knowledge but also found a way of making use of it in managing their own lives.

## Facilitating learning

Some people have rejected the use of the term 'teaching', since to many it has implications of an expert passing on knowledge to a pupil. Rogers (1983), for example, suggests that he has no use for a word which implies imparting knowledge or skill to another and prefers to use the term 'facilitating learning' and this phrase has been widely adopted by others. Indeed, its use may be justified if teaching is confined solely to helping people to learn new facts about a given topic. However, if teaching is viewed more broadly – as providing the facilities under which another may learn – then maybe Rogers' view is a little harsh since there are times when it is entirely appropriate for an expert to share his or her knowledge with another. The difference may be in what the expert expects the recipient to do with the knowledge. If the expectation is that the recipient will accept the information in blind faith then maybe such an approach can be criticized. If, however, there is an understanding of sharing and debate about the relevance of that knowledge to a person at a given point in his or her life then it can be argued that teaching is entirely appropriate. What can be called into question is the style of teaching which is used to impart knowledge from one person to another. While 'didactic' teacher-led lectures can, in fact, make a contribution to patient/client education there is also a case to be made for nurses having sufficient discrimination to know both the advantages and the limitations of such an approach. It must be remembered that not every person has the same learning styles and while some people find a degree of safety and group support in the more impersonal and anonymous formal learning situation, others will find that same impersonal approach unhelpful. Thus, as in all other areas of nursing, practitioners need to have sufficient knowledge not only of their specific subject area but also of the variations in people's learning styles in order to be able to practise well.

## Experiential learning

Following a humanistic approach, Carl Rogers (1969) suggests that for learning to be effective, the drive and impetus must come from the learner him or herself. In defining significant or experiential learning, he has identified the essentials as:

1  A quality of personal involvement – the whole person in both his feeling and cognitive aspects being in the learning event
2  It is self-initiated – even when the impetus comes from the outside the sense of discovery, of reaching out, of grasping and comprehending comes from within
3  It is pervasive – it makes a difference in the behaviour, the attitudes, perhaps even the personality of the learner
4  It is evaluated by the learners – they know whether it is meeting their needs, whether it leads towards what they want to know, whether it illuminates the dark area of ignorance they are experiencing.

Inherent in Rogers' view of learning is the humanistic belief that there is potential in all people to develop and grow and that by facilitating learning, a teacher can help in this process. However, unless there is personal commitment and involvement from the learner, efforts to help are fruitless.

Experiential learning has provoked considerable interest in recent years, particularly in helping people to develop the human skills of self-knowledge or self-awareness. Burnard (1985) sees it as a valuable way of helping nurses to learn those skills which, according to Peplau (1952) and many others since, are a prerequisite to therapeutic nursing. The argument is that without knowledge of self, one cannot empathize with others in order to help them to learn from new experiences.

Burnard (1985) suggests that learning can occur both through current experiences and from past experiences, the emphasis always being on action. Some of his suggestions, which are primarily aimed at nurse education, may be equally applicable for patient education. For example, recall (an intentional action) of a previous hospital admission may help a patient to understand his or her fears of a current hospital admission. Similarly, giving patients the opportunity to handle their own drugs and self-medicate prior to discharge from hospital (a positive action) may lead to a better understanding of the need to continue taking the drugs and more accuracy in their use following discharge.

While the use of experiential learning methods can be of great value to nurses, it is also necessary to add a word of warning. Many people, but particularly those who underwent their general education a long time ago, will not be familiar with experiential methods of learning, their recall of a teacher being someone who told them what was 'right and proper'. Indeed, they may believe that it is the responsibility of health-care workers to 'tell me what is good for me' without apparently being concerned with the reasons why. Furthermore, some people find the very involvement of some experiential learning methods extremely uncomfortable and disconcerting. This does not mean to say that they cannot be employed when working with patients. It does, however, raise a note of caution again over the importance of matching teaching methods to the individual needs of patients rather than becoming overenthusiastic about a particular approach which may not be right for everyone.

### An unconditional service

A further note of warning concerns how nurses themselves feel about this approach to learning. Because of their expert knowledge and their privileged position of access to personal information about patients, there may be times when they feel that a patient's own actions are harmful and should be stopped. Thus, they can feel an obligation to try to influence a patient's behaviour when the patient is neither motivated nor ready to learn. If Rogers' thesis is accepted, such actions are unlikely to have a lasting effect. Furthermore, it has to be added that in some instances patients are censured for non-compliance regardless of the underlying circumstances. This raises the interesting issue that nurses have a responsibility to offer an unconditional service. There are some who believe that if a patient's own actions are not appropriate then the obligation of the health-care worker to offer a service is no longer applicable, the obvious example being of someone who continues to smoke despite being given information about its harmful effects. The question which has to be raised is whether the service which nurses offer is, in fact, unconditional. Nurses themselves need to have self-knowledge of how they feel about such situations. Working with a patient in anger and resentment is unlikely to be effective yet there are times when these feelings are very real. There is no easy answer to problems of this kind which nurses face so often. However, it does raise very important issues in relation to their own learning needs, using experiential methods of reflection and debate so that they may increase their understanding of themselves and therefore their skills in supporting appropriate learning methods which are geared to individual needs.

## ALTERNATIVE APPROACHES

Watson (1985) suggests that the tutorial method of teaching is probably the one seen most commonly in clinical practice where teaching is an isolated event in the pattern of care on offer. However, she also advocates the promotion of what she called 'interpersonal teaching/learning' as a major caring factor. In this instance, the interaction can be seen as a much more personal experience with growth and understanding occurring for both the nurse and the patient. Teaching and learning in this sense go well beyond the traditional expectations of an expert imparting knowledge to a learner about a specific isolated event. In this situation, both parties will play the roles of both teacher and learner throughout their interaction. Thus, the nurse will learn from the patient of past experiences, previous coping strategies or personal perceptions of a given situation while in turn the nurse will share both cognitive and perceptual information which may help the client to manage his or her own health. In turn, both have the opportunity to develop their understanding of a situation and extend the repertoire of information which can be used to solve problems both currently and in the future.

This view of nursing, as a developmental process in which patient and nurse grow, was described by Peplau (1952) as far back as the early 1950s. However, she argues that there is a difference between the way in which peers may learn together and the way in which a nurse and a client will both develop. She describes the relationship between a skilled nurse and a client as one of **professional closeness** where the nurse has developed sufficient empathy to be able to manage her own behaviour in such a way as to help a client to develop and learn through a personal health crisis. Such a relationship is differentiated from **interpersonal closeness**, where the needs of each party take mutual precedence, **physical closeness**, which is of a more personal nature, and **pseudocloseness** where false sympathy can deny true empathy and be used as a barrier to professional support by the nurse (Peplau 1969). With professional closeness one of the major functions of nursing can be seen as the creation of environments in which clients can feel safe and learn more about themselves which can be of both short- and long-term benefit to them. This does not, however, negate the fact that in each new nursing situation the nurse will also learn something new which can be added to her total repertoire of knowledge for future practice.

Ideas such as this comply well with the way in which Benner (1984) has identified levels of nursing competence ranging from that of a novice to an expert practitioner. Using a care study example, she describes how the expert practitioner, who has gained advanced formal knowledge as well as a wealth of practical experience, is not only able to recognize the learning needs of a patient but also the time at which that patient is most ready to learn. It is her premise that the less experienced nurse, while knowing what it is that she should be teaching, will be much less skilled in knowing when and how to share information. The reasoning behind this view is partly based on the fact that until any nurse has a considerable length of experience in a given situation, she is not able to be sufficiently sensitive to the cues to be able to react to individual differences between people. She therefore has to rely more heavily on either formal theories or personal life experiences which cannot be the same as those of the person with whom she is working. Thus if she knows that information can lead to a reduction in stress her major goal will be to share that information regardless of the contextual circumstances, particularly if she has found this approach helpful personally. There are, however, some instances when sharing of information at the wrong time can make a situation more, rather than less, stressful. It is the mark of an expert to be able to discern not only what to tell but when to tell it.

The skill of making judgements of this kind takes patient education well beyond the realms of routine practice and reinforces Watson's premise of relating the degree and depth with which a nurse is involved with her level of education, provided that the formal education is matched with clinical experience.

## Teaching and stress reduction

There is now a considerable body of knowledge supporting the notion that patient education can lead to a reduction in stress levels in patients, thus enhancing their recovery. Limited information, on the other hand, can lead to a feeling of lack of control which in its turn can lead to a feeling of helplessness and stress. While this principle has been well accepted in some areas of care, such as before surgery (Boore 1978, Hayward 1975) it is questionable as to how widely it is accepted in other areas. For example, it is not unusual for patients to know that they will be having some form of investigation on a given day but not to know the time. In consequence there is no way that they can plan their own day with regard to simple things such as visiting the shop or even going to the bathroom, for fear of being absent at the crucial moment when they are needed. Waiting seems to be the order of the day. Such conditions are not accepted by most people in other areas of their lives and can give rise to considerable annoyance yet they are commonplace in health care.

While it is often not possible to know the exact time of forthcoming events it is sometimes feasible to give people some explanation of the need for delay or waiting which may reduce the amount of anxiety or anger they feel. For example, there is anecdotal evidence that there seems to be less disturbance in the waiting area of an accident department if people know the reason for the delay, such as the fact that an emergency is being dealt with elsewhere. Similarly, there are times when all people need to know is that they will not 'miss their turn' if they disappear to the bathroom for a few minutes, provided they let someone know where they will be. It is often just a case of saying that it is all right to do these things, of 'giving permission' and freeing people to do things for themselves rather than having to wait passively and compliantly for things to happen to them. Actions of this kind may seem to be simplistic and obvious but in reality they are often omitted, simply because the need for information has not been recognized. Furthermore they do not fall into the formal category of health-care teaching since they are not directly related to a specific health problem. However, it is often small things such as these which become the focus of attention and cause the greatest worries. Waiting and boredom are common factors which people complain about when they are receiving health care, which can all add to the total accumulation of stress.

In talking of interpersonal teaching/learning, Watson (1985) has identified factors, supported by research from the psychosocial fields as well as from clinical studies, which suggest that information:

- promotes accurate expectations and reduces discomforting discrepancies between the degree of stress expected and the degree of stress experienced
- increases the ability to predict what will happen, leading to a feeling of being in control and reducing associated fears
- fosters the realistic worry and mental rehearsal necessary for emotional acceptance of stress
- changes beliefs and reduces the dreadful fantasies that may be caused by the impending stress
- leads to information that may constitute a method of dealing with the illness and conceptualizing it in a less stressful way
- is intimately involved in the evaluation of situations as threatening and the evaluation of ways of reducing threat.

In reviewing these factors, it is interesting to see how familiar they are to most people in their everyday lives and are not unique to health-care situations. Feeling out of control because one does not know what is happening is a common enough experience to most of us and it often arises out of simple lack of information. Furthermore, how many people have discovered that the fantasy of a dreaded trip to the dentist, often arising from unreal worries, was not nearly as bad in reality? Our imaginations can play disconcerting tricks at times.

There is some evidence to suggest that sharing information prior to an event can, in fact, increase the initial amount of anxiety experienced (e.g. Wilson-Barnett 1978) and some people have used this as a reason for not talking with patients about what will happen. However, to counter this argument there is also considerable evidence to suggest that if people do not undergo the 'work of worry' prior to an event their actual experience of that event is considerably worse at the time as they are unprepared for what will happen (Janis 1974). If they are unrealistic about the forthcoming event, for example not acknowledging that surgery will cause a degree of pain, then the actual pain experience can come as a much greater shock and be more difficult to manage. Without prior knowledge, people are not in a position to prepare coping strategies from their repertoire of past experience. While a caregiver may be able to make suggestions of ways in which stressful situations could be coped with, it is only the individual himself who will know what has worked for him personally in past situations. For example, it is customary to use opiates in the management of postoperative pain but there is now a growing number of people who prefer to reduce the amount of analgesia taken and use relaxation or distraction to help themselves. If there is no knowledge that pain may occur, then such actions cannot be prepared for.

In the same way, there may be others who have extreme fantasies about the degree of pain they will have to undergo following surgery. In this situation false promises that there will be no pain can be just as harmful as leaving the patients with their fantasies. But honest discussion about the degree of pain and the strategies which can be employed to control it can only be helpful. Furthermore, patients may justifiably lose faith in those who are trying to help them if they are perceived as less than honest.

## Teaching and quality of life

The degree of disruption which people will accept in their daily lives because of a health-care difficulty is a constant source of amazement. Yet in many instances patient education can make a significant difference to the way in which they can adapt to either short- or long-term disabilities. For example, in early data collection in a study relating to information given to patients prior to discharge following surgery, one highly intelligent patient reported that he had not had a bath for two weeks (it was the height of summer) because no one had told him that it didn't matter too much if he got his wound wet. While in the long term this would not affect his recovery from surgery, in the short term it would make a considerable difference to the quality of his everyday life! In the follow-up to this study there was very positive response from patients who had been given written information supported by personal teaching of how to cope at home in the early days following surgery (Vaughan 1988).

Similarly, Pearson (1987) has found that if people are given written information with suggestions about how they can adapt their lifestyles when wearing a below-knee plaster their degree of independence in activities of daily living is significantly enhanced. Even more importantly, in his studies of nursing beds Pearson found that independence in living was considerably higher at the time of discharge and at a point six weeks after discharge in those patients who had been cared for in a unit where therapeutic teaching was fundamental to nursing practice (Pearson 1992, Pearson *et al.* 1989, 1992). These important studies go some way to demonstrating the vital contribution which nurses can make to the welfare of patients, measurable more in terms of the quality of their lifestyles indicated by their ability to be independent and to have some say in the control of their own lives than in terms of actual care.

### Teaching and personal growth

Much has already been said about the way in which sharing of information, teaching or facilitation of learning can enhance the lives of both patients and nurses. However, it is also important to recognize that this is not an easy thing to achieve. Inherent in the notion of teaching and learning is the need to change since unused, new knowledge is fruitless. However, change requires energy and commitment. It is, in many instances, easier to maintain the status quo than to introduce a new order of things. Suggestions of change can pose personal threats to individuals as well as creating a fear of the unknown, of failure or of error of judgement.

The action of sharing or imparting information to others and of giving people choice in how they handle that information on a personal basis can, in itself, be a threat to the power of the holder. Basically, it means that there is a shift in control of what happens from the person who holds the resources, in this instance knowledge gained through professional education, to the recipient. Similarly, there is a shift away from a model of creating dependency to one of creating a greater degree of independence. While considerable emphasis is laid on the importance of nurses in helping patients to gain independence, there are still some who see nursing as caring and interpret caring as doing things for others. In reality, this is far from the truth.

Thus, sharing knowledge with patients not only puts nurses in a position of having less control than has been the case in the past but, in many instances, asks them to make fundamental changes in the way they practise. It has already been said that lack of control is one of the factors which create stress in patients and it has to be acknowledged that the same holds true for nurses themselves. However, stress does not always have to be seen in negative terms. Instead, it can be seen as the necessary stimulus to growth, provided that support is given during the period of development and learning, which for a professional practitioner should continue throughout his or her career. Access to both continuing education and support groups on either a formal or an informal basis becomes vital to good practice since it can be suggested that nurses cannot be asked to care for patients unless they are cared for too.

**Prerequisites to therapeutic teaching**

While there is a huge amount of evidence to support the fact that sharing knowledge with patients can make a considerable difference not only to the degree of stress which they experience but also to their ability to live independently, teaching is still not an everyday activity in clinical practice. This raises questions as to why such a situation should have arisen. It can be suggested that a large number of nurses do not acknowledge the extent and importance of their teaching function. When priorities have to be set in a busy clinical area, 'visible work' often gets done at the cost of the less visible but arguably more important invisible work of helping people to learn. There also appears to be some confusion over who is responsible for what. A small study carried out with nurses working with leukaemic patients highlighted that, while nurses acknowledged that they were in the best position to teach patients about both their clinical condition and ways of adjusting their lifestyles, they neither felt it was their responsibility nor had the knowledge to do so. They did not perceive health education, the focus of this study, as part of their role (Preston 1988).

A further concern is that, to date, knowledge about teaching and learning has not played a high profile in the curriculum for basic nurse education, these skills often being 'tagged on' either as part of a postbasic course or as a separate learning activity. In this instance, the emphasis is often on teaching students rather than patients. Hopefully, this situation will improve with the development of our understanding of the relevance of patient teaching in nursing and the development of a new curriculum but this still leaves the vast body of nurses already in practice and emphasizes the essential need for continuing education.

So what are the areas in which a nurse requires competence in order to participate effectively in patient teaching? Ellis (1989) has suggested that many practitioners work from an 'understanding within the privacy of one's own head' and suggests that they 'survive in practice through the application of imperfectly articulated intuitive knowledge'. While the importance of intuition should never be denied, such a position is unacceptable if knowledge is to be shared with others. Thus, the first prerequisite to teaching is an indepth understanding of the subject to be taught. As Manthey (1980) suggests, for nurses this is not confined to matters which can be clearly classified as nursing but also requires a clear understanding of the disease processes which are affecting the patient. This does not mean that nurses need to have the depth of knowledge which doctors have in relationship to disease but they do require a working knowledge of the disease processes which may affect the specific client group with whom they work, since lack of understanding about the aetiology and prognosis of the disease and the possible courses of treatment would lead to a danger of false or unhelpful teaching. For example, teaching skills of mobility to someone who has a progressive motor neurone disease will be quite different from working with someone who is paraplegic but whose clinical condition is not likely to alter or deteriorate.

A second area of competence for the expert practitioner lies in developing an understanding of the way in which people learn. Such knowledge will guide them not only in deciding what to teach but also in using their clinical discretion in making decisions about when and where to teach it. Linked with this is a knowledge of how to teach. Having expert knowledge alone is not the same as being able to share that knowledge with others. Indeed, we have all suffered from time to time as a result of experts using terms with which we are not familiar, making false assumptions of what we already know or moving on to a new topic too quickly for us to be able to grasp a new concept. There are skills in teaching which, like most other things, can be learned and to rely on inborn skills is not sufficient. Thus, both learning and teaching become key components in any basic nursing curriculum.

Finally, if it is accepted that teaching is an interpersonal activity occurring between two or more people rather than simply an expert passing on knowledge didactically, then it becomes essential that teachers develop self-knowledge. Without exploring how we perceive and interact with the world around us on a personal basis, it is unlikely that we can offer help to others.

## CONCLUSION

The arguments which have been put forward in this chapter are that patient education in therapeutic nursing goes well beyond the realms of didactic teaching and is, in fact, an integral part of everyday nursing. While it has been suggested that there is a legitimate place for 'experts to teach', the process is in fact much more complex than simply imparting knowledge to another since if that knowledge is not seen as being relevant or important, it will not be understood. Furthermore, in any teaching situation learning can and should occur for all the people concerned, including the so-called teacher. Thus, it is not seen as a separate and isolated function but as an integral part of practice.

For the future it has been suggested that there are two paths which nurses could follow (Orlando 1987). They may choose to follow a path of advanced technology and enhance their roles in attaining ever more complex technical skills. In this instance, maybe teaching has a lesser part to play as the role would become essentially technical in nature and dependent on medicine. Alternatively, there is an option to expand the nursing function of working with people to assist them in the management of their own lives by helping them gain a greater understanding of the knowledge and skills which will equip them to live independently. Here there is a clear independent function of nursing. In this case patient education is an essential component of therapeutic nursing. Much work is still needed in developing our understanding of how patient education in therapeutic nursing can help others to develop and grow but if the belief in the value of this work is upheld, it is a path well worth exploring.

## REFERENCES

Bendall, E. (1975) *So You Passed, Nurse*, Royal College of Nursing, London.

Benner, P. (1984) *From Novice to Expert – Excellence and Power in Clinical Nursing Practice*, Addison-Wesley, California.

Bergen, A. (1987) in *Elderly Care* (ed. J. Easterbrook), Hodder and Stoughton, London.

Boore, T. (1978) *Prescription for Recovery*, Royal College of Nursing, London.

Burnard, P. (1985) *Learning Human Skills – a Guide for Nurses*, Heinemann, Oxford.

Ellis, R. (1989) *Professional Competence and Quality Assurance in the Caring Professions*, Chapman and Hall, London.

Friedson, E. (1975) *Profession of Medicine*, Dodd, Mead, New York.

Hayward, J. (1975) *Information – A Prescription Against Pain*, Royal College of Nursing, London.

Janis, I. L. (1974) *Psychological Stress*, Academic Press, New York.

King, I. M. (1981) *Toward a Theory of Nursing*, John Wiley, New York.

Levin, L. 1978. Client education and self care: how do they differ? *Nursing Outlook*, **26**(3), 170–175.

Manthey, M. (1980) *Primary Nursing*, Blackwell, Oxford.

Neuman, O. (1982) *The Neuman Systems Model*, Appleton-Century-Crofts, Norwalk.

Orem, D. (1980) *Nursing – Concepts of Practice*, (2nd edn), McGraw-Hill, New York.

Orlando, I. (1987) Nursing in the 21st century – alternative paths. *Journal of Advanced Nursing*, **12**(4), 405–412.

Pearson, A. (1987) *Living in a Plaster*, Royal College of Nursing, London.

Pearson, A. (1992) *Nursing at Burford. A Story of Change*, Scutari Press, Harrow.

Pearson, A. and Baker, H. (1992) *Compliance or Alliance? A Case Study on an Attempt by Nurses to Introduce Self-administration of Medication in The Geelong Hospital Professorial Nursing Unit*, Research Paper Series 6, Deakin Institute of Nursing Research, Geelong.

Pearson, A., Durand, I. and Punton, S. (1989) Determining quality in a unit where nursing is the primary intervention. *Journal of Advanced Nursing*, 269–273.

Pearson, A., Durand, I. and Punton, S. (1992) *Nursing Beds. An Evaluation of the Effects of Therapeutic Nursing*, Scutari Press, Harrow.

Peplau, H. (1952) *Interpersonal Relations in Nursing*, G.P. Putman, New York.

Peplau, H. (1969) Professional closeness. *Nursing Forum*, **8**(4), 342–360.

Preston, R. (1988) *Nurses as Health Educators*, Burford Nursing Development Unit, Burford.

Rogers, C. (1969) *Freedom to Learn*, Bell and Howell, Ohio.

Rogers, C. (1983) *Freedom to Learn for the Eighties*, Merrill, Ohio.

Roper, N., Logan, W. and Tierney, A. (1985) *The Elements of Nursing*, (2nd edn), Churchill Livingstone, Edinburgh.

Roy, C. (1976) *Introduction to Nursing – an Adaptation Model*, Prentice-Hall, Old Tapping, New Jersey.

Vaughan, B. (1988) Homeward bound: discharge following surgery. *Nursing Times*, **84**(15), 28–33.

Watson, J. (1985) *The Philosophy and Science of Nursing*, Associated University Press, Colorado.

Wilson-Barnett, J. (1978) Patients' emotional responses to barium X-ray. *Journal of Advanced Nursing*, **3**, 37–46.

Wilson-Barnett, J. (1989) Patient teaching, in *Further Research for Nursing*, (eds J. Macleod-Clarke and L. Hockey), Churchill Livingstone, Edinburgh.

# Therapeutic nursing: emerging imperatives for nursing curricula

# 6

John Field and Mary FitzGerald

## INTRODUCTION

The concept of therapeutic nursing has proven very durable. Its tenacity is largely attributable to its inherent appeal as the epitome of a caring that contributes to positive health outcomes. Those who practise nursing know intuitively that this is the end to which nursing aspires. Thus, although caring is itself a human activity that is inherently prized, it is the association of caring with curing that makes nursing so obviously effective. Just as the ethic of caring has been used to develop nursing and nursing curricula, so too can the idea of therapeutic nursing make an important contribution. Indeed, we would argue that therapeutic nursing can be a source of inspiration for the developers of curriculum to advance the work of caring by supplementing it with an intentionally productive dimension. This development may well serve to ensure that the practical nature of nursing will remain its reference point and help nursing to survive in the current climate.

Therapeutic nursing draws upon nursing theory but it is here that we would add a cautionary note – nursing needs to learn from past experience. It is a truism that curriculum is inherently dynamic. It is organic by nature – it reacts and adapts to environmental pressures and in turn it effects change in the environment that is the catalyst for further curricular reaction and adaptation. However, if one accepts this cyclical nature of curriculum development, then for those involved with nursing curricula the alarm bells should be ringing. Like any discipline trying to make its way in the world of academia, nursing has struggled through successive curricular vogues in the search for its Holy Grail – a curriculum that will produce the ideal nurse. Laudable though this aspiration is, the pursuit has been confounded and frustrated by the ephemeral nature of what is regarded as the ideal nurse at any given time and by the changing demands and expectations of equally rapidly changing, bureaucratized health services. Perhaps the objective should be a nurse who is able to contribute in a positive and practical way to the health and well-being of the people he or she nurses.

As the role and expectations of the nurse have evolved over time, nursing curricula have endeavoured to accommodate these changes. Thus, over time we have swung from the nurse as 'doctor's handmaiden' – who was educated accordingly – through to current conceptions of the nurse as 'professional practitioner', educated in the university. Alongside and underpinning curricular development has been the debate about the true nature of nursing. This debate, however, has moved from its origins within nursing practice. It is now a debate engaged in almost exclusively by academics, albeit nursing academics. This historical development can be seen in constructions of nursing as 'doing' (Nuffield 1953), nursing as 'being' (Paterson and Zderad 1976), nursing as reflective practice (Powell 1991) and nursing as 'caring' (Bevis and Watson, 1989). We have also seen curricula designed to develop nurses who could satisfy these various constructions. None of this, however, has quarantined those involved in the design of nursing curricula from the protestations of health services that the graduates from their courses are not, at the time of graduation, what they regard as competent nurses. Neither has it enabled those same graduates to feel that they are competent nurses.

In many respects this outcome might be regarded as inevitable. Those who have been charged with the responsibility of curriculum design in nursing have generally been in the vanguard of developing the discipline. They have had a position on the nature of nursing and a vision of where nursing needed to go both professionally and as an academic discipline. However, this development of curricula by those in the vanguard has led to an almost inevitable disjuncture between the product of those curricula and the practice setting.

Whilst the development of this disjuncture may have been inevitable, there is no compulsion for it to be regarded as a permanent feature of nursing. Therapeutic nursing holds the potential to bring about a sea change here. There is an emerging conceptualization of nursing as therapy which offers the possibility of building on the work of those pioneers of nursing curricula to capture both the *essence* of nursing as caring and the *necessity* of nursing as therapy. In so doing, a space may be created where nursing students can learn to nurse effectively through the internalization of an ethic that prizes the client's need for a positive outcome of the care nurses provide. This imposes upon nurses an obligation to acknowledge the contribution to client outcomes of the practice of nursing and the need for that contribution to incorporate inextricably linked elements of cure and care.

In this chapter we demonstrate the impacts of this conceptualization of nursing as therapy upon nursing curriculum and consider the imperatives for the design of such curricula. We contend that for nursing curricula to be effective, it is incumbent upon the designers of those curricula to achieve a synchronism between the service demands on practitioners and the intellectual ideals of the discipline. That is to say, the purpose of the curriculum should be to afford students the opportunity to become contemporary practitioners. It is not the role of the curricula to prepare students for an ideal world that simply does not, and which for the foreseeable future will not, exist.

The contributions to the first edition of *Nursing as Therapy* in most instances were associated with and derived from nursing practice in the nursing development units in Oxford. That work was heavily influenced by Hall (1963, 1964, 1969) and Pearson (1983, 1988). Pearson led a practice-driven movement that subsequently influenced two important nursing curricula, these being the Oxford Polytechnic nursing undergraduate programme in the UK and the nursing curriculum developed at Deakin University in Australia. These curricula establish the link that we wish to explore in this chapter between nursing therapy and the learning of nursing.

## CURRICULUM CONTENT

Let us be clear about what we mean by nursing curriculum and curriculum content. By nursing curriculum, we mean the entire range of learning experiences that form part of the nursing course and which are intended to contribute to the preparation of the nursing student for the practice of nursing. This definition of nursing curriculum should signal our view that the content of the curriculum will very much influence the nature and quality of the practitioner of nursing who emerges from the particular curriculum. It is this view which underpins our contention that curriculum design is of central importance in achieving therapeutic nursing. The history of nursing curricula supports this view.

### Nursing models

Classically, the developers of nursing curricula have relied upon nursing theory and models as the determinants for the framework and content of curricula. These theories and models, on the whole, are claimed to have been developed inductively from the practice of nursing although they rely heavily upon theoretical frameworks from other disciplines. However, their almost universal rejection by practitioners of nursing may well be related to the fact that they are not susceptible to testing in practice. The evolution of this reliance upon the theories of nursing for construction of curricula by teachers of nursing and the rejection of those same theories by practitioners are circumstances that are both understandable and predictable, given the different and competing pressures that each party experiences. That is to say, on the one hand there is the imperative to develop a distinctive disciplinary focus to establish credibility for nursing in the universities and on the other, the relentless demands for increased productivity in service areas. In each case, these pressures have originated outside nursing, notwithstanding that they have often been embraced by many nurses. There is some irony in the fact that practice is almost untouched by these theories yet the curriculum intended to prepare nurses for practice is so steeped in them.

Logic would suggest that the content of any nursing curriculum should be guided by the things that practitioners are required to do in the practice of nursing. Even so, the framework of the curriculum should be capable of remaining relatively constant over time provided that it takes account of all the dimensions of therapeutic nursing. In the context of this discussion, that also means it should be guided by a conception of those things that a practitioner is required to do in the practice of therapeutic nursing. It has already been established in other parts of this book that therapeutic nursing needs to be understood both as an integrative way of nursing (i.e. where the therapeutic relationship is the foundation of all practice) and also as discrete therapeutic techniques to be learned and practised within the *context* of the therapeutic relationship.

## Therapeutic nursing

The notion of nursing as therapy was developed by Hall (1963, 1964, 1969) at the Loeb Center in New York. She took the view that nursing was itself a distinct therapy and at the time this was highly innovative – some would say even presumptuous – but Hall took the debate beyond this. She recognized that there were times when a person's primary need was for nursing therapy over and above any other available therapy. Her writing is not steeped in philosophy, sociology or any other discipline – just the practice of nursing. As a result, it is refreshingly touching, simple and practical.

Hall did not concentrate upon the psychosocial aspects of nursing care. Rather, she celebrated the physical. She believed that nurses are privileged to care for people in intimate physical ways and that through this type of contact it is possible to create therapeutic relationships. Through her observation of practice Hall proposed that the central feature of nursing practice

which made it 'healing' or 'therapeutic' related to the use of intimate physical touch. For her, only nurses were given the opportunity to care for and
about the intimate physical needs of patients. It was the nurses who used
this opportunity to generate closeness with the patient, who were able to
use this to therapeutic effect. Hall (1964) refers to this as the care component of nursing and describes this as one of three overlapping circles from
which therapeutic nursing can be modelled (Figure 6.1).

The care component of therapeutic nursing is largely seen to be the
province of nurses although other health professionals at times engage in
caring processes. The core component of nursing relates to an understanding of the human condition which stems from the experience of being
with people in need of care and from the study of the behavioural sciences.
The third component within Hall's description is a cure component which
relates to all those activities that nurses engage in alongside their medical
and paramedical colleagues with the explicit goals of treating disease and
illness and the achievement of a cure.

Hall derived her understanding and vision for nursing from her hands-
on experience in establishing and running a nursing unit where nursing
was considered to be the chief therapy (Tiffany 1977). She differentiated
between two types of nursing – 'caretaker' nursing and 'healing' or professional nursing (Pearson 1991). The former is task centred while the latter
is seen to be patient centred. Hall was convinced that the nurses who
were healing were those who reached an understanding that patients are
the achievers.

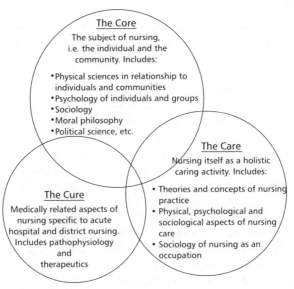

**Figure 6.1** A model of therapeutic nursing (based on Hall (1969)).

Hall's theory of nursing influenced the development of the Oxford Nursing Development Units and the 1988 Deakin curriculum. Her ideas were used as seeds for further development of therapeutic nursing. The concept of therapeutic nursing has the potential to be developed in many interesting ways, as the second edition of this book attests. Curriculum developers who wish to create optimal opportunities for nursing students to learn to apply their nursing in a therapeutic manner will find guidance in the works of the practitioners who have built on Hall's original ideas, refined them for their own practice and developed new ideas as well. Whilst most of these theorists were referred to in the first edition of this book, a significant new work is that of Ersser (1997) *Nursing as a Therapeutic Activity: An Ethnography.* In his work, Errser concludes that there is still a need to examine and determine the therapeutic nature of nursing. He has, however, identified three core concepts of nursing (Ersser 1997:280): the presentation of the nurse, relating to the patient and the specific actions of the nurse. The actions of nurses relate to many of the tasks and procedures undertaken in the course of nursing. These actions need to be underpinned by evidence in order to ensure that nursing is as effective as possible. The type of evidence nurses need to gauge effectiveness tends to be empirical rather than interpretive and herein lies an important opportunity for the designers of nursing curricula to equip students of nursing with the tools to appreciate all forms of evidence and its importance.

**Research**

Knowledge and understanding of the nature, processes and outcomes of nursing generated by research are used to define the discipline and to guide nursing practice and curriculum. Nursing has been disadvantaged in the research stakes relative to other disciplines such as medicine because some of the methodologies most appropriate to the study of nursing have been interpretive and critical in nature, using qualitative data, and these approaches to research have only recently begun to find favour with funding bodies. This enthusiasm for interpretive methodologies in nursing research, coupled with the protracted struggle to establish their credibility, may have contributed to a somewhat negative perception among nurses of quantitative studies. In part, this is probably also a reaction to the dominance in the early days of nursing academia of the traditional scientific paradigm which is so closely aligned to the biomedical model (Meleis 1997). Therapeutic nursing necessitates an eclectic approach to research generally insofar as nursing generates a range of questions that are most suitably answered through different research perspectives. The research perspectives are presented here in the classic arrangement of interpretive, critical and positivistic paradigms. It is, however, acknowledged that the boundaries of these paradigms may become blurred and there is a degree of critique and interpretation in all research.

Some of the interpretive nursing research is legendary and has contributed positively to the morale and pride of nurses generally. Benner's landmark investigations of nursing expertise (Benner 1984) and caring (Benner and Wrubel 1989) established practice as the bedrock of nursing knowledge. The therapeutic benefits that emanate from the nurse–client encounter are graphically described and their meanings extrapolated. Any student of nursing would do well to read existential accounts of nursing and illness in order to be able to consider and come to a better understanding of the world of nursing as it is lived.

The links between nursing practice, the establishment of a therapeutic relationship and phenomenological enquiry have been identified (FitzGerald 1997). On the whole, nurses make good collectors of qualitative research data because the skills required in nursing are similar to the ones that help a researcher to establish the kind of relationship with research participants that encourages them to feel safe and divulge information. As nursing students gain more expertise in learning from and listening to patients, so they will also develop skills to become researchers of nursing in the interpretive paradigm.

Research in the critical paradigm creates the opportunity for questions to be asked regarding the status quo. It enables us to look sceptically at the power relationships that hold a system together and control its future directions and to bring about radical change that redresses inequality and oppression. Although action research projects are notoriously difficult to manage, again the skills required to conduct this research are also those required to nurse. Inherent in critical theory are the skills to access, to collaborate and to communicate as well as the moral intent to be just. Each of these is necessary for critical research and for nurses who wish to practise in a therapeutic manner.

Earlier we noted that there has been a preference among nursing researchers for interpretive and critical research stances over the past decade. In reality, nursing therapy is an extremely broad concept and all research perspectives have to be embraced if all questions regarding nursing therapy are to be answered. The clinician needs to know which therapy is proven to be best just as much as she or he needs to know what it means to be ill. It is also possible to see that the skills of the experimental researcher are skills inherent in therapeutic nursing. That is, the skill to observe objectively and to make logical deductions and rational decisions based upon the most reliable evidence.

The evidence-based practice movement has a great deal of support (Pearson *et al.* 1997) because it is so very practical. For years nurses have needed research that gives a clear mandate for decision making. Systematic reviews of the literature and meta-analysis provide clinicians and teachers alike with the kind of condensed factual information they require for certain therapeutic techniques used in nursing.

The overlap between the skills required to nurse therapeutically and the skills to research in the different paradigms has been mentioned because it is always a moot point as to where in any nursing curriculum to put nursing research. In order to learn to nurse in a therapeutic manner, the nursing student needs to be able to appreciate and evaluate nursing research and to be able to discriminate in the choice of evidence to guide practice. The ability to conduct research comes later in most careers but the basic foundation of core skills makes this acquisition much easier.

### Practice-led curricula

The obvious corollary of therapeutic nursing is the development of practice-led curricula. Some very significant work has already occurred in this area, most notably in the form of the curriculum developed at Deakin University in Australia in 1988, Oxford Brookes University in the UK in 1989 and the Tasmanian School of Nursing, in Australia in 1994. The underlying assumption of a practice-led curriculum is that nursing practice is of itself an intellectual pursuit worthy of academic attention. Examples of this intellectual work can be seen in the writing of Pearson and the teams in the Burford Nursing Development Unit (1981–1987), the Oxford Nursing Development Unit (Pearson 1988, McMahon 1991) and Deakin University (1988). The Deakin curriculum has been extremely influential in Australia and many schools are encouraged to use elements of it to this day.

The practice-led curriculum in these two cases focused upon practice and the work that had been done in the nursing development units to establish the therapeutic nature of nursing care. Boundaries between the academic and service providers were broken down as far as possible with practitioners working in the university and academics practising regularly. The significant element of these early appointments, which is often overlooked and shed in similar roles, is the acceptance of responsibility and authority for standards of nursing practice and the standard of the curriculum. Examples of such collaborations are few and far between largely because of the attendant complex difficulties related to the establishment and operation of crossinstitutional organizational arrangements (Lathlean 1997). Examples of collaborative appointments abound but few of them have endured beyond the pioneering stage for reasons which are well documented elsewhere (Cox *et al.* 1994, FitzGerald 1988, 1994b, Lathlean 1997) but lie beyond the scope of this discussion.

Strategies such as the inclusion of practitioners on curriculum development working parties and course advisory teams are unlikely, of themselves, to result in practice-led curricula. Similarly, the inclusion of practitioners in the supervision of students in the clinical setting is unlikely to contribute substantially to this end unless they feel they are suitably enfranchised. Experience suggests that it is most likely that they will feel uncomfortable in situations where they feel dominated by academics. It is perhaps noteworthy that the idea that a curriculum should be practice led is not accepted universally and there would be considerable opposition to these ideas in some schools of nursing. These opponents do not see practice as the legitimate source of nursing knowledge which, of course, is the underlying assumption that supports a practice-led curriculum.

## METHODS TO FACILITATE LEARNING

Just as the emphasis in therapeutic nursing is for the client to be as independent as humanly and humanely possible, the proponents of a humanistic curriculum (Bevis and Watson 1989) and professional nursing practice (Titchen and Binnie 1993) concentrate upon the learner and the practitioner becoming responsible for and capable of controlling his or her own learning and practice. That is, of course, within certain boundaries. There is no such thing as complete freedom. The boundaries referred to are to do with an overall professional responsibility held by nurses, nursing teachers, managers and licensing boards to protect the public, by ensuring first that nurses are prepared and then continue to be safe practitioners (FitzGerald 1994) and second that practitioners practise within the limits of their knowledge and skills (FitzGerald 1990).

### Independent practitioners

In this chapter we wish to concentrate upon the advantages that professional practice has for the client rather than the usual focus upon the need for nurses to be recognized and remunerated as a professional group. Manthey (1980) proposed that primary nursing was a means of enabling nurses to offer a professional service to clients and there is now considerable evidence that primary nursing is conducive to the establishment of therapeutic relationships between nurses and clients (Black 1992). It has already been established, in this book and elsewhere (Ersser 1997), that therapeutic nursing is dependent upon the good relationship between the nurse and the nursed. There are different versions of primary nursing but the underlying principles of authority, responsibility and accountability remain constant. That is that one nurse accepts responsibility for the planning and delivery of nursing from the admission of a client until his or her discharge (whether this be in hospital, a nursing home or the community). The continuity of care that comes with primary nursing is one of the more obvious advantages for clients.

It is our contention that the health service today is so complex and specialized that newly registered nurses cannot be expected to function at the level of primary nurse. The level of autonomy that primary nurses have requires them to have commensurate practical knowledge and skills. Further postgraduate education that is practically orientated is wise before this type of responsibility for independent nursing practice is accepted. As nurses gain more experience in practice, they learn to recognize the knowledge embedded in their practice. It is reasonable to expect that through further education combined with constantly accumulating experience of practice, they will confidently seek the challenges and rewards that come with further responsibility (Figure 6.2).

At Adelaide University the Department of Clinical Nursing, set up by Pearson in conjunction with the Royal Adelaide Hospital, has designed a range of graduate diplomas in speciality nursing (intensive care, peri-op, orthopaedic, cardiac, general practice nursing, etc.) (Pearson and FitzGerald 1997). Preparation for specialist clinical practice is the highest priority and all students are encouraged to appraise and to use theory in the light of their experiences in practice. The courses are designed for clinicians who are working in speciality areas and study focuses upon practice.

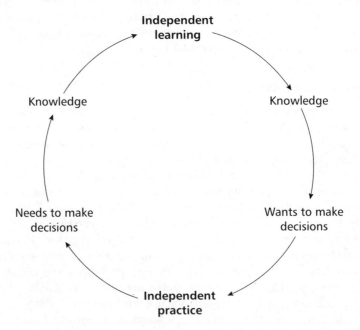

**Figure 6.2** Mutual support of independent learning and practice (FitzGerald 1991: 50).

## Independent learners

The theory that introduces the concepts of adult learning, independent learning and humanistic learning, is well documented (Bevis and Watson 1989, Jarvis 1983, 1987, Knowles 1970). The educational trends that go hand in hand with these philosophies of education are: student-centred learning, self-evaluation, student autonomy and education as a lifelong, self-directed process. These processes have been talked about for a long time in nursing and it is rewarding to see some good results. Graduate nurses are praised for their ability to adapt, to think critically and to solve problems.

It is perhaps still worth referring to Knowles' (1970) assumptions regarding adult learning because they do relate well to nursing students*. He proposed that: as adults learn they change their self-concept and become more independent in their learning; adults need to have prior experience acknowledged; adults' willingness to learn is associated with what they need to do socially and adults like to learn about things that are immediately useful to them. The experience with the graduate diploma nursing students in Adelaide completely concurs with these assumptions. It is a constant challenge to the lecturers to present theories of nursing and professional issues as having currency for students in their contemporary practice. Wherever possible, prior learning and experience in nursing are given status and in order to be relevant to immediate practice, 50% of the course is spent with students immersed in clinical practice alongside clinical title holders of the university. These clinical title holders are clinicians with the requisite expertise in their speciality to supervise and encourage the nursing students undertaking the graduate diplomas. The reality of practice ensures that as soon as they are able, the students become progressively more independent in their practice.

## Learning from experience

Although it is acknowledged that different students will favour one or another teaching technique, all nursing students are likely to learn most nursing through their own experience in practice. In our opinion, there is no substitute for clinical experience in both undergraduate and postgraduate programmes. In many instances the clinical hours in undergraduate programmes have been eroded because the curriculum is full of theoretical subjects or the cost of supervising students becomes prohibitive. Postgraduate courses may have no practice component at all. The paucity of practice in some postgraduate courses runs counter to Benner's proposition that nursing knowledge is embedded in practice and relegates this premise to mere rhetoric.

*(By 'nursing students', we are referring to all those who study nursing)

There are problems associated with the supernumerary status of students, especially when this status is accompanied by sporadic attendance and working days are interrupted by lectures, tutorials or library time. Nursing students need to experience the same working lives as the more experienced nurses if they are to appreciate and emulate the therapeutic actions of the nurses they are learning with in practice.

Oxford undergraduate nursing students worked alongside mentors for the full range of shifts and gradually became more independent as their course progressed and their ability and confidence to nurse increased. In return for guidance and time from the mentor, the students contributed to the workload of the various practice areas. By working with one nurse and the patients assigned to him or her, the students experienced the benefits of continuity of care both for the client and for themselves. They began to form therapeutic relationships with clients and were able to see nursing therapies through to productive ends.

Another important aspect of immersing students in realistic practice is that they learn the culture of clinical nursing (hospital or community), they become familiar with the environment, how to communicate with the multi-disciplinary team and how to cope with being busy. 'Business' and confusion come almost naturally in most nursing spheres and learning to prioritize and keep calm is a necessary nursing skill (Cox and Moss 1988). Too many nursing students are underexposed to the realities of everyday practice and find it difficult to transfer learning in a protected and artificial environment to the stark realities of the first six months of practice as a registered nurse. It is ironic that the reality shock (Kramer 1974) of beginning RN practice, described so many years ago, is likely to be worse now than it was when first identified. The quick adaptation that nurses have to make must surely detract from their ability to nurse therapeutically – how much better and less stressful for the nursing student to learn gradually.

## Learning through critical reflection

Once students learn the technique of crtical reflection on and in practice they can begin to discover the wealth of knowledge embedded in practice and learn to link this with extant theories. The work of Schön (1987) and Boud et al. (1985) provides useful educational perspectives on critical reflection and Cox et al. (1991) and Palmer et al. (1994) give excellent practical examples of critical reflection in the ongoing development of nursing expertise.

Holmes and Stephenson (1994) give a good account of their increasing ability to reflect critically upon and learn from their practice as undergraduate nursing students in Oxford. In the same volume, Reid (1994) describes the supervision process of nursing students, balancing the amount of support she gave students to make them feel comfortable in practice with challenges she put their way to encourage them to learn more. Nursing students obviously need a degree of help to become reflective practitioners and FitzGerald (1994) has warned elsewhere that this method of learning should not be regarded as requiring fewer resources than other learning strategies. Burns (1994) describes how critical reflection was an integral part of the assessment of learning processes in the Oxford undergraduate programme.

Critical reflection upon one's own performance is commonly accepted as an essential part of professional nursing practice. The ability to reframe problems and draw upon experience to solve practical problems is surely an essential skill for the nurse who wants to deliver care that is therapeutic in nature.

## Learning through the arts

The ability to develop a nurse–patient relationship which has a therapeutic effect is by no means an ordinary skill. While some nursing students have an abundance of social skills, it is not easy to learn to empathize with clients and to help them achieve optimal independence. Communications skills are an integral part of all undergraduate nursing programmes and curriculum designers should continually strive to find techniques that are the most conducive to the learning of these skills. The arts as a medium for both understanding the human condition and communicating with each other at an emotional level has a great deal to offer nursing students and other caring professions in terms of establishing caring relationships with therapeutic intent and effect.

Early work between nurses at Burford Nursing Development Unit and a group of professional actors is a good example of a creative way of learning how to become close to patients and to use this closeness therapeutically (Pearson 1992). The actors took on the roles of clients and the nurses nursed them. Staying in role, the actors then gave feedback in response to the care they received from a lay perspective. This process gave the nurses '. . . an opportunity to actually see themselves in practice; and to develop a degree of empathy . . .' (Pearson 1992), thereby improving their awareness of themselves as helper to the client and their understanding of the client's perspective. The actors were independent in this process. As a group, they developed patient characters and as individual performance artists, grounded in the Stanislavsky school of method acting, they 'became' the characters.

This approach to learning about 'being' with patients to enhance therepeutic effect has a number of interesting and important features.

- The leadership in terms of teaching is vested in the hands of non-health professionals.

- The 'action' component moves beyond the somewhat artificial and superficial process which characterizes role play between peers.
- The actors, as pseudo-patients, are quite different to simulated patients used commonly in medical and nursing programmes. Simulated patients follow a 'script' written by professionals and present a classic, stereotypical portrayal, rather than an emotional being.
- The use of skilled, professional actors creates opportunities for the actor to eventually shed the patient role and to provide an informed critique of the interaction as a kind of third person.
- The focus is on *what happened here*, rather than on the mechanics of technique or the dominant values of health professionals.

This approach became an integral component of the Deakin University undergraduate nursing curriculum (Deakin University 1988) and a further development of it is being incorporated into curricula at the University of Adelaide (University of Adelaide 1997).

Campbell (1994) writes of work he did at Deakin with nursing students encouraging them to understand the experience of illness through various art media: writing, drama and mask making. He writes:

Artistic accounts of the experience of a mastectomy can be extremely moving through their graphic, sensitive, emotive, inquisitive and personal nature. They may also show within their work the necessity of expression and its therapeutic potential. (Campbell 1994:3)

The range of potential opportunities to enrich the nursing student's understanding of therapeutic nursing through art is still open for further development in the curricula.


**CONCLUSION**

In this chapter we have argued for the objective of nursing curricula to be therapeutic nursing because we believe that the overriding imperative for nursing curricula is to prepare students to nurse. We have not sought to prescribe curricula in terms either of content or method and clearly curricula designed by nurses that concentrate upon nursing as therapy will still include much of the conventional content. However, curricula can become too full and unfortunately this crowding all too often results in reductions in clinical placements. Some choices do need to be made about allowing certain subjects to be reduced or dropped from the curriculum in order to accommodate the things that bear most relationship to the immediate requirements of the students to practise therapeutic nursing.

What we are advocating, however, is that current content together with any modifications be assembled in a manner best suited to emphasize those aspects of the curriculum germane to therapeutic nursing. This requires that the curriculum be practice led. For curriculum to be practice led, it must value experiential learning and the experience through which this learning occurs must be 'real' insofar as it occurs in the actual milieu of current health services. Even this will be insufficient to guarantee that the curriculum is practice led for just as important as the acquisition of experience is a culture that both understands the processes of experiential learning and supports students as they engage in critical reflection.

For students to emerge as effective therapeutic nurses, it is necessary that the curriculum be informed but not dominated by theories of nursing. This chapter has been about the challenges for the nursing curriculum to ensure that the graduating student of nursing has been afforded the opportunity to develop the skills, attitudes and knowledge necessary for the practice of therapeutic nursing. The imperatives as we see them are:

- for curriculum designers to recognize that curriculum is a means to an end rather than an educational icon, however superbly crafted it may be
- for there to be some better balance between theoretical ideals and the reality of the practice setting
- for an acceptance that nursing is learned through experience as long as that experience is critically reviewed with help and guidance and as long as the learning is guided and supervised by experienced nurses
- the eclectic nature of research
- a tangible acknowledgement of the coexistence and usefulness of art and science in nursing.

In order to encourage therapeutic nursing, protracted experience in practice is an essential component of any learning programme. This experience, however, needs to be made meaningful and related to theories through critical reflection on and in practice. Clinicians who are themselves reflective practitioners are best positioned to facilitate and encourage this process in students.

A particular school of thought regarding therapeutic nursing and the means by which this is orchestrated in practice has been used in this chapter. These theories have arisen from practice and despite the theories relied upon or used in any curriculum, it is proposed here that the guiding force for nursing curricula should be practice and what goes on there. A case has also been made for facilitators of the learning of nursing to be responsible in the practice institution and the educational institution. For too long the nursing spheres of education and practice have been divided.

Those who are engaged in the design of nursing curricula have before them an opportunity to review existing curricula. The utilization of therapeutic nursing – an inherently integrative approach – as the object of nursing curriculum has the potential to overcome the traditional theory–practice divide through bringing together theory and practice in the practice setting. At the same time, the needs of both service and academia can be met. This is an inspiring prospect.


## REFERENCES

Benner P. (1984) *From Novice to Expert: Excellence and Power in Clinical Nursing,* Addison-Wesley, Menlo Park.

Benner, P. and Wrubel, J. (1989) *The Primacy of Caring: Stress and Coping in Health and Illness,* Addison-Wesley, Menlo Park.

Bevis O. and Watson J., (1989) *Towards a Caring Curriculum: A New Pedagogy for Nursing,* National League for Nursing, New York.

Black, F. (1992) *Primary Nursing: an Introductory Guide,* King's Fund, London.

Boud, D., Keogh, R. and Walker, D. (1985) *Reflection: Turning Experience into Learning,* Kogan Page, London.

Burns, S. (1994) Assessing reflective learning, in *Reflective Practice in Nursing: The Growth of the Profesional Practitioner,* (eds A. Palmer, S. Burns and C. Bulman), Blackwells, Oxford.

Campbell, I. (1994) *Through Elephant Eyes: Communicating the Experience of Illness Through the Arts,* Monograph, University of New England Press, Armidale.

Cox, H. and Moss, C. (1988) Promiscuous knowledge: the chaos of practice. The Olive Anstey Nursing Foundation International Conference, Perth.

Cox, H., Hickson, P. and Taylor, B. (1991) Exploring reflection: knowing and constructing practice, in *Towards a Discipline of Nursing,* (eds G. Grey and R. Pratt), Churchill Livingstone, Melbourne.

Cox, H., Hanna, B. and Peart, K. (1994) The joint appointment, in *Unifying Nursing Practice and Theory,* (eds J. Lathlean and B. Vaughan), Butterworth Heinemann, Oxford.

Deakin University School of Nursing (1988) *Diploma of Nursing: Curriculum Document,* Deakin University, Geelong.

Ersser, S. (1997) *Nursing as a Therapeutic Activity: An Ethnography,* Avebury, Aldershot.

FitzGerald, M. (1988) Lecturer practitioner: action researcher, unpublished MN thesis, University of Wales, Cardiff.

FitzGerald, M. (1990) *Limits to Autonomy,* paper presented to the Nursing Times Ward Sister Conference, Manchester and London, UK.

FitzGerald, M. (1990) Autonomy for practising nurses. *Surgical Nurse,* **Dec,** 24–26.

FitzGerald, M. (1991) Educational preparation for primary nursing, in *Primary Nursing in Perspective,* (eds S. Ersser and E. Tutton), Scutari Press, London.

FitzGerald, M. (1994a) Theories of reflection for learning, in *Reflective Practice in Nursing: The Growth of the Professional Practitioner,* (eds A. Palmer, S. Burns and C. Bulman), Blackwells, Oxford.

FitzGerald, M. (1994b) Lecturer Practitioners: Creating the Environment, in *Unifying Nursing Theory and Practice* (eds J. Lathlean and B. Vaughan), Butterworth Heinemann, Oxford.

FitzGerald, M. (1997), Nursing and researching. *International Journal of Nursing Practice,* **3**(1), 53–57.

Hall, L. (1963) A centre for nursing. *Nursing Outlook,* **11**, 805.

Hall, L. (1964) *Project Report. The Solomon and Betty Loeb Center at Montefiore Hospital,* Loeb Center for Nursing, New York.

Hall, L. (1969) The Loeb Center for Nursing and Rehabilitation, Montefiore Hospital and Medical Center, Bronx, New York. *International Journal of Nursing Studies,* **6**, 81–95.

Holmes, D. and Stephenson, S. (1994) Reflection – a student's perspective, in *Reflective Practice in Nursing: The Growth of the Professional Practitioner,* (eds A. Palmer, S. Burns and C. Bulman), Blackwells, Oxford.

Jarvis, P. (1983) *Professional Education,* Croom Helm, Worcester.

Jarvis, P. (1987) Lifelong education and its relevance to nursing. *Nurse Education Today,* **7**, 49–55.

Knowles, M. (1970) *The Modern Practice of Adult Education: from Pedagogy to Andragogy,* Cambridge Book Co., Cambridge.

Kramer, M. (1974) *Reality Shock: Why Nurses Leave Nursing,* Mosby, St Louis.

Lathlean, J. (1997) *Lecturer Practitioners in Action,* Butterworth Heinemann, Oxford.

Manthey, M. (1980) *The Practice of Primary Nursing,* Blackwell Scientific, Oxford.

McMahon, R. (1991) *Therapeutic nursing in practice,* in *Nursing as Therapy,* (eds R. McMahon and A. Pearson), Chapman and Hall, London.

Meleis, A. (1997) *Theoretical Nursing: Development and Progress,* Lippincott, Philadephia.

Nuffield Provincial Hospitals Trust (1953) *The Work of Nurses in Hospital Wards: Report of a Job Analysis,* (ed. H. Goddard), Nuffield Provincial Hospitals Trust, London.

Palmer, A., Burns, S. and Bulman, C. (eds) (1994) *Reflective Practice in Nursing: The Growth of the Professional Practitioner,* Blackwells, Oxford.

Paterson, J. and Zderad, L. (1976) *Humanistic Nursing,* National League for Nursing, New York.

Pearson, A. (1983) *The Clinical Nursing Unit,* Heinemann, London.

Pearson, A. (1988), *Primary Nursing: Nursing in the Burford and Oxford Nursing Development Units,* (ed A. Pearson) Chapman and Hall, London.

Pearson, A. (1991) Taking up the challenge: the future for therapeutic nursing, in *Nursing as Therapy,* (eds R. McMahon and A. Pearson), Chapman and Hall, London.

Pearson, A. (1992) *Nursing at Burford: A Story of Change,* Scutari Press, London.

Pearson, A. and FitzGerald, M. (1997) Establishing a clinically-based nursing department in partnership with a university faculty of medicine and an acute hospital. *Journal of Higher Education, Policy and Management,* **19** (1), 53–60.

Pearson, A., Borbasi, S., FitzGerald, M., Kowanko, I. and Walsh, K. (1997) Evidence based nursing: an examination of nursing within the international evidence based health care practice movement. *Nursing Review,* Royal College of Nursing, Deakin, ACT, February, 1–4.

Powell, J. (1991) Reflection and the evaluation of experience: prerequisites for therapeutic practice, in *Nursing as Therapy,* (eds R. McMahon and A. Pearson), Chapman and Hall, London.

Reid B, 1994, The mentor's experience – a personal perspective, in *Reflective Practice in Nursing: The Growth of the Professional Practitioner*, (eds A. Palmer, S. Burns and C. Bulman), Blackwells, Oxford.

Schön, D. (1987) *Educating the Reflective Practitioner*, Basic Books/HarperCollins, San Francisco.

Tiffany, D. (1977) Nursing organisational structure and the real goals of hospitals, unpublished PhD thesis, Indiana University.

Titchen, A. and Binnie, A. (1993) What am I meant to be doing? Putting practice into theory and theory back into practice in new nursing roles. *Journal of Advanced Nursing*, **18**, 1054–1065.

University of Adelaide, Department of Clinical Nursing, (1997) *Bachelor of Nursing Science/Bachelor of Nursing Science (Honours), Draft Curriculum Document,* University of Adelaide.

# Facilitating therapeutic nursing and independent practice

**7**

Stephen Wright

If nursing is to be therapeutic, then nurses must be able to recognize the breadth and potential they have in such a role. At the same time, the need to work in organizations which enable them to nurse therapeutically is paramount. Nightingale (1859) considered nursing as 'putting the patient in the best condition for nature to act'. How can nurses be put in a condition whereby nursing can act? Just as there are responsibilities laid at the feet of nurses constantly to re-examine and improve the mode of individual practice, so there is a need to examine the 'milieu' in which the nurse works.

## THE INDIVIDUAL, THE ORGANIZATION AND THERAPEUTIC NURSING

The UKCC (1992) has provided a code of conduct which maps out the nurse's role in maintaining and developing standards of practice. Yet nursing which aspires to therapeutic values needs more than the commitment of the individual; it also needs a supportive climate in which to practise. The two are inseparable.

Historically, when nursing has failed, the trend has invariably been to seek out the scapegoat. Identifying and dismissing the 'bad' nurses is seen as resolving the problem. However, as Martin (1984) succinctly points out:

> Individual psychopathology may have a part, but the issues are both broader and deeper. They are broader in the sense that much turns

on the attitudes of society to its weakest members (i.e. the ill and vulnerable). They are deeper in that what may occur is a perversion both of individual motive and of social institutions.

Thus, to facilitate therapeutic nursing it is necessary to look at what nurses believe about and do in nursing (the 'individual motives') but also the context (the 'social institutions', be they health-care systems, hospital or nursing organizations) in which nursing is carried out.

Martin (1984), who surveyed over 30 major government and health authority enquiries into situations where health care had failed, suggests that a number of key factors are significant.

1  The values which nurses hold depend not just upon those acquired while being socialized into nursing, but also those brought in from the wider culture in which they are raised
2  The quality of leadership of the team in which nurses work
3  The knowledge base which nurses and colleagues possess for practice and the extent to which this is developed
4  The resources available (funding for salaries, equipment, staffing levels, etc.) to carry out nursing
5  The degree to which nurses, and patients, are involved in the decision-making process on matters affecting care
6  The facilities available for nursing practice, e.g. buildings and design for the working environment.

A more recent report commissioned by the government of the day, and for very different motives, sought to explain the exodus of nurses from nursing (Price Waterhouse 1988). Interestingly, much of their findings mirrored the work of Martin (1984) and of the American 'Magnet' study (McLure *et al.* 1983). Fears related to demographic changes have led many to wonder where the nurses of the future will be recruited from (UKCC 1986). Yet even a changing structure of the population could not explain the difficulties of recruiting and retaining nurses. What had gone so terribly wrong with a profession in which the attrition rate was so great that nursing was having to reproduce itself every ten years, simply to keep enough nurses working 'at the bedside' with patients (RCN 1986)? Ten years later, and despite the implementation of a radical new educational programme for nurses, midwives and health visitors, the recruitment problems of nursing have not abated. While the education system has changed, some deeper issues concerned with the working context for nurses appear to have been largely unaffected. Government attempts to reform National Health Service (NHS) systems also appear to have had little impact on the working environment for nurses, with over a decade of argument between government and unions. The former tend to believe that the reforms have been good for the service and nursing, the latter taking the opposite view. The independent sector has continued to expand its employment of nurses, but there is little evidence of any improvements in recruitment and retention or nursing morale from this quarter either (*Nursing Times* 1995). The Price Waterhouse Report (1988) pointed to a number of key areas of dissatisfaction, which can be summarized thus:

1 Inadequate pay
2 Lack of support and involvement in the decision-making process, on the part of managers
3 Feeling undervalued at work, with little attention given to personal and professional development
4 Feeling unable to carry out nursing in the way that it should be done.

While the loss of nurses from nursing is influenced by matters of pay and conditions, of equal if not greater importance to the nurse is the sense of personal worth and of 'doing a good job'. Indeed, an air of 'martyrdom' seems to pervade many avenues of nursing, as nurses continue to practise and struggle to maintain standards in spite of poor conditions of work and salary. While pay remains a factor in recruiting and retaining nurses (and the clinical regrading exercise began in 1988 sought to improve remuneration for clinical nurses), there are also a number of other key factors at work which must be considered. Even if clinical nurses achieve remarkable improvements in pay, the effects upon the loss of nurses from nursing are uncertain. Nurses will continue to leave nursing (or be discouraged from entering it) while they feel that the climate for practice is absent. For nurses to take on their therapeutic role requires more than just attention to financial rewards; they also demand the facility to place themselves in the best conditions for nursing to act.

## THE CONDITIONS FOR THERAPEUTIC NURSING

From the above discussion, a number of significant factors can be identified which govern nursing practice. These factors not only determine whether nurses come into and remain in practice, but whether features prevail which enable them to develop that practice into something which moves beyond 'getting through the work' (Clark 1978). For nursing practice to become holistic, healing and humane, i.e. therapeutic, it requires a fertile ground in which to grow.

### The nurse: commitment and values

Becoming and remaining a therapeutic nurse demands a (nursing) lifetime of commitment from each individual nurse. In moving from novice to expert and becoming a 'connoisseur' of nursing (Benner 1984), the time is filled with the acquisition of new kinds of knowledge and skills and the testing of old ones. To some degree, the organization has a commitment to develop nursing and nurses, but this does not abrogate the responsibility of each nurse to become expert by their own efforts. Keeping up to date through reading books and journals and attending workshops, courses and conferences when possible are one side of the bargain which each nurse makes with the organization in which he or she works.

However, if each nurse takes on the commitment to expertise and excellence, then this raises a further question – to what end is this effort being applied? To suggest that each nurse should work for high standards of practice is simplistic unless the nature of that practice and the values which underpin it are explored and defined.

In order to practise therapeutically, each nurse has to have a very clear vision of what nursing is – a healing art and science in its own right. Such nurses share positive values about all human beings, regardless of age, race, beliefs or sexuality. Elder (1977) believes that those who enter positions of caring for others must have a 'belief in the species, which is an integral part of the will to survive, and therefore a belief in life' which presupposes 'an acceptance of the doctrine that all individuals count and have a right to a full life'.

Therapeutic nurses must have taken on board such values about people. As such, they will not countenance alternative approaches which at best tend to reduce patients to what the Briggs Report (1972) called 'the production line of care'. Patients are divided into a series of tasks to be completed, carried out by varying levels of staff according to status and experience and no one is left to care for the patient as a whole. The Ombudsman's Reports (1994 *et seq.*) alone testify to the many problems this brings for patients as they come to feel isolated and ignored in the hands of those who are ostensibly there to care for them. Hall (1969) regards such nursing as having declined beneath the level of professionalism and derides it as having become a 'trade'. Beyond this lie the extremes of the 'total institution' (Goffman 1961) where patients become mere dehumanized objects peripheral to nursing activity. In such places, graphically summarized in Martin's (1984) survey, the reductionist approach achieves its nadir. Nursing becomes the antithesis of therapeutic caring. The needs of individual human beings are ignored as the nursing system strives to create a routinized and ritualized approach to 'care' which preserves the status quo. The system is served, but not the patient. It seems that nursing continues to be bedevilled by the tragedy of the institutional mindset. Since Martin's survey, the reports of dehumanized care in hospitals and homes continue unabated and are regular features of the popular and professional media. Complaints about care, to some extent fuelled by the rights of patients enshrined in *The Patient's Charter* (DoH 1991) continue to escalate and nursing remains a central source of the dissatisfactions (Ombudsman's Reports 1994, 1995).

The therapeutic nurse recognizes not only the value of each person, but also that of nursing. To suggest that nursing is valuable may seem like a statement of the obvious. However, the question has to be asked as to *what kind* of nursing is valuable. For many nurses, there is still a tendency to dismiss some elements of their practice as 'basic' or 'menial'. Instrumental skills are deemed to be more important and have greater status attached to them. Such nurses, in Oakley's (1984) view, have come to see themselves in the narcissistic mirror offered by medicine. Thus 'clever', skilled', 'real' nursing is usually closely associated with medical 'cure', with acute illness and a high degree of medical-technological intervention. The therapeutic nurse does not entirely reject such roles, for such instrumental activities are indeed a part of nursing support, but only a part. They are peripheral to the core of nursing and, indeed, might be considered valueless unless they are combined with certain other elements. Otherwise, the nurse seen in the narcissistic mirror is a medical helper, a doctor's handmaiden or biological plumber's mate – anything but a nurse.

Therapeutic nursing may include many medicotechnical or 'instrumental' skills, but at its heart lies the 'expressive' skills. It is the latter which the patient often sees as 'real' nursing and about which he or she complains most bitterly when it fails (e.g. Ombudsman's Report 1994). These expressive skills include the ability to 'be with' the patient – sharing plans of care, teaching, comforting, informing. The therapeutic nurse works as a partner with the patient and acts as advocate when the patient is unwilling or unable to participate in choices about care. Campbell (1984) sees the nurse as expressing a form of 'moderated love' by acting as a form of 'companion' to the patient who seeks to share care with the patient, rather than imposing nursing upon him or her. These expressive skills lie at the very centre of nursing and are part of the way in which therapeutic nurses are seen to act out their values. For them, there is no such thing as 'basic' nursing. Helping an elderly man to use the washbasin again successfully, comforting the distressed child at night, relieving the pain of the postoperative patient where the drug is but a small part of the therapy – these are tasks which some have dismissed as menial and therefore the territory of the nursing auxiliary or support worker. Yet these activities, and others like them, are the 'high-touch' skills of nursing without which the 'high-tech' skills have little meaning. Without them, the patient may be treated but is not healed and feels alone and abandoned as a person.

The therapeutic nurse has a very clear idea of what constitutes nursing and recognizes that those acts often dismissed as basic are actually complex, intricate and high-value elements in their own right. Without them, the essence of nursing is lost. It is nursing of a sort but it is not therapeutic nursing. The challenge is to combine both facets, the instrumental and the expressive, into a healing whole which serves the patient.

When nurses succeed in this they have come to terms with the value of nursing, and created a unique form of professionalism. If the functional, reductionist and institutional approach is the nadir of nursing, then its zenith is the therapeutic nurse.

## The nurse as a change agent

Much of health care and particularly nursing is still organized along hierarchical and bureaucratic lines. To work professionally in such a system may in some way be seen as a contradiction in terms. The nurse may seek to exercise professional autonomy and make decisions about patient care (and, indeed, the organization may seem to be encouraging him or her, at least superficially, to do so). Yet at the same time the nurse receives conflicting signals as others, such as doctors, managers, finance directors and so on, endeavour to exercise control over nursing practice.

The struggle between the twin poles of professionalism and bureaucracy is mirrored in that between the holistic, therapeutic approach in nursing and that which is reductionist and functional (e.g. the task-centred approach to care). To work successfully in such a climate demands considerable skills of nurses, for they must seek to change the nature of the organization, or at least to neutralize its effects so that they can concentrate on therapeutic practice. Amongst these skills must be those of change agency.

Nursing has tended to experience a power-coercive approach to change in health care. Policies determined at higher levels are passed down through the hierarchy, with the nurse expected to put them into practice (Keyser 1989). This top-down approach is flawed. It leads to resistance and possibly ultimate failure of the proposed changes, because the nurses at the clinical level may not feel committed to or 'own' the new norms. Alternatives such as the normative re-educative style ('bottom-up') of change enable nurses actively to participate as change agents in their own practice, and is argued to be more successful (Pearson 1992, Wright 1989a).

All nurses are change agents. It may be at the level of helping a patient to adapt to a different lifestyle or educating for self-care or teaching students and colleagues to achieve mastery of nursing. In a grander sphere, it may be that they act to influence decisions in their health organization or their professional associations.

Perhaps nurses know 'what' needs changing, but it seems that they are less certain of 'how' to change. Many authors have recently argued for a planned approach to change (Pearson 1992, Pearson *et al.* 1996, Salvage 1988, Turner-Shaw and Bosanquet 1991, Turrill 1988, Wright 1989a) and particularly for the development of the skills of nurses as change agents. A full discussion of change agency and strategies is beyond the scope of this chapter, but from the work of the authors cited above, a few key points can be suggested.

Figure 7.1 shows a few of the key features in a successful change strategy. However small or grand, the approach to change needs to be as planned and systematic as possible. Therapeutic nurses recognize their role as change agents, whether this involves working with individual patients, with larger groups or in much more wide-ranging activities. The implications for nurses recognizing and making greater use of their role are enormous. Nurses can not only help to produce an organizational climate where change is accepted as a way of life; they can also transport the effects way beyond the boundaries of the workplace. There are over half a million nurses in the UK. If a majority, if not all, were to become self-aware, knowledgeable, skilled change agents, then the implications are enormous, not just for nurses or for health care but for society as a whole.

**Providing the knowledge base**

Having a knowledge of nursing and its value and knowing how to work in it as a change agent are essential to the role of the therapeutic nurse. While to some degree each nurse has an obligation to attend to their own development, there is also an obligation on the part of the organization in which he or she works. Nursing development units, such as those in Oxford and Tameside, have shown how the development of nursing is intimately linked to the development of nurses (Bamber *et al.* 1989, Punton 1989, Salvage 1989, Salvage and Wright 1995).

Developing nursing and nurses is, however, not the exclusive province of nursing development units, nor can it be abrogated to the school or nursing as its responsibility. It is also the province of the service sector in which the nurse works. The reputation of the latter in offering further education to nurses has initially been poor (Price Waterhouse 1988, RCN 1986). In a hardpressed and often underresourced service, an ethos has tended to develop that funding and time off for nurses cannot be afforded. However, the argument can be developed that the service cannot afford not to. High-quality nursing needs high-quality nurses. An investment in nurses in terms of time and money for their development is therefore an investment in the quality of patient care. However, despite the many recent changes in health services organization and the adoption in the 1990's by the UKCC of a mandatory continuing education strategy, nurses in many areas seem to be struggling to obtain support for ongoing development. For every enlightened organization which cares for its staff, there is another which sees this as a much lower priority. For over a decade, the emphasis in government thinking in relation to the NHS, for example, has focused very much on patient outcomes which can be measured. These have been the subject of patient's charters and the annual publication of 'league tables' of the performance of individual trusts (a title introduced

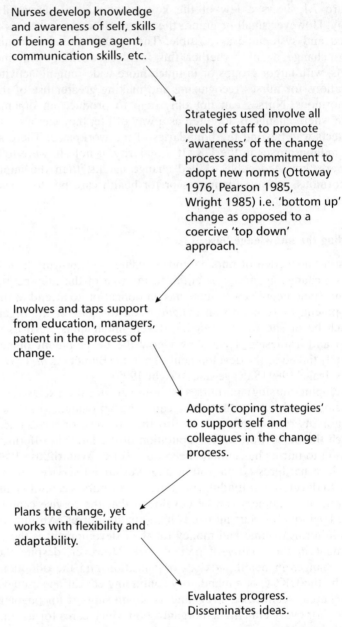

Nurses develop knowledge
and awareness of self, skills
of being a change agent,
communication skills, etc.

Strategies used involve all
levels of staff to promote
'awareness' of the change
process and commitment to
adopt new norms (Ottoway
1976, Pearson 1985,
Wright 1985) i.e. 'bottom up'
change as opposed to a
coercive 'top down'
approach.

Involves and taps support
from education, managers,
patient in the process of
change.

Adopts 'coping strategies'
to support self and
colleagues in the change
process.

Plans the change, yet
works with flexibility and
adaptability.

Evaluates progress.
Disseminates ideas.

**Figure 7.1** Elements of a change strategy.

into the NHS reforms of the 1980s for service delivery organizations, such as hospitals and community units, as opposed to the purchasers of health services – the 'health authorities'). While these give some indicators of performance, they offer a very limited perspective, others suggesting that greater emphasis should be laid on giving the public information about their local trust's performance in relation to staff support and morale (Cohen 1994). While patient's charters have laid the foundations of the patient's rights in relation to health care, others have argued that every trust should also have a staff charter. One organization has defined such a charter (National Association for Staff Support 1992) embracing rights on access to study leave, creche facilities, independent counselling and so on. Thus far, there has been little systematic uptake by health-care organizations of the challenges it set.

The Price Waterhouse Report (1988) illustrated how nurses' feelings about being valued by the organization (in terms of being encouraged to develop) are strongly linked to recruitment and retention rates. However, it seems that large parts of health care have yet to accept this notion fully, although the benefits to both nursing and the organization are clear. Therapeutic nursing can grow when the organization supports it and the development needs of nurses are thus satisfied. When nurses are developed, they feel more valued and reduce costs attributed to high staff turnover, sickness and absenteeism (Dean 1986).

The organization can provide on-site development or may tap the resources of local colleges and universities or encourage participation in the enormous range of courses and workshops provided for nurses. Pearson (1988) and Purdy et al. (1988) have illustrated the direction such nursing developments should take – focusing on communication skills, assertiveness, self-awareness, research skills, complementary therapies, etc. which assist nurses in the move along the trajectory from novice to expert (Benner 1984). Recognizing the financial difficulties which many settings experience, Purdy and Wright (1988) have suggested ways in which the organization can generate income to enhance the limited funds which might otherwise be available. At the same time, it has to be recognized that development does not just take place in formal programmes such as courses or study leave. There is increasing awareness of the complexity of nursing knowledge (Benner 1984, Watson 1988) and how the day-to-day world of nursing practice underpins its development. This has led to some recognition of the importance, even at government level (DoH 1992) of the need to support this learning through clinical supervision and reflective practice (Butterworth and Faugier 1992, Palmer et al. 1994). However, such recognition has yet to be translated into widespread action at clinical level.

The facilitation of therapeutic nursing does not, therefore, rely only on the personal commitment to development by the nurse. It also requires a whole-hearted commitment by the organization to support the nurse. It is in their mutual interest to do so. Every setting should be a nursing development unit.

## The organizational aspects

The development and support of the therapeutic nursing requires a particular organizational climate. It is characterized by being non-hierarchical and allowing nurses to be involved in the decision-making process (McLure *et al.* 1983). Managers tend to have an open and supportive style and demonstrate qualities of leadership with which the staff feel at ease, free to develop, to criticize, to change and to ask questions. At ward level, this style of leadership is crucial for the clinical leader/ward sister (Christian and Redfern 1996, Ogier 1981, Pembrey 1980) whose behaviour is so crucial to the generation of a therapeutic nursing climate.

Sparrow (1986) has illustrated how the ward sister/charge nurse role shifts from being autocratic controller of the nursing staff to supporter, teacher and encourager of nursing colleagues. Individual nurses, meanwhile, assume a greater autonomy and accountability for their practice over a limited caseload of patients, resulting in the practice of primary nursing.

This management style and the squashing of the hierarchy where care is devolved to individual nurses is essential to liberate them to practise therapeutically. It is a management style which permits methods of organizing care which can put nurses in a position where they can develop the 'partnership' relationship with patients. Many traditional approaches such as task allocation (Merchant 1985) and team nursing (Waters 1985) have tended to reduce nursing to a functional, reductionist approach. Patients become a series of tasks to be performed by varying nurses according to skill and status (aptly illustrated in Pearson and Vaughan 1986). The most senior nurse sits at the pinnacle carrying out the 'important' tasks (e.g. the ward sister and the doctor's 'round'), while other activities are delegated down, with the most junior dealing with the most 'menial'. Thinking about and organizing care in the primary nursing (Pearson 1988, Wright 1989b) approach is a radical shift away from these ideas. An individual (registered) nurse is accountable for the assessing, planning, implementing and evaluating of the care of a limited caseload of patients from admission through to discharge.

The development of primary nursing is highly complex and contentious, but it seems to be an approach which puts nurses in a position where they can act therapeutically. Nursing in this fashion requires a considerable degree of understanding between nurse and patient. Primary nursing facilitates this by enabling the nurse to work as a partner with the patient. The nurse gets involved. Methods such as task allocation limit nurse–patient involvement and, indeed, it has been argued, are actually used to prevent it, so that the nurse can cope more easily with the anxiety of nursing (Menzies 1961).

It has to be remembered, however, that systems of patient-centred care such as primary nursing, latterly given a boost with the advent of the 'named nurse' (Wright 1993) concept in the patient's charters, are no guarantee that nursing will be therapeutic. Having the right system of care in place also seems to require the development of 'right relationships' between employees and their organization, amongst the multidisciplinary team members, within nursing teams and, last but not least, for the nurse to be in right relationship with the self. This chapter is concerned with organizational relationships but there is strength in the argument that nurses must also be developed as persons, coming to terms with their personal values and motivations, spiritual beliefs, strengths and weaknesses and the healing of old childhood wounds and traumas if they are to help and heal others more effectively (Snow and Willard 1991).

If task allocation became a defence mechanism to protect nurses in the fraught world of their practice, then primary nursing, which involves the nurse with the patient much more intimately, requires other methods to support the nurse. The morality of unleashing nurses into this type of relationship with patients is questionable, if it is not concurrently backed up with a personal and managerial commitment to develop the nurse and the climate in which the nurse works. If the defensive props of tasks are removed, what is put in their place so that the nurse is not physically and psychologically exhausted by the work?

There appear to be two key areas for consideration. The first relates to the commitment to develop the nurse (referred to in 'Providing the knowledge base' above). The second relates to the creating of support mechanisms for nurses. Manthey (1988) has discussed how the multidisciplinary team can outline their roles, responsibilities and relationship boundaries with each other. Purdy et al. (1988) identified examples in their nursing development unit.

1  The formation of on-site peer groups and forums for mutual support
2  Setting up a support team (consisting of the nurse manager, consultant nurse and nurse specialists) to provide counselling, development and clinical expertise
3  Involving clinical nurses in quality assurance methods (patients are also included in this strategy), ward audits, standard setting, shared governance, staff appraisal and appointments, budget management and so on
4  Reviewing and revising skill mixes to enable primary nursing to develop and review the work of the support roles (e.g. ward clerks)
5  Setting up an extensive staff development and research programme involving all grades of staff and planned on a continuous basis

**6** Facilitating 'quality circles' (Christie 1986) which enable problem solving on day-to-day working practices and difficulties to be developed to clinical level

**7** Applying maximum resources to improving the working environment (e.g. furnishings, decorating, facilities) or to equipment needed to facilitate nursing practice (e.g. modern beds, revised nursing documentation, etc.).

The general aims of these and other principles suggested is to devolve the maximum power, control and accountability of nursing to those nurses who are in practice and enable them to develop their roles at minimal risk to themselves and their patients. Thus, the organizational structure needed to support therapeutic nursing has to be reviewed from the traditional hierarchical mode to a structure such as that shown in Figure 7.2. For nurses to act therapeutically, they need not only a method of organizing care to do so, but a supportive organizational structure which facilitates them. Thus a picture emerges of several contexts of support for therapeutic nursing. The first is the wider organizational support network, the second is that concerned with the team at clinical level. The third is how nurses develop and support themselves in terms of their own personal growth, awareness and well-being.

A shift in nursing practice which emphasizes the healing role of the nurse and additionally assumes a degree of independent practice has significant implications for interdisciplinary relationships as well as for patients and relatives.

MacDonald (1988) and Bowers (1988) have suggested numerous conflicts for nurses who develop primary nursing. Expectations of patients, relatives and members of the multidisciplinary team may be in conflict with the traditional role of the nurse. Strong and Robinson (1988) and Young *et al.* (1981) suggest there may be worries for managers about containing the costs of nursing or even of keeping it firmly under control in the widest sense. In developing their role, nurses disrupt the status quo of established 'role sets' and 'role' expectations' (Argyle 1978).

The development of nurses – their awareness of themselves, of the organization and of their capacity as change agents – is essential in the move towards therapeutic nursing. The changeover of roles puts nurses on a collision course with the establishment and ultimately they may need all the skills at their disposal to minimize the shock of the repercussions which occur in other roles.

Some colleagues may be willing supporters of nurses in their change of role while others may resist, become hostile or obstructive or actively seek to destroy nursing innovation (Salvage 1985). The term 'multidisciplinary team' conjures up an image of mutual respect and authority within the team, each member being committed to the benefit of the patient. The

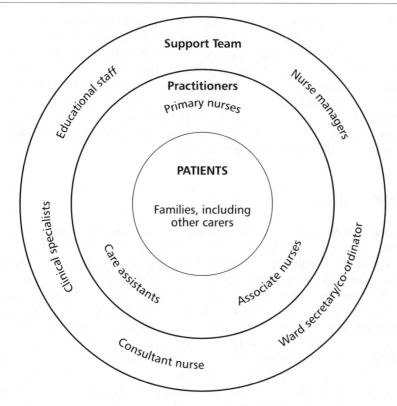

**Figure 7.2** An organizational structure supportive of therapeutic nursing.

reality may be somewhat different, particularly for nurses (predominantly female) who must deal with (predominantly male) doctors and senior executive managers.

While nurses must work with a variety of disciplines, there has been relatively little work undertaken on evaluating multidisciplinary teams. Does the ideal of a team of equals, with each contributing to the patient's needs according to skills (rather than one discipline ruling the others), work in reality?

McFarlane (1980) claims that the narrow disease orientation of the NHS, coupled with undue emphasis on medical function, has served to concentrate attention on the role of the doctor and minimize the contribution and potential of other health workers. The extent to which doctors will relinquish their traditionally dominant role in the team is debatable. While some doctors appear to accept the development of the nurse's therapeutic role, others (Rastan 1989) have shown a marked hostility and have contributed to a reversal of nursing innovation (Naish 1989).

Recognizing the potential for conflict is an important aspect of the role of the therapeutic nurse, for it will occur in varying degrees with all levels of the multidisciplinary team. Awareness of these difficulties and the possibilities of managing them can contribute significantly to the skills of the therapeutic nurse in defusing them. In time, if the therapeutic role of the nurse survives and spreads, then a corresponding adjustment of role perceptions by those in other disciplines must ensue. It will be the generations of nurses in the future who will be in a position to judge the success or failure of the role of therapeutic nurses.

## CONCLUSION

The success or otherwise of the therapeutic role of the nurse will be determined not only by nurses themselves but also by the nature of the organization in which they work and the degree of support they receive from their colleagues. Many of the obstacles and potential conflicts can be overcome by examining the way each nurse is prepared and what each setting can do to support nurses in the development of their practice. Financial rewards, re-examining values, education, learning change agency, improving the environment, reorganizing patterns of care and creating support structures – these are some of the key features in enabling therapeutic nursing to happen. Such nurses are out on the boundaries of professional practice. They are testing the territory of traditional practices. They cannot be left to take such risks alone.

## REFERENCES

Argyle, M. (1978) *The Psychology of Interpersonal Behaviour,* Penguin, Harmondsworth.

Bamber, T., Johnson, M. L., Purdy E. and Wright, S. (1989) The Tameside experience. *Nursing Standard,* **22**(3), 26.

Benner, P. (1984) *From Novice to Expert,* Addison-Wesley, London.

Bowers, L. (1988) The significance of primary nursing. *Journal of Advanced Nursing,* **14,** 13–19.

Briggs, A. V. (1972) *Report of the Committee on Nursing* (Chairman: Professor Asa V. Briggs), HMSO/DHSS, London.

Butterworth, A. and Faugier, J. (1992) *Clinical Supervision,* Chapman and Hall, London.

Campbell, A. V. (1984) *Moderation Love,* SPCK, London.

Christian, S. and Redfern, S. (1996) *Clinical Leadership in NDU s. Nursing Times,* **92**(47), 36–37.

Christie, H. (1986) Quality circles – staff ideas are your richest resource. *Health Service Options,* **1**(4), 17.

Clark, M. (1978) Getting through the work, in *Readings in the Sociology of Nursing*, (eds R. Dingwall and J. McIntosh), Churchill Livingstone, Edinburgh.

Cohen, P. (1994) Star Treatment. *Nursing Times*, **90**(27), 22–24.

Dean, D. (1986) *Manpower Solutions,* Scutari, London.

Department of Health (1991) *The Patient's Charter*, DoH, London.

Department of Health (1992) *A Vision for the Future*, DoH, London.

Elder, G. (1977) *The Alienated – Growing Old Today,* Writers' and Readers' Publishers' Co-operative, London.

Goffman, I. (1961) *Asylums,* Penguin, Harmondsworth.

Hall, L. E. (1969) The Loeb Centre for Nursing and Rehabilitation. *International Journal of Nursing Studies, 6,* 82–83.

Keyser, D. (1989) Meeting the challenge: strategies for implementing challenge, in *Changing Nursing Practice*, (ed. S. Wright), Edward Arnold, London.

MacDonald, M. (1988) Primary nursing: is it worth it? *Journal of Advanced Nursing,* **13** 797–806.

Martin, J. P. (1984) *Hospitals in Trouble*, Basil Blackwell, Oxford.

Manthey, M. (1988) *A Commitment to Each Other*, CNM Ltd, Minneapolis.

McFarlane, J.K. (1980) *Multi-disciplinary Clinical Teams*, King's Fund, London.

McLure, M. L., Poulin, M. A., Sorie, M. D. and Wandelt, M. A. (1983) *Magnet Hospitals – Attraction and Retention of Professional Nurses,* American Academy of Nursing, Kansas City.

Menzies, I. (1961) The functioning of social systems as a defence against anxiety, reprinted in Menzies-Lyth, I. (1988) *Containing Anxiety in Institutions,* Free Association Books, London.

Merchant, I. (1985) Why task allocation? *Nursing Practice*, **1**(2), 67–71.

Naish, J. (1989) Picking up the pieces. *Nursing Standard*, **25**(3), 13.

National Association for Staff Support (1992) *A Charter for Staff Support*, NASS, London.

Nightingale, F. (1859) *Notes on Nursing* (republished 1980), Churchill Livingstone, Edinburgh.

*Nursing Times* (1995) Editorial – Dying for Support. *Nursing Times*, **91**(13), 3.

Oakley, A. (1984) The importance of being a nurse. *Nursing Times*, **80**(50), 24–7.

Ogier, M. (1981) *An Ideal Sister*, Royal College of Nursing, London.

*Reports of the Parliamentary Liaison Officer (Ombudsman) for the Health Service* (1994 et seq.) Department of Health, London.

Ottoway, R. N. (1976) A change strategy to implement new norms, new styles and new environment in the work organization. *Personnel Review*, **5**(1), 13–18.

Palmer, A., Burns, S. and Bulman, C. (1994) *Reflective Practice in Nursing*, Blackwell, Oxford.

Pearson, A. (ed.) (1988) *Primary Nursing*, Croom Helm, London.

Pearson, A (1992). *Nursing at Burford: A Story of Change*, Scutari, London.

Pearson, A. and Vaughan, B. (1986) *Nursing Methods for Practice*, Heinemann, London.

Pearson, A., Vaughan, B. and FitzGerald, M (1996) *Nursing Methods for Practice*, 2nd edn, Butterworth Heinemann, Oxford.

Pembrey, S. (1980) *The Ward Sister – Key to Nursing*, Royal College of Nursing, London.

Price Waterhouse (1988) *Nurse Retention and Recruitment,* Price Waterhouse, London.

Punton, S. (1989) The Oxford experience. *Nursing Standard,* **22**(3), 271–278.

Purdy, E. and Wright, S. G. (1988) If I were a rich nurse. *Nursing Times,* **84**(41), 36–38.

Purdy, E., Wright, S. G. and Johnson, M. L. (1988) Change for the better. *Nursing Times,* **84**(38), 34–36.

Rastan, C. (1989) Angels who are more than guardians. *The Independent,* June 26th.

Royal College of Nursing (1986) *The Education of Nurses: a New Dispensation,* Royal College of Nursing, London.

Salvage, J. (1985) *The Politics of Nursing,* Heinemann, Oxford.

Salvage, J. (1988) Facilitating model-based nursing, unpublished paper, Nursing Models Conference, Gateshead.

Salvage, J. (1989) Nursing development units. *Nursing Standard,* **22**(3), 25.

Salvage, J. and Wright, S. (1995) *Nursing Development Units,* Scutari, London.

Snow, C. and Willard, P. (1991) *I'm Dying to Take Care of You,* Professional Counsellor Books Redmond.

Sparrow, S. (1986) Primary nursing. *Nursing Practice,* **1**(3), 142–147.

Strong, P. and Robinson, J. (1988) *New Model Management: Griffiths and the NHS,* Nursing Policy Studies, University of Warwick, Warwick.

Turner-Shaw, J. and Bosanquet, N. (1991) *A Way to Develop Nurses and Nursing,* King's Fund, London.

Turrill, T. (1988) *Change and Innovation: A Challenge for the NHS,* Management Series 10, Institute of Health Service Management, London.

United Kingdom Central Council for Nursing, Midwifery and Health Visiting (1992) *Code of Professional Conduct for the Nurse, Midwife and Health Visitor,* UKCC, London.

United Kingdom Central Council for Nursing, Midwifery and Health Visiting (1986) *Project 2000,* UKCC, London.

Waters, K. (1985, Team nursing. *Nursing Practice,* **1**(1), 7–15.

Watson, J. (1988) *Nursing: Human Science and Human Care, A Theory of Nursing,* NLN, New York.

Wright, S. G. (1985) Change in nursing: the application of change theory to practice. *Nursing Practice,* **1**(2), 85–91.

Wright, S. G. (1989a) *Changing Nursing Practice,* Edward Arnold, London.

Wright, S. G. (1989b) *My Nurse: My Patient – Primary Nursing in Practice,* Scutari, London.

Wright, S. G. (1993) *The Named Nurse, Midwife and Health Visitor,* NHS Executive, Leeds.

Young, J. P., Giovanetti, P., Lewison, D. and Thoms, M. L. (1981) *Factors Affecting Nurse Staffing in Acute Care Hospitals: a Review and Critique of the Literature,* DHEW Publication No. HRP0801801, Department of Health Education and Welfare, Hyattsville.

# Quality discourse and nursing as therapy | 8

Michael Clinton and Sioban Nelson

## INTRODUCTION

The increasing pressure on health-care budgets in OECD countries has led to significant reforms. Resource allocation systems have been revised, management arrangements have been reorganized and lines of account-ability have been strengthened. These trends are associated with the rise of the consumer movement and a growing preoccupation with quality. The quality movement in turn has impacted on structural reforms, management practices and the accountability of health professionals.

But what is meant by quality? And what are its implications for nursing as therapy? Rather than restrict the discussion to formal definitions of quality and descriptions of methods of quality assurance, this chapter proposes to answer these questions from a number of perspectives. The concept of quality will be considered but equal attention will be paid to the assumptions and arguments of its proponents and critics. The polarity between these two will then be examined and opened up for analysis by contrasting what will be defined broadly as the 'rational-instrumental' and 'critical-humanist' perspectives on quality. The 'rational-instrumental' approach will then be considered in detail before considering the 'critical-humanist' critique. These approaches will then be examined at a discursive level using the concepts of 'systematic and 'edifying' discourse. The intro-duction of the concept 'discourse' leads on to consideration of the language used to discuss quality in nursing. Finally, the implications of the functions of discourse will be considered from the perspective of Wittgenstein's (1971) views on language.

## WHAT IS MEANT BY QUALITY?

Quality is assured, controlled, evaluated and managed in the health-care systems of today (Attree 1993: 355). But what is meant by quality? And what are these processes? There is much confusion about the word 'quality'. According to Attree (1993: 359–360) it can mean: excellence (Pfeffer and Coote, 1990); the ideal (Berwick 1989); fitness for purpose (Pfeffer and Coote 1990); conformance to standards (Crosby 1979); meeting the customer's requirements; satisfying needs (Pfeffer and Coote 1990); or giving customers value (Statland 1989). To complicate matters, the meaning of quality was generally taken to mean conformance to standards. The 1980s was the decade of quality assurance. This era was dominated by a perspective on quality seen from the standpoint of the professional or expert. The producer/provider view came a close second. In the 1990s the emphasis has shifted to the perspective of the consumer (Attree 1993: 360–361). However, it is fair to say that nursing has lagged behind the quality movement by as much as a decade in applying these different perspectives.

Confusion is added by the growing number of concepts associated with quality. The concepts **structure**, **process** and **outcome** are used to distinguish between categories of criteria against which a service is compared (Donabedian 1980). The term 'standard', although central to the development of quality assurance systems, is also the subject of confusion as it has been applied to adequate, acceptable and optimum levels of quality (Attree 1993: 361). Similar confusion has arisen about whether quality refers to the standards of service that exist or standards of service as they should be. Standards have also been linked to both the quality and effectiveness of care. Attree (1993) distinguishes between **effectiveness**, doing the right things; **efficiency**, doing things right; and **economy**, the frugal use of resources. Other terms are equally important. **Quality assurance** is generally taken to refer to programmes intended to ensure the quality of service received by the customer. **Quality circles** are groups formed with the intention of identifying and solving quality problems (Kinlaw 1992). **Quality management** is the process of quality control achieved through strategic planning, resource allocation and reporting systems (Berry 1991).

As health-care organizations have become increasingly concerned about quality, it has become clear that quality cannot be considered in isolation from the management of health-care systems. Increasing costs, competition for scarce resources and structural reforms have challenged managers to strive for management arrangements that support quality assurance. Among the changes in management arrangements that have increased the preoccupation with quality is the growing trend for purchasers and providers to be split in the health-care systems of OECD countries (Clinton and Nelson 1995). Total quality management (TQM), continuous quality improvement (CQI), quality improvement (QI) and continuous improvement (CI) have become commonplace terms in hospitals and health agencies (Sherman and Malkmus 1994: 37). Progress with these initiatives has been dependent on the commitment of leaders to reorientate their organizations to a consumer focus. It has been important also for priorities to be set and for resources to be allocated to enable them to be achieved. Equal effort has gone into merging the drive for quality into the mission statements of organizations, often encouraged by the accreditation requirements of organizations such as the Joint Commission on Accreditation of Health Care Organizations in the United States and the Australian Council on Healthcare Standards (ACHS). Such initiatives have required a process of change management that is as yet incomplete. For example, employees are now more involved with quality assurance as the focus changes from performance of individuals toward work processes. This emphasis on quality-driven daily activities and formal problem-solving processes using statistical data to inform decisions is intended to ensure that services of the highest quality and maximum benefit are delivered at reasonable cost (Sherman and Malkmus 1994: 37).

Therefore, 'The main concern in today's health care environment is preserving or enhancing quality while delivering services in a more efficient and cost effective manner' (Jones 1993: 145). The really hard task is to connect the concern for quality with outcomes for the consumer. Any amount of energy can be put into improving the quality of care but if the cost is to be justified, it must be possible to relate quality, productivity and cost to outcome. Patient outcome approaches to quality are among the most challenging in today's climate of health care. In Lohr (1985) outcome is defined as the end-result of care or measurable changes in the health status of behaviour of patients (Lohr 1985).

Health status, functional status, reduced pain, improved mobility, return to work or normal activities and patient satisfaction are measures of patient outcome. Outcome measures in general can be categorized according to their focus. Hegyvary (1991) has proposed:

- *Clinical* – patient response to medical and nursing interventions
- *Functional* – maintenance or improvement in physical functioning
- *Financial* – outcomes achieved with efficient use of resources
- *Perceptual* – patient satisfaction with outcomes, care received and providers.

Jones (1993: 146) proposes the following more specific typology of patient outcomes:

- Mortality in the hospital or shortly after discharge
- Adverse events and complications during hospitalization
- Inadequate recovery or complications requiring readmission

- Prolongation of a medical problem that was not adequately assessed because of treatment of an unrelated condition
- Decline in health status because of problems or situations that lead to delay or denial of admission
- Decline in quality of life, including poorer physical, emotional or mental function.

Thus, not only has the debate over quality shifted in its 30-year history, but the concepts developed shift in meaning between ideal and adequate, outcomes and consumer perspectives, resource allocation and best practice. Meanwhile the political will to implement comprehensive quality measures in health care throughout OECD countries has fired the debate on the purpose of quality, the appropriateness of the model in use and the role of nurses and their clients in the process. This discussion will now turn to examine the polarized views of the proponents and critics of the quality movement.

## PROPONENTS OF QUALITY

### Accountability

Predictably, the quality movement has its proponents and critics. First, we will examine the arguments of those who believe in the value added to health care by quality improvement processes. One argument is that these processes ensure that patients are not denied available services (WHO Working Group 1989). Another argument is that they protect patients from injury by excessive or inappropriate services (WHO Working Group 1989: 79). Both arguments are supported by the belief that public accountability is a major goal of quality assurance. They also imply that identifying variations requiring corrective action in a continuous process of change leads to more efficient resource allocation. This view stems from a rational-instrumental perspective that views quality as a process for widening access to health services, as a means of protecting patients from harm and as a mechanism for resource allocation, goals which have become major foci for quality improvement in the health-care systems of OECD countries. The health-care systems of these countries differ in important respects, but the fundamental concern remains the same: how to ensure cost-effective services that are sensitive and responsive to the needs of patients. From this perspective, quality is a mechanism for regulating health care, at the macro level of the health-care system and at the micro level of the individual provider. This imperative is central to the accountability perspective on quality in health care.

## Transformational perspectives

More radically, proponents argue that the quality agenda is a means to achieve paradigm shifts in health care (Decker *et al.* 1994: 18). One of the major paradigm shifts mooted is the move from a provider-oriented to a patient-centred approach. Proponents of this view stress the notion that consumer expectations are increasingly regarded as having priority over the convenience of staff. It is also argued that the concern for quality encourages health professionals to become less interested in their activities *per se* and more interested in the outcomes of care. A third paradigm shift moves away from a focus on quality assurance to a focus on the performance of major processes in organization-wide activities. Quality from this perspective requires of organizations a systematic assessment and improvement of performance through the use of outcome measures and techniques for continuous monitoring (Decker *et al.* 1994: 18). Such trends are claimed to encourage an increased multidisciplinary focus on performance improvement as accreditation processes require evidence of collaboration across the health professions. The empowerment of employees to cross professional boundaries in problem solving and the breaking down of professional subcultures are related gains. These arguments are taken as representative of the transformational perspective on quality in health care.

To recap, the accountability perspective stresses the role of quality in regulating the behaviour of health-care providers. The transformational perspective is concerned with deeper organizational reform achieved by changing the way health-care providers think. The first perspective focuses on individual behaviour aggregated to the unit, organization or health-care system as a whole. The second focuses on the performance of organizational systems aggregated to the same levels of analysis. The two perspectives are not discrete. Arguments based on patient outcomes are justified by assumptions about individual preferences (Johannesson 1994: 1623). Whereas arguments about the value of the patient-centred framework (Robinson 1991: 29) are justified by reference to resource allocation models such as DRG-based prospective payment systems, the logic of the accountability perspective is that of rational change. The metaphor is that of the living organism that needs regulating to achieve optimum performance. The logic of the transformational perspective is that of the collective conversion experience. The relevant metaphor is that of metamorphosis. Later in this chapter the language of the two perspectives will be taken up as distinctive forms of discourse.

## Quality

The accountability perspective on quality is associated with measurement, statistical analysis and rational decision making to protect the interests of the consumer and the wider community. This perspective is the dominant one in health care today, but it is not confined to the health industry. Everywhere from manufacture to the public service the drive for quality is found. Scarcely any commercial or public organization of any size is without quality assurance processes and procedures. In the past three decades quality has grown from the inspection of manufactured goods on the factory bench to an integral part of almost all manufacture and service industries. The obsession with quality has become so pervasive that it has spawned the growth of specialized organizations and a specialist literature. Why? Because in the competitive societies of the OECD, cost reduction through quality improvement is essential if organizations are to stay in business. This trend is not confined to manufacture; there is increasing competition for resources among health-care providers. Public hospitals vie with each other to attract resources and to avoid closure, private hospitals compete for funds from third parties and individual providers compete to maintain their client base. The fundamental imperative in the quality movement is that of economic rationality, the drive to do more with less to achieve significant improvements in outcome by doing everything better than before.

## TQM

Total quality management (TQM) is one of the approaches to quality that demonstrates this imperative (Oakland 1989). The approach reflects a systems perspective in which process is an intermediary between inputs and outputs. Figure 8.1 shows a simple model of TQM applied to the health-care industry.

In TQM quality processes are driven by an obsession with the needs of consumers, the 'cult(ure) of the consumer' in fact (Du Gay and Salaman 1992). The approach requires quality in all functional areas of an organization and commitment from all employees to promoting service efficiency and effectiveness. This imperative requires a comprehensive approach from management. TQM is the combination of strategic and operational management that ensures that commitment to quality pervades every functional department. In the health-care industry the health professions can be regarded as functional departments, alongside other hospital and community services. TQM is about achieving a mindset that ensures quality in every aspect of service delivery. This mindset is built around a fundamental restructuring of organizational and individual values. Building the capability for quality is one of the resulting priorities for the organization. This process is often presented as building a commitment to excellence (Pinkerton and Schroeder 1988).

Nurses have embraced the quality movement and have developed approaches to quality assurance and evaluation (Katz and Green 1992,

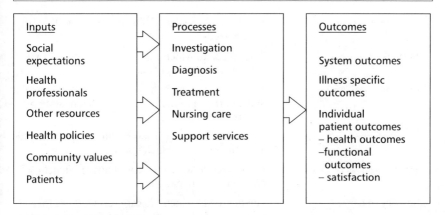

**Figure 8.1** Simple model of TQM applied to the health-care industry.

Pearson 1987, Schroeder, 1991a,b,c). The focus on process in the TQM model has encouraged some authors to define quality as a process. For example, Katz and Green (1992: 10) define quality assurance in nursing as 'an orderly series of activities designed to corroborate the defined attributes of quality'. Some of the factors that determine the quality of patient care are listed in Figure 8.2.

Standards are required for each of these factors if quality in nursing is to be assured. Standards are sets of rules, actions or conditions that determine the structure of nursing care, the care to be given and the outcomes to be achieved (Katz and Green 1992: 9). Nurses are guided in these activities by their professional education, by the policies of their employers and by the codes of conduct of their professional organizations. Other influences are the requirements of accrediting organizations, such as the Australian Council on Healthcare Standards, published research findings and the innovations achieved by such initiatives as the introduction of clinical nursing units (Pearson 1983, Pearson *et al.* 1992) and nursing practice units (Wright 1991) in the United Kingdom. With the development of computerized databases, it has become possible for nurses to consider performance indicators for their areas of practice where such systems are in place. Performance indicators are statistical indicators of performance, measured in units of service that facilitate comparisons among services.

## Performance measurement

The really hard question to answer about quality in the health-care industry is: What outcomes do health services achieve? Any acceptable answer must recognize that health care is more than the short-term care of the sick in hospitals and the treatment of disease (Mitchell 1993: 2).

| | |
|---|---|
| Accessibility to care | The ease with which a patient can obtain the care he/she needs. |
| Timeliness of care | The degree to which care is made available to a patient when it is needed. |
| Effectiveness of care | The degree to which the care rendered is provided in the correct manner, given the current state of the art. |
| Efficacy of care | The degree to which a service has the potential to meet the need for which it is used. |
| Appropriateness of care | The degree to which the care received matches the needs of the patient. |
| Efficiency of care | The degree to which the care received has the desired effect with a minimum of possible effort, expense or waste. |
| Continuity of care | The degree to which the care needed by the patient is co-ordinated effectively among practitioners and across organizations and time. |
| Privacy of care | The rights of a patient to control the distribution and release of data concerning his/her illness, including information provided to health care professionals and any additional information contained in the medical record and/or other source documents. |
| Confidentiality of care | Information the health care team obtains from or about a patient that is considered to be privileged and thus, except in specified circumstances, that may vary by illness and jurisdiction, cannot be disclosed to a third party without the patient's consent. |
| Participation of patient and patient family in care | Patient (or patient family) involvement in the decision-making process in matters pertaining to his/her health. |
| Safety of care environment | The degree to which necessary spaces, equipment, and medications are available to the patient when needed. |

**Figure 8.2** Factors that determine quality of patient care (from Katz and Green 1992).

A further complication is that a comprehensive approach to health-care outcomes would have to take account of the influence of housing, income, education and environmental policies. Therefore most recent definitions of health-care outcomes have shifted from the five Ds – death, disease, disability, discomfort and dissatisfaction – toward survival (clinically specific endpoints), health status (including emotional health), satisfaction, functional status, general well-being and satisfaction with care (Mitchell 1993: 4). Even the latter list of health-care outcomes is restrictive because it focuses primarily on the individual consumer and ignores the interests and perspectives of families, friends and communities. System-level outcomes are those achieved by co-ordinated hospital- and community-managed care systems. The outcomes of mainstream integrated mental health services are examples of system-level outcomes. Another example is the outcomes achieved by emergency departments and critical care units considered as a 'production line' of services (Mitchell 1993: 4).

## Outcomes

Two measures developed to look at condition-specific outcomes of health care are QUALYs (quality-adjusted life years) and HYEs (healthy years equivalents). Further work is required, however, to develop the best assumptions to make when applying these measures (Johannesson 1994). A still more difficult area is that of identifying the extension of life gained through medical treatment. Bunker et al. (1994) estimate that for the population of the United States, gains in quality of life are made for 70–80% of people with unipolar depression, although less than 50% of people affected receive treatment. Near complete pain relief is achieved in people with terminal cancer, but only an estimated 40–50% of those affected are treated. Another example is the treatment of hypotension which reduces the incidence of non-fatal stroke by age 70 in 50% of those at risk, but the proportion of people treated is 50%. Such figures vindicate taking access to services as an indicator of accountability in health care.

Buchanan (1994) has identified outcome measures for advanced practice in nursing. The tools Buchanan suggests for this purpose are shown in Figure 8.3.

However, outcomes should not ignore processes (Mitchell 1993: 5). Process criteria for quality in nursing care have been proposed (Attree 1993: 365). The categories suggested by Attree (1993) are listed in Figure 8.4.

## Instruments

Redfern and Norman (1990) note that the process quality assurance instruments that have received most attention from practitioners and nurse researchers are Qualpacs (Wandelt and Ager 1974), the Phaneuf Nursing Audit (Phaneuf 1976) and Monitor, the Rush-Medicus Nursing Process methodology (Jelinek et al. 1974), modified in the United Kingdom by Goldstone et al. (1983). Qualpacs and Monitor are concurrent audits of nursing practice. The Phaneuf Nursing Audit is a retrospective assessment of nursing care. The choice facing clinical nurses is that between using one or other of the preformulated scales, of which these are examples, or

| Suggested tool | Content of tool |
| --- | --- |
| Physical and psychosocial assessment tool | Skills checklist which measures basic cognitive, affective, and psychomotor skills necessary for performance of phases of the nursing process as related to the therapeutic nursing interventions. |
| Art of nursing questionnaire | Measures the affective domain of therapeutic nursing interventions such as patient comfort, communication, sense of worth, and respect during care given (Source: Curl & Koerner, 1991). |
| Therapeutic nursing interventions outcome abilities tool | Measures basic cognitive, affective, and psychomotor skills necessary for performance of the steps of the nursing process with integration of models for research utilization, use of the steps of the scientific research method and methods of research critique. |
| Advanced therapeutic nursing interventions outcome abilities tool for advanced practice roles | Measures cognitive, affective, and psychomotor skills necessary for performing advanced nursing therapeutic interventions and the nurse's ability to utilize research in practice and disseminate research findings, conduct clinical studies, prescribe therapy and evaluate individual and family response to treatment. |
| Quality of life and health status improvement tool | Measures changes in individual and family health status outcomes and perception of quality of life as a result of therapeutic nursing interventions. Links nursing actions, interactions to changes in individual and family health status. |

**Figure 8.3** Suggested tools for measuring nurse ability and individual and family outcomes related to therapeutic interventions (from Buchanan 1994).

of developing local methodologies through such techniques as quality circles or peer review (Redfern and Norman 1990: 1267).

To summarize, the proponents of quality focus on the regulation of the health-care industry to improve efficiency and effectiveness. TQM and QI are related concepts that underpin the quality imperative. Accountability for the use of resources is an overriding concern in this perspective. The approach is associated with measurement, large computerized databases, statistical analysis and the use of performance indicators to compare organizations and providers. Service outcomes are highly regarded as indicators

| Criteria type | Examples |
| --- | --- |
| (a) Health/wellness level | Death, disease, disability, discomfort and dissatisfaction; Improvement/maintenance of health; morbidity; mortality; peaceful; death; problem resolution, goal attainment; rehabilitation; survival rates; symptom control; control of illness. |
| (b) Functional ability | Physiological, psychological, social functioning; self-care ability; patient health knowledge; motivation; skill; low stress levels. |
| (c) Patient satisfaction | Access; availability complaints; compliments; co-ordination; communication; timing. |
| (d) Resource utilisation/cost effectiveness/efficiency | Benefit v harm; cost of correction, repetition, or compensation; compliance; patient return rate; effect for individual patients; quality of life. |
| (e) Undesirable events | Accidents and incidents; falls. Complications; contractures, nosocomial infections, pressure sores, iatrogenic diseases; readmission; return to theatre, patient self-harm; suicides, postmortems, untimely deaths. |
| (f) Undesirable processes | Medication and recording errors; unco-ordinated services; unmanaged pain. |

**Figure 8.4** Consequences of outcome criteria of quality nursing care (from Attree 1993).

of quality in this perspective, but it is also concerned with issues of access and process. However, the really hard question to answer is: What does the health-care industry achieve? Conceptual progress has been made towards answering this question by the development of the concepts of QUALYs and HYEs. However, the value added by health care to the quality of human life is compromised by the inability of large numbers of people to access the services they need. The issue of outcome has been of equal concern to nurses, but until recently more attention has been paid to the quality of the process of nursing. Methods are available for practitioners to evaluate nursing practice and a choice has to be made between the use of preformulated scales or locally developed methods. The former have the advantage of enabling comparisons to be made among units and organizations. The latter have the advantage of local involvement and, perhaps, commitment to using the results. However, it is difficult to conceive of the quality of nursing as something separate from the quality of health care as a whole because the outcomes of nursing care are limited by system-level outcomes. Nurses cannot add value beyond what is achieved by the health-care industry as a whole.

## DISCOURSES ON QUALITY

In examining the models of quality and debates concerning the quality movement, it is useful to turn to the work of Max Weber (1864–1920) and place the quality debate in the context of social action. One way of doing this is to draw on the distinction between *zweckrationality* (instrumental rationality) and *wertrationality* (value rationality) proposed by Max Weber in *Economy and Society* (1978) as a way of understanding social behaviour. For Weber, *zweckrationality* is that form of rationality given by social action intended to attain rationally pursued and calculated ends. *Wertrationality* is that form of rationality determined by belief in the value of some ethical or other form of behaviour for its own sake, irrespective of its prospects of success (Weber 1978: 25).

The logic of *zweckrationality* underpins the rational-instrumental perspective on quality. This perspective uses what Rorty (1980) has called 'systematic' discourse to promote the need for accountability and regulation in the health-care industry. The goals of the quality movement in this paradigm are to regulate health care to protect the interests of the consumer and to ensure public accountability. The underlying ideology is that of economic rationality. This perspective depends on measurement to provide information to support rational processes of change. The approach as a whole is concerned with large-scale unitary systems of performance that depend on surveillance and bureaucratic structures for implementation. Such systems are characteristic of managerialism and implicit forms of domination.

In contrast, *wertrationality* (Weber 1978: 25) underpins the critical-humanist perspective on quality in health care. This perspective substitutes reflective critical action for performance in an ideology drawn from humanist and left-based critical reasoning. Within this perspective, 'nursing as therapy' can be understood as an example of what Rorty (1980) calls an 'edifying' discourse, in that it seeks to transform nursing into something more than it currently is.

Although the two perspectives have been disentangled and will be shown to belong to separate domains, they are intertwined in the everyday reality of nursing practice. Importantly, these two forms of life are not presented as two halves of the divided whole, somehow dialectically brought into resolution. Rather, the delineation of these two ethical domains (*Lebensführungen*), formal and substantive, is not to suggest that they are the *only* possible forms of life, merely two influential types (Weber 1978: 85). The section that follows further distinguishes between those two substantive (i.e. driven by adherence to some ultimate value system) forms of opposition to the quality movement: critics who argue that the quality movement threatens to distract nursing from its concern to humanize health care and those motivated by the more radical concern to resist all forms of power and surveillance that inhibit autonomy and the right of the individual nurse practitioner to decide what is best within the constraints of a therapeutic relationship in which the client (or patient) is sovereign, not only as an individual but as a symbol of the human dignity that nursing takes as its mission to enhance. For heuristic purposes the forms of discourse typical of the two perspectives will be considered separately. In practice, many readings of social processes are possible and commentators differ in the extent to which they give equal attention to what will be called humanist and critical perspectives. What differentiates commentators is not so much their primary concern with this or that aspect of the quality debate but the implicit privilege claimed for their arguments. Ian Hunter argues in the case of education that:

> ... liberal [humanist] philosophy tends to identify ... with individual judgement, while sociological and historicist approaches invest in it a collective process leading to humanity's 'complete' development. ... the principle to which [both] ... accounts ... are committed is contained in a certain image of the moral personality. (Hunter 1994: 2).

For the critics of the quality movement, therefore, resistance is a form of defence of the moral personality of the subject. The subject, whether the individual or the collective, the nurse and/or the profession of nursing, is deemed to be threatened by the ordering, monitoring and regulating of practice.

Claims to privilege in discourse can be fruitfully examined by the application of the concept of 'language games' developed by the later Wittgenstein (1971). Wittgenstein argued that meaning is attached not to arguments and not even to words, but to the uses to which language is put, both as a means for talking a particular conception of nursing (nursing as therapy) into existence and as an expression of resistance to what is seen as a process (the quality movement) for disempowering nurses by splitting their practice from their values for the crass purpose of measurement. The views of the critics of the quality movement will now be examined in detail.

## CRITICS OF QUALITY

As we have seen, arguments against the quality movement fall into one of two camps: 'humanist critics' (Redfern and Norman 1990) and 'left-based critics' (Balogh 1992). As with the proponents of quality, at times the distinction between these two groups is far from clear. Nonetheless, the objections raised by the two groups of critics derive from different analyses of the nature of nursing, organizations and change and thus should be examined in turn.

### Humanist concerns

Humanist concerns over organizational change implemented through processes of quality management rest upon one issue – whether nursing care can and should be measured. For those who believe very strongly that nursing is implicitly a humanist mission (Gadow 1988, Benner 1984), in other words where the focus of nursing care stresses the subjectivity and intersubjectivity of the client, then the rationalist measures of the quality movement could be construed as missing the point. The concern generated by such critics questions the locus of nursing. Is good nursing care about efficiency? Is good nursing care the same to all clients? Clearly, for those who see nursing practice as the expression of skills that nurture and enhance the distinctiveness of clients and stress the ineffable nature of humanity, there is a concern that the quality movement threatens to undermine this conception of practice.

There is a widely held perception that humanist nursing is under assault from the 'reductionist' threat (see Dzurec and Abraham's (1993) review of this extensive literature). Empirical methodologies, including those intended to contribute to quality, are seen to present a narrow picture of nursing practice (Allen and Hall 1988, Gadow 1984, McKee 1991, Redfern and Norman 1990). The analysis and interpretation of data are limited by the methodology that frames its collection and interpretation (Dzurec and Abraham 1993, McKee 1991). Some authors (Allen and Hall 1988, Gadow 1984, Redfern and Norman 1990) construe a polarity between qualitative and quantitative methodologies in nursing. The fear that the 'special' nature of nursing is lost in these analyses underpins this tension (Redfern and Norman 1990). Central to this concern is a fixed belief in the importance of unrestricted creativity in the practice of nursing. Consequently, one finds calls in the humanist literature for interpretative or qualitative methodologies to be applied in the evaluation of nursing practice.

The debate concerning methodological approaches is not simply concerned with methods and analyses. Crucially, it concerns the question under study. As Ersser (1991: 44) states, 'Qualitative designs are used when attempting to understand rather than measure phenomena of concern to nurses and allow richly descriptive data to be collected on the meanings situations have for people'. For the proponents of qualitative research, the question of quality centres upon the nature of care, the quality of care, improvements to care. Care in this perspective is a patient-centred process (Robinson 1991). Nurses too are a focus with the personal/ professional development of the nurse seen as axiomatic in improving care and patient outcomes (Manthey 1992).

Such arguments are, however, posited within the context of wide-ranging reforms to the organization and delivery of health care. Prominent among the foci for opposition is the managerialism perceived to typify the corporatization of health. Within this paradigm, strategies of reform—strategic planning, the creation of internal markets within the health sector, the separation of funders and providers, quality assurance and the like – are thought to create structural controls that reduce professional autonomy to a means of economic rationality. The one source of opti-mism in this perspective is the possibility of resistance through forms of practice, such as therapeutic nursing, that context centralized policy decisions and bureaucratic processes by elevating the issues to the moral domain of what is in the best interests of the consumer.

Therefore, the response of humanist nurses to the quality movement must be contextualized with the wider debates over the essential nature of nursing. Encompassed within these debates are a number of antino-mies: holism/technical care (Benner 1984, Gadow 1984), medical/nursing model (Allen and Hall 1988, Berry and Metcalf 1986, Reed and Watson 1994), male/female approaches (Pearson 1991), central/local or top-down/ bottom-up regulation of nursing (Redfern and Norman 1990, Wright 1991). These antinomies provide the crux of the debate about the nature of nursing and function as value statements for the marshalling of argu-ments. They represent, however, a great deal more about what nurses think of themselves and rather less about what nursing in fact is. The polarity of technical versus holistic care, like its close relative medical versus nursing model, carves out a discursive rescripting of the nursing domain. Just as heaven needs hell to balance the order of the cosmos, the definition of nursing in opposition to medicine or science (as though these in fact exist as singular entities) enables nurses to script their practice in a discursive space that is more balanced, kinder, humanistic and more value oriented.

These concerns form the nexus of the power/resistance struggle between humanist practice and organizational ends as represented in the imple-mentation of standards for practice and measures of outcome. Rational schema for improved resource allocation and management, for achieving minimum standards of care, for implementing programmes and policy changes efficiently are viewed with suspicion on the wards and by some authors (Redfern and Norman 1990). A good part of this suspicion is derived from concerns over resource allocation and local resistance to any moves that would undermine resources at the unit level. As Redfern and Norman (1990: 1261) state: 'Traditionally, these quantitative data have been used by planners to set budgets and by managers seeking to justify unpopular cost-cutting decisions'. This pragmatic resistance should not be confused with a principled resistance against central organizational efforts to regulate or measure practice which is viewed as an assault on professional autonomy (Redfern and Norman 1990). Much of the problem in that latter case stems from the humanist proclivity to adopt a subject-centred analysis of organization change (Clegg 1988: 194, 1993: 28). In other words, organizational ends are viewed as the personal objectives of management. Bureaucratic goals, which are by definition impersonal, are seen as a personal threat. In the second form of opposition to the quality movement, left-based critique, this confusion over bureaucratic goals is even more evident.

## Critique

For those who adopt a stance of critique, based upon post-Marxist and Habermasian notions of emancipatory political activity, bureaucratic means for the implementation of organizational goals are to be resisted *ipso facto*. The position is described by Wright (1991: 107) as a 'struggle between the twin poles of professionalism and bureaucracy'. Schön (1983) provides weight to this argument, depicting the technical rational domain as inherently limited in its application to the domain of practice. An alternative view is provided by Ian Hunter's (1991, 1994) analysis of the critique position in education. For Hunter, the critical perspective can be understood as the self-conscious stance of virtue against the stance of instrumentalism (Hunter 1994: 146–147). Inherent in this stance is the assumption of a wide ethical disparity between these two *Lebensordnungen* or forms of life – the principled critic and the bureaucrat. And while Weber (1978) described this distinction in his delineation of instrumentally rational and value-laden social action when he conceived of the issue as formal and substantive rational domains, he argued that rather than one domain achieving a higher level of ethical comportment, they each represented *distinct* domains, although the concept 'substantive' is itself in a certain abstract sense formal. The ethical nature of the critic, which enshrines the striving for social change, empowerment of democratic communities, social justice and their parallels the advancement of nursing, the empowerment of nurses, equality in the patient–nurse relationship and so forth, is simply a different form of ethical comportment to the bureaucrat or administrator who values impartiality, implementation of policy, commitment to the application of procedure. Thus to frame the issue of quality, power and autonomy in ethical terms that claim to have the 'true' interests of nursing at heart is to misrepresent an issue of power for an issue of ethics.

For it is power indeed that is at issue here. The extension of techniques for the measurement of practice and the management of nursing facilitated by the quality movement could be argued to represent an extension of the mechanism of government surveillance (Foucault 1991). Foucault's view of government is not to be confused with parliamentary office. Rather, government here refers to the broad category of regulation and management of conduct. Some areas of government are unproblematic, such as sanitation controls or traffic regulations, other are often problematized as 'invasive', such as information required by Social Security from its recipients or accountability measures within professions. An unsophisticated reading of Foucault could use the notions of government and surveillance as a platform to extend the critique of the quality movement. In fact, Foucault argued that power was not a single conduit from the oppressor to the oppressed; on the contrary, power is a circuit, it has no stable form but generates the forms of its resistance (Foucault 1991, Hindess 1996). In this reading of power/surveillance with respect to the quality movement, resistance to the quality movement and top-down imperatives can be seen as a locus of power. The connection between power and knowledge, observed by both Weber (1978) and Foucault (1991), can be seen in the emergence of the nursing as therapy discourse. Here, professional advancement is linked with the development of the knowledge base measuring the therapeutic effect of nursing (Pearson 1991). The challenge is to satisfy the criteria of the many contenders in the power/knowledge nexus of health care – consumers, nurses, administrators, doctors, service providers, politicians. . . . The list is a long one!

While this discussion may appear remote from the concerns of nurses engaged in therapeutic practice confronting the challenge of the implementation of quality procedures and the development of standards of practice, it is in fact central to the response(s) of nurses to these challenges. Despite the fact that these debates are largely occurring beyond nursing, the intellectual flow-on effect can allow us to anticipate the turn of the debate as quality and outcome review comes increasingly to dominate practice. It can be seen, therefore, that critique offers a number of analyses *vis-à-vis* organizational reform and processes of professional regulation.

One such analysis centres on accountability. As has been argued above, an essential aspect of the quality movement is the issue of accountability. This point provides a difficult challenge for critics of the quality movement. Consumer input into the evaluation process is a cornerstone of quality, yet it relies upon access to data and processes for review of procedures. To some extent this issue has been framed in methodological terms. The reductionist model of accounting for practice is seen as the wrong approach, the wrong method, rather than a flawed notion *per se*, with methodologies that focus upon meanings for the subject a more valuable tool. However, the limitations of this approach are obvious and even acknowledged by researchers, as Price declares in the summary of her study on parent responses to nursing of their children: '... this study is based on a small sample size hence generalization and subsequent appli- cation of findings may be limited' (Price 1993: 40).

If the correct response to consumer feedback participation and so forth were to rely on subjective measures of satisfaction/dissatisfaction rather than on global measures such as infection rates or length of stay, then the ability of the interpretive, subjective assessment of care to provide data pertinent to, for example, national comparisons would be severely limited. This is not to say the matter is straightforward. To delineate the effect of nursing in these measures presents an enormous challenge to nurse researchers. But without such measures the consumer movement and nursing as therapy movement are severely hampered in their ability to assess data that would form the basis for political action. As Pearson (1991: 206) argues: 'Politically, hard, quantifiable data is needed to demon- strate that nursing does make a difference in terms of outcomes'. Mitchell (1993: 1) goes further, calling on nurses to 'replace our obsession with individual outcomes with a recognition that outcomes exist and must be defined at the local and national care system level as well'. Mitchell adds a plea for outcomes that encompass system-level outcomes. This position is in contrast to the argument of Redfern and Norman (1990) which expresses deep scepticism at the utility of most quality measures. Balogh (1992) is more than sceptical; in fact, this author argues that the existing instruments are based upon unrealistic assumptions about scientific method's ability to validate areas such as clinical decision making. Kitson *et al.* (1994) identify the conflict as one between 'expert' approaches and 'practitioner' approaches. Consequently, the resolution of issues of accountability, consumer and service provider access to data at the service level all too easily becomes bogged down in the circular debate of quan- titative versus qualitative methodological approaches in nursing.

## AN ALTERNATIVE ACCOUNT

A different way of conceptualizing the issue moves away from the view that sees the implementation of quality measures as part of a singular programme implemented by a singular entity known as management or government. Similarly, nursing is not served by its depiction as a single entity, opposed to a contingent and complex set of practices, bent on a humanizing mission. To move away from the resultant polarity offers the opportunity both to review the manner in which nursing therapy is

conducted and understood and to examine the agenda of the quality movement with a cool head.

Nursing as therapy depicted in this text centres upon the therapeutic
effect of nursing care. This focus achieves two things: it raises the value
of the process of nursing by making its intrinsic worth manifest and it
articulates the aim of nursing care. The constraints that operate against
this therapeutic process are variously interpreted. There is the perception
that the mission of the hospital or of medicine (singularly assumed) or of
management may militate against therapeutic nursing. This may well
be the case. However, it is important to distinguish between the actuality
of this occurrence and the philosophical assumption that this is so.

The focus of the quality movement, on the other hand, is more tangible
and less overarching. The movement is driven by imperatives that are
external to health. The belief in the need for formal procedures to frame
and evaluate services is not driven by specific nursing goals. Nursing goals
have certainly been articulated by proponents of the quality movement
but this is a far cry from the essentialist movement of nursing as therapy.
Quality processes can aim to ensure a minimum standard of service – in
this case, nursing care. The nursing therapy advocates want to enhance
practice to achieve the highest level of practice. The fit between the two
movements therefore is not an easy one.

The disparity lies in the gaps between a model of ideal practice and a
model of minimum practice. The quality assurance movement (although
it too aims at best practice models in TQM, etc.) in general is concerned
with the appropriate and even distribution of services. For example, there
is little benefit to the taxpayer if there is a wide disparity in services
between one district and another. The development of best practice
in one area cannot be achieved at the expense of minimum practice in
another. This rather brutal piece of realism amidst an idealistic discourse
may appear shocking. However, it does underwrite the view that these
discourses function in different domains.

Rather than examine these discourses on their own terms and thus suffer
the risk of being caught up in the circular argument of rational versus
substantive domains, it may be useful to consider a Wittgensteinian
approach to the issue. For the later Wittgenstein (1971), meaning was not
a function of truth. Rather, meaning lies in the use of language.
Wittgenstein held the view that words did not own their meanings but it
was in what he called the language games that attended their usage that
meaning was given to a word or term. The meaning attached to a language
game was inherent, it was understood by all players, it could change as
the game changed. This view of language provides an insight into the
function of discourses. The focus of examination should not be the truth-
value of the discourse, but its use. What role do the discourses of quality
movement, of the 'nursing as therapy' movement, play in nursing?

One function of 'nursing as therapy' could be described as 'edifying' discourse (Rorty 1980). Edifying discourse nominates those discursive activities
that serve to enhance the esteem and credibility of the user of the discourse.
Foucault (1982) distinguishes between discourses that operate as authoritative discourses and 'ordinary' discourses. The role of the therapeutic
discourse is both edifying and authoritative. It operates to create the notion
of nursing, within nursing, as a distinctive therapeutic practice. By introducing the language of therapy it engenders the notion, on a discursive level, that
nursing is or should be something more than it has considered itself to be
in the past. Thus, it operates as an edifying discourse, elevating nursing
practice, talking into existence the level of practice that it strives towards.

Contrast this with the function of the quality movement discourse.
While it must be stressed that the quality movement is heterogeneous and
the various schools of thought within it should be conceptualized distinctly,
the general thrust of the movement evidenced in health services world-
wide can be sketched. The thrust of the quality movement is that of
organizational efficiency and reform. The basic premise that data about
organizational processes and employee practices can be examined,
reviewed and refined with resulting improved efficiencies in costs and
outcomes is constant throughout the quality movement. The related expectation that organizational change can be achieved by changing the way
members of the organization think is another strong assumption. The
extent to which organizations can be transformed or the precise mechanism by which this is attempted varies with the different models of quality
systems and modes of discourse. Consistently, however, the quality movement perceives change as a function of organizational processes. Here
organizations are projected as solid, constant edifices and reform as the
procedural implementation of policy. The danger with this view is that it
reifies organizational structure. Not only does it ignore the complexities
and uncertainties of circuits of power within organizations, but it belies
the contingent nature of both organizations and the development and
implementation of policy.

A far more limited view, but one with a firmer grasp of reality, is offered
by the idea that organizations represent multiple rather than singular interests. Indeed, organizations should not be viewed as the external
manifestation of some inner logic – such as rationalism or economic
exploitation – but rather as the 'locus of decision and action' (Hindess
1986). Furthermore, power is not held by anyone or any group. Rather,
power is exercised through the 'deployment of those intellectual and
political technologies that render reality calculable as an object of administration' (Hunter 1991: 55).

The same applies to nursing. The conceptualization of nursing as a
singular edifice with clear functions and epistemological bases clouds the
reality of a contingent set of historical practices. It is far easier to grasp

the multiplicity of nursing, its rough assemblage of historical practices and newly adapted technologies of care if one abandons attempts at totalizing conceptualization (Nelson 1995). In order to make sense of the multi-farious aspects of nursing, its various expressions and its relations with quality issues, one should realize the likelihood that local contingencies will usually dominate, whatever their standing within the overarching discourse. In other words, the political will behind quality moves, the level of morale within the organization and the perspectives of nurses as therapists will provide the boundaries of the language game that gives both nursing as therapy and the quality movement their meaning.

## CONCLUSION

Arguments have been presented in this chapter that draw on a diverse range of perspectives and concepts. How can they all be brought together to present a coherent statement on the relationship between the drive for quality in health care and nursing as therapy? The starting point has been to place the quality debate in the context of social action. The distinction between *zweckrationality* (instrumental rationality) and *wertrationality* (value rationality) has been used to contrast approaches to quality. Weber (1978) has also offered insight into the connection between knowledge and power and this connection has been explored by drawing on the analysis of Foucault (1990). Consideration of Foucault introduced the notion of authoritative discourses and Wittgenstein's (1971) idea of language games has been applied to turn the discussion from meaning to use.

The question of use brings in Rorty's (1980) notion of 'edifying' dis-courses. Here, the 'quality of nursing' discourse is argued to be a discursive attempt to transform nursing into something more than it currently is. The process is one of empowerment through metamorphosis. Emancipation is substituted for control in this perspective, holism for technical care and humanist values for efficiency. At the same time, autonomy replaces surveillance and the power to resist contests bureaucratic control.

On the other hand, instrumental aspects of the quality movement are part of a 'systematic' discourse which seeks to promote the need for accountability and regulation in the health-care industry. The goals for the quality movement in this paradigm are to regulate health care to protect the interests of the consumer and to ensure public accountability. The underlying ideology is that of economic rationality. This perspective depends on measurement to provide information to support rational processes of change. The approach as a whole is concerned with large-scale unitary systems of performance that depend on surveillance and bureaucratic structures for implementation. Such systems are characteris-tics of managerialism and implicit forms of domination.

The various discourses that operate on and constitute nursing are inter-twined at the level of everyday nursing practice, hence both the confusion about what is meant by quality in nursing and the uncertainty over how far the concept should be embraced by clinical nurses. The contributors to this book are worthy advocates of nursing as therapy and nursing needs its edifying discourses if anything is to change, but the harsh reality is that the dominant perspective on quality in health care today is that of instru-mental rationality. Efficiency and effectiveness are the watchwords and this is the climate in which the proponents of nursing as therapy must seek to make ground.

## REFERENCES

Allen, J. D. and Hall, B. A. (1988) Challenging the focus on technology: a critique of the medical model on a changing health care system. *Advances in Nursing Science*, **10**(3), 22–34.

Attree, M. (1993) An analysis of the concept 'quality' as it relates to contemporary nursing care. *International Journal of Nursing Studies*, **30**(4), 355–369.

Balogh, R. (1992) Audits of nursing care in Britain: a review and a critique of approaches to validating them. *International Journal of Nursing Studies*, **29**(2), 119–133.

Benner, P. (1984) *From Novice to Expert*, Addison-Wesley, Menlo Park.

Berry, A. J. and Metcalf, C. L. (1986) Paradigms and practices: the organization of the delivery of nursing. *Journal of Advanced Nursing*, **11**(5), 587–597.

Berry, T. H. (1991) *Managing the Total Quality Transformation*, McGraw-Hill, New York.

Berwick, D. (1989) Continuous improvement as an ideal in health care. *New England Journal of Medicine*, **320**(1), 53–56.

Buchanan, L. M. (1994) Therapeutic nursing intervention knowledge and outcome measures for advanced practice. *Nursing and Health Care*, **15**(4), 190–195.

Bunker, J. P., Frazier, H. S. and Mosteller, F. (1994) Improving health: measuring effects of medical care. *Millbank Quarterly*, **72**(2), 225–259.

Clegg, S. (1994) Power and institutions in the theory of organizations, in *Towards a New Theory of Organizations*, (eds M. Parker and J. Hassard), Routledge, London, pp. 24–52.

Clegg, S. (1988) *Frameworks of Power*, Sage, London.

Clinton, M. and Nelson, S. (1995) Issues and trends in nurse management, in *Management in the Australian Health Care Industry*, (eds M. Clinton and D. Scheiwe), HarperEducational, Sydney.

Crosby, P. (1979) *Quality is Free: The Art of Making Quality Certain*, New American Library, New York.

Curl, E. D. and Koerner, D. K. (1991) Evaluating students' esthetic knowing. *Nurse-Educator* Nov–Dec **16**(6), 23–27.

Decker, P. J., Moore-Greenlaw, R. C. and Strader, M. K. (1994) Functional stan-dards: the walls come tumbling down. *Journal of Nursing Administration*, **24**(7/8), 18–20.

Donabedian, A. (1980) Criteria, norms and standards of quality: what do they mean? *American Journal of Public Health*, **71**(4), 409–412.

Du Gay, P. and Salaman, G. (1992) The cult[ure] of the customer. *Journal of Management Studies*, **29**(5), 615–633.

Dzurec, L. C. and Abraham, I. L. (1993) The nature of inquiry: linking quantitative and qualitative research. *Advances in Nursing Science*, **16**(1), 73–79.

Ersser, S. (1991) A search for the therapeutic evaluation of experience: prerequisites for therapeutic practice, in *Nursing as Therapy*, (eds R. McMahon and A. Pearson), Chapman and Hall, London, pp. 192–210.

Foucault, M. (1982) On a genealogy of ethics: an overview of work in progress, in *Foucault: Beyond Sructuralism and Hermeneutics* (eds H. L. Dreyfus and P. Rabinow), Harvester Press, Brighton.

Foucault, M. (1990) *History of Sexuality* Vol 3, Penguin, London.

Foucault, M. (1991) Governmentality, in *The Foucault Effect: Studies in Governmentality* (eds G. Burchell, C. Gordon and P. Miller), Harvester Wheatsheaf, Brighton.

Gadow, S. (1984) Touch and Technology. *Journal of Religion and Health*, **23**, 63–69.

Gadow, S. (1988) Clinical subjectivity: advocacy with silent patients. *Nursing Clinics of North America*, **24**(2), 535–541.

Goldstone, L. A., Ball, J. A. and Collier, M. (1983) *Monitor: An Index of the Quality of Nursing Care for Acute Medical and Surgical Wards*, Newcastle on Tyne Polytechnic, Newcastle on Tyne.

Hegyvary, S. T. (1991) Issues in outcome research. *Journal of Nursing Quality Assurance*, **5**(2), 1–6.

Hindess, B. (1986) Interests in political analysis, in *Power, Action and Belief*, (ed. J. Law), Routledge, London.

Hindess, B. (1996) *the Discourses of Power*, Routledge, London.

Hunter, I. (1991) Accounting for the Humanities, *Cultural and Policy Studies*, Griffith University, Brisbane.

Hunter I. (1994) *Rethinking the School*, Allen and Unwin, St Leonards, NSW.

Jelinek, R., Haussman, R. K. D., Hegyvary, S. T. and Newman, J. E. (1974) *A Methodology for Monitoring Quality of Care*, US Department of Health, Education and Welfare, Bethesda.

Johannesson, M. (1994), QALYs, HYEs and individual preferences: a graphical illustration. *Social Science and Medicine*, **39**(12), 1623–1632.

Jones, K. R. (1993) Outcomes analysis: methods and issues. *Nursing Economics*, **11**(3), 145–152.

Katz, J. and Green, E. (1992) *Managing Quality: a Guide to Monitoring and Evaluating Nursing Services*, Mosby, St Louis.

Kinlaw, D. C. (1992) *Continuous Improvement and Measurement for Total Quality: A Team-base Approach*, San Diego Pfeiffer, Homewood.

Kitson, A., Harvey, G., Hyndman, S. and Yerrell, P. (1994) Criteria formulation and application: an evaluative framework. *International Journal of Nursing Studies*, **31**(2), 155–167.

Lohr, K. N. (1985) *Impact of Medicare Prospective Payment on the Quality of Medical Care: A Research Agenda*, The Rand Corporation, Santa Monica.

McKee, C. (1991) Breaking the mould: a humanistic approach to nursing practice, in *Nursing as Therapy*, (eds. R. McMahon and A. Pearson), Chapman and Hall, London.

Manthey, M. and Spirlet, L. E. (1992) Nursing Kaleidoscope: clinicians as teachers. *Nursing Management*, **23**(6), 14–16.

Mitchell, P. H. (1993) Perspectives on outcome-oriented care systems. *Nursing Administration Quarterly*, **17**(3), 1–7.

Nelson, S. (1995) Holistic Nursing: the Re-emergence of the Light, in *Nursing Inquiry*, **2**, 36–43.

Oakland, J. S. (1989) *Total Quality Management*, Butterworth Heinemann, Oxford.

Pearson, A. (1983) *The Clinical Nursing Unit*, Heinemann, London.

Pearson, A. (1987) *Nursing Quality Measurement: Quality Assurance Methods for Peer Review*, John Wiley, Chichester.

Pearson, A. (1991) Taking up the challenge: the future for therapeutic nursing, in *Nursing as Therapy* (eds R. McMahon and A. Pearson), Chapman and Hall, London, pp. 192–210.

Pearson, A., Punton, S. and Durant, I. (1992) *Nursing Beds: An Evaluation of the Effects of Therapeutic Nursing*, Scutari Press, Harrow.

Pfeffer, N. and Coote, A. (1990) *Is Quality Good For You?* Social Policy Paper No. 5, IPPR, London.

Phaneuf, M. (1976) *The Nursing Audit*, Appleton-Century-Crofts, New York.

Pinkerton, S. and Schroeder, P. (1988) *Commitment to Excellence: Developing a Professional Nursing Staff*, Aspen, Rockville.

Price, P. J. (1993) Parents' perceptions of the meaning of quality nursing care. *Advances in Nursing Science*, **16**(1), 33–41.

Redfern, S. J. and Norman, I. (1990) Measuring the quality of nursing care: a consideration of different approaches. *Journal of Advanced Nursing*, **15**, 1260–1271.

Reed, J. and Watson, D. (1994) The impact of the medical model on nursing practice. *International Journal of Nursing Studies*, **3**(1), 57–66.

Robinson, N.C. (1991) A patient-centred framework for restructuring care. *Journal of Nursing Administration*, **21**(9), 29–34.

Rorty, R. (1980) *Philosophy and the Mirror of Nature*, Blackwell, Oxford.

Schön, D. (1983) *The Reflective Practitioner*, Basic Books, New York.

Schroeder, P. (1991a) *The Encyclopedia of Nursing Care Quality. Volume I: Issues and Strategies for Nursing Quality Care*, Aspen, Gaithersburg.

Schroeder, P. (1991b) *The Encyclopedia of Nursing Care Quality. Volume II: Approaches to Nursing Standards*, Aspen, Gaithersburg.

Schroeder, P. (1991c) *The Encyclopedia of Nursing Care Quality. Volume III: Monitoring and Evaluation in Nursing*, Aspen, Gaithersburg.

Sherman, J. J. and Malkmus, M. A. (1994) Integrating quality assurance and total quality management/quality improvement. *Journal of Nursing Administration*, **24**(3), 37–41.

Statland, B. (1989) Quality management: watchword for the '90s. *Medical Laboratory Observer, **21**(7), 33–40.*

Wandelt, M. and Ager, J. (1974) *Quality Patient Care Scale*, Appleton-Century-Crofts, New York.

Weber, M. (1978) *Economy and Society: An Outline of Interpretive Sociology* (reissue), (eds G. Roth and C. Wittich), University of California Press, Berkeley.

WHO Working Group (1989) The principles of quality assurance. *Quality Assurance in Health Care*, **1**(2/3), 79–95.

Wittgenstein, L. (1971) *Philosophical Investigations*, Blackwell, Oxford.

Wright, S. (1991) Facilitating therapeutic nursing and independent practice, in *Nursing as Therapy* (eds R. McMahon and A. Pearson), Chapman and Hall, London, pp. 102–118.

# 9

# Tailoring research for therapeutic nursing practice

## Jillian MacGuire

Kitson (1986) has appealed for a methodology to validate the hitherto intangible and elusive qualities of caring. 'Intuition and experience' are daily used to justify action, but since a hit-and-miss attitude is morally and professionally indefensible where persons of value are concerned, this mystique of the nurse demands to be brought to consciousness and clarity, and a place in the research base and methodology of practice. Once achieved not only can its essence be communicated and taught but its influence may *inform* caring by providing guidelines for the selection of methods and a frame of reference for prescriptive choices for action and interaction. ...
Muetzel (1988)

## INTRODUCTION

This chapter looks in a broad way at the contribution of research to nursing practice and, more specifically, at how therapeutic nursing might be advanced through research. Key questions to address are whether the study of nursing practice demands the use of particular research methodologies, what these might be and whether resources for such research are likely to be restricted because of the very methodologies advocated. Finally, consideration is given to some of the difficulties associated with isolating what might be regarded as nursing outputs and with the adoption of research-based knowledge into clinical practice.

Though there is now an extensive body of work that may be labelled nursing research and a growing number of nurses, as well as people from other disciplines, are directly engaged in research activity, it is doubtful if nursing can as yet sustain the claim to being a research-based profession. In part, this is because not all nurses engaged in patient care fully accept the arguments for research-based practice. Many do not feel that research necessarily has relevance to their own work and fail to seek a role for themselves in the development of practice through research (Luker and Kenrick 1992). Research, for a variety of reasons, has not always addressed the concerns of clinical nurses and frequently does not produce the kind of reliable guide to practice that practitioners require. The research process is clouded in mystery and the results are sometimes couched in impenetrable language (Buckledee and McMahon 1994).

Nursing research as an identifiable and separate discipline has a relatively short history. That of research into practice is even briefer (Hunt 1987). Since therapeutic nursing is only on the edge of the consciousness of the profession it might be anticipated that relevant research into its practice is limited. This may be, as McMahon (1989) suggests, because it is still a character in search of an author and, therefore, lacks an accepted definition and partly because it is difficult to see how the process and outcomes of such practice might be researched.

Nursing research cannot so far lay claim to the invention of any methodology peculiar to itself. Instead, it draws on a wide range of methodologies from other disciplines; an eclectic approach which offers a wealth of possibilities but no single, definitive pathway. In principle, the choice depends on the proclivities of the researcher and the nature of the research question. In practice, things are not that simple.

The main distinction is between quantitative methodologies, which have their origins in the natural sciences and are concerned with proof and prediction, and qualitative methodologies which have been developed in the social sciences and are concerned with the knowledge, understanding and perceptions people have of their worlds and how this affects their actions. The difference is not just one of methods of investigation but of philosophical dispute about the nature of knowledge, the purpose of research and the relationship between investigator and subject.

It is tempting to try to resolve the qualitative/quantitative debate by arguing that 'the problem dictates the method of investigation' (Trow, quoted in Lathlean and Farnish 1984) but this apparently simple solution obscures two associated difficulties. The first is that the conceptualization of research as a 'problem-solving activity' suggests that there is a 'problem' and that the problem has been properly identified, a potential pitfall identified by Menzies (1966) in her work on student nurses. The second is that it implies that there must be an answer that can underpin policy initiatives and practice guidelines. Moreover, it appears to deny the converse of the proposition which is that a particular methodological approach may itself be used to determine the research question. This may result in the formulation of inappropriate questions and misguided research effort.

What is it that leads both practitioners and researchers to question the applicability of available methodologies? First, there is the pervading myth of the 'uniqueness' of nursing which, while often not brought into the open in discussions about methodology, underpins the search for a 'nursing' research methodology. Second, there is a defensiveness which seeks to protect nursing research from criticism by incorporating and misappropriating other methodologies. 'Ethnonursing research' is an example of this tendency. Workers in the nursing field ought to be able to take an ethnomethodological approach without needing to create a specifically *nursing* version. There is a very real danger that this process may lead to nurse researchers being inadequately prepared in the rigours of the particular methodology and thus to using it in ways which do not stand comparison with the work of the experts in the discipline. Third, there is a propensity to jump on the latest methodological bandwagon in order to demonstrate that nursing research is out there in the forefront. Fourth is the view that nursing is both art and science and can, therefore, be studied neither as pure science nor pure art without misrepresentation. This standpoint is sometimes used to devalue all research and as an excuse for not subjecting practice to enquiry.

Fifth, and this must be seriously considered, there is the argument that nursing is a *practice* discipline and as such requires that research be contextual, related to and carried out in the workplace, whether this be home, hospice or hospital. 'The centrality of practice to nursing mandates a bond between nursing research ... and nursing practice' (Jennings and Rogers 1988). This suggests that one of the characteristics of nursing research is that it should be small scale and practice related and, therefore, may not be generalizable beyond the immediate situation. Finally, there is the idea that research should be focused primarily on the interaction between nurse and patient because this relationship mediates all nursing activity. Integral to such a view is the idea of the primacy for nursing research of the viewpoints, perceptions, understandings and intentions of the participants.

It is suggested that available methodologies do not enable us to understand patients as actors and initiators of their own strategies for dealing with illness, pain, discomfort or stress or to grasp the meanings that they attribute to the actions of nurses. Nor do they help to make clear what it is that nurses and nursing are about; the meaning of caring or nurturing or the essentially therapeutic nature of nursing interventions.

In Chapter 1 therapeutic nursing is defined as nursing that *deliberately* has beneficial outcomes for patients. This definition suggests not only that all nursing activities should be planned but that the only legitimate activities are those which can be shown to have a positive effect for patients. This, indeed, would constitute research-based practice.

Can therapeutic nursing be defined and practised in ways that make it possible to research? What evidence is there that nurses and researchers are interested in this concept of nursing? Are there genuine problems about methodology or are the difficulties more to do with ethics, access, training and resources? How are we to look at outcomes for patients and how are we to know that they are beneficial?

## FUNDING, ACCESS AND ETHICAL COMMITTEE APPROVAL

Muetzel (1988) has stated that nurse researchers have neglected certain areas of research and certain forms of research in favour of the 'scientific' methods associated with medical research. We need, first, to ask whether this contention is true and second why this should have happened. While it may be fashionable to talk about the art and science of nursing, nursing as it has entered into the academic arena in the UK has tended to be associated with existing faculties, whether of biological sciences, social sciences, medicine or education. Both the social sciences and education, as academic disciplines, have had to make their own bids for academic and scientific recognition. We should not, therefore, be surprised if the research methodologies current in those departments have also tended to be adopted by nursing research. One strand lies in the search for academic respectability in general and in the bid for medical recognition in particular. From its origins, nursing research has had to assert itself as being something other than a handmaiden to medical research. Until recently professional relevance and clinical credibility have been seen as of lesser importance.

Medicine has developed a very powerful research design in the randomized crossover clinical trial and there is an extensive literature on its development and use. The design should not be undervalued in nursing research nor denigrated because it is derived from medicine. It has been used effectively (Luker 1983) but may also be used inappropriately.

The social sciences have made great use of large-scale sample surveys based on carefully constructed and pretested questionnaires. A great deal of nursing research has drawn on this tradition. At the same time, much of this work has been criticized for being small scale, unrepresentative and thus not generalizable.

All research costs money; large-scale research requires large-scale financing. Even small-scale exploratory work requires money to employ appropriately qualified staff and additional cash for the running costs of a project. Universities are no longer willing or able to carry the hidden costs of research and grant applications to funding bodies have to take this into account. Nursing research, like all other research, is becoming more expensive at the same time as research funding from all sources is becoming more restricted. Emphasis on value for money and the ascendancy of policy-driven research must inevitably have some effect on the kinds of research project that ultimately secure funding. This is true for all areas of research and not just for nursing.

Nursing research can call on no separate, identifiable budgets at national, regional or local level within the structure of NHS financing nor is there specific funding within the university or educational sectors. Since the review in Britain of NHS-funded research (the Culyer Report) in 1994, all funds have been centralized and are being distributed in a planned way against long-term bids submitted by health providers. These bids have to be supported by an alliance of the bidder with academic institutions with first-class research credentials. However, at the present time few British university departments of nursing score high ratings for their research activity and there is a genuine concern that nursing may get 'tagged on' to medically led projects.

The main financing of nursing research has been through the Department of Health's directly managed projects. In 1988 about 7% of the £13.6 million spent under this heading went to programmes which are clearly identifiable as 'nursing research' in that they are about some aspect of the organization of nursing, the recruitment and education of nurses or the delivery of nursing care. While it is not always possible to tell from the title the exact nature of the research approach adopted, the emphasis would appear to be on large-scale survey research though other approaches are by no means excluded.

Major funding for nursing research from this source can only be obtained by adherence to the Rothschild principles. These require that the customer, which is the Department of Health, should commission such research. Proposals have to fall within the current priorities established by the Department of Health and to provide 'objective information for Ministers on ways of improving the efficiency and effectiveness of the HPSS and Social Security by promoting improvements in organization, operation and administration' (DHSS 1989). Clinical nursing research may not have a high priority on these agendas and may be seen as a more narrowly professional matter for which funding should be sought elsewhere.

Small amounts of money have been available for research which does not have an identified customer. In addition, postgraduate and post-doctoral awards have been made by the Department of Health to support nursing research activities. These proposals, too, have had to fall within stated priority areas though, in practice, there seems to be considerable flexibility. Finance for clinical work can be obtained. The strength of the research design rather than the specific theoretical or methodological approach is probably the major determinant of success.

Non-governmental research-funding bodies and charitable organizations also support nursing research. They will also have their own priorities which are bound to be reflected in the nature of the projects they are prepared to finance. Research which is perceived as having immediate practical applicability or which addresses some major current concern is likely to be seen as more attractive than more theoretical work or, indeed, more basic work.

The development of clinical nursing research depends in part on the ease with which individuals can move between clinical and research settings and the degree of autonomy they are allowed in choosing what research to undertake. Increasing numbers of nurses are being funded by their employing authorities to register for higher degrees on a part-time basis. Most of such courses require students to prepare a research dissertation or to carry out small-scale research projects. Some of this work is clinically orientated and innovative but, inevitably, limited by the time constraints imposed. Courses currently being developed in research for practitioners place a high premium on tailoring teaching of research methodology to the practice concerns of the participants, not all of whom are likely to be nurses. These innovations are productive in so far as they allow clinical nurses to get a grounding in research but restrictive if the research undertaken has to fit into the agenda of the employing authority or the researchers run into difficulties over ethical approval and access simply because of their dual status.

Funding for nursing research is closely tied up with questions of access and ethical committee approval. Those who control access and those who give ethical committee approval may also seek to influence research methodology and study design. The more nearly the research touches clinical issues and focuses on sensitive areas such as pain or patients' feelings about surgery, sexual behaviour or the perceived value of treatment regimens, the more likely it is that difficulties will be encountered in keeping these issues separate. Embargoes on funding and access can sometimes be issued from very high places, leaving researchers with very little room to manoeuvre.

Pressure to adopt a quantitative rather than a qualitative approach and to employ an experimental research design frequently comes directly from the members of ethical committees. Medical researchers are themselves critical of the way in which ethical committees seek to control access and research design (Institute of Medical Ethics Bulletin 1989) but can ignore real ethical issues.

Funding is often dependent on prior agreements about access and ethical committee approval. Nurses sometimes experience difficulties with ethical committees but rarely report on such problems in their research papers because of the understandable fear that any future research proposals might be in jeopardy were they to put their criticisms and experiences on record.

Some of the difficulty arises because the idea of nurses doing research at all is still unfamiliar and partly because qualitative methods are not entirely understood within such committees, which may only rarely include a sociologist or anthropologist. Criteria more applicable to experimental work are applied and proposals are inevitably seen to fall short. A few medical clinicians try to use their position on such committees to block access to their patients. In such a context, nurse researchers may well feel that proposals which fit medical design canons and which do not concentrate on patients' experience of their treatment are more likely to succeed.

Clinical medical research is in part legitimated by the clinical position and therapeutic orientation of doctors. Nurses undertaking research are often recently qualified or hold marginal positions in the nursing hierarchy. As more clinical nursing research is undertaken by practitioners in clinical nursing career posts and as nursing is seen to have an independent therapeutic contribution, it may become easier to get access to patients in medically dominated areas.

While such clinical nurse researchers employed in practice settings are in no way absolved from seeking ethical approval for their research and, indeed, have special responsibilities to their patients because of such a dual role, access to patients is legitimated by their clinical position. Also, because they are participants in the clinical situation by right, they may be able more readily to use qualitative approaches in their work and to undertake research in aspects of clinical work which have previously seemed too difficult or too dangerous.

Much of the more qualitative research is currently carried out by nurses in the course of their higher degree work. Because many of them go back into clinical, teaching or management posts rather than continuing in research, this work is often not published and is therefore not developed by other researchers. A lot of valuable work lies buried in theses which practitioners and even researchers may never think to access.

## CLINICAL NURSING RESEARCH

Pearson's (1988) prophetic statement that 'The future of practical, hands-on nursing obviously lies in the hands of clinical nurses – who need to assert the potential of nursing as a means of healing' is a good starting point for the consideration of the relationship between practice and research. One vehicle for asserting the value of nursing as healing is research which demonstrates the efficacy of nursing intervention.

Clinical nursing covers a broad spectrum of nursing activity. Any part of that activity may be called into question, through research, in terms of the contribution it makes to the well-being of patients, to the recovery process, to rehabilitation and to the maintenance of health. It is not self-evident that *nursing* and *nurses* make a difference to outcomes for patients. Until relatively recently, nurses have worked in a climate in which their work has been tacitly accepted at its face value. Both overtly and covertly, the value of nursing is being brought into question. It is now becoming increasingly urgent to evaluate independent nursing interventions both as a means of describing the essential core of nursing work and as part of the justification of the continued employment of highly trained professionals in the care of patients.

The concepts of *independent* nursing intervention and of *healing* are both crucial in determining the direction of research into clinical nursing practice. In what sense can nursing be regarded as independent? And how may nursing be understood as healing? It is only when we are able to define these terms satisfactorily that it is possible to design and undertake research which will support or refute the proposition that independent nursing intervention promotes healing.

Hockey's (1989) typology of nursing activities as consisting of autonomous, derived and delegated elements suggests we should focus on the interventions which are initiated as well as undertaken by nurses. This is the core of nurses' work. It is what nurses do which is not done by other people. Nursing has always found it difficult to describe this core. Goddard's (Nuffield Provincial Hospitals Trust 1954) choice of the term 'basic' to describe this element of nursing work has had a disastrous influence not only on nurses' perceptions of the value of their work but also on the way in which nursing is regarded by other professional groups. It has been suggested that the term was used as a shorthand for 'fundamental' or 'essential' and that it has been systematically misinterpreted over the last four decades by those who wish to use it to justify the horizontal division of nursing labour. Goddard demonstrated that basic nursing was undertaken by the least qualified and the lowest skilled. This observation might have sparked off a revolution in the delivery of nursing care but instead it has been and is used to justify the continued employment of unskilled labour in direct patient care. The competencies being outlined for the support worker suggest that this process will be extended yet again. As Robinson *et al.* (1989) put it: 'Debate about the role of support staff undoubtedly disguises debate about the future of nursing itself'. The substitution of the terms 'direct patient care' or 'hands-on care' for 'basic care' gets slightly closer to the heart of the matter but we still remain in the realms of an instrumental understanding of nursing.

Smith (1988) has explored the relevance of the concept of emotional labour to nursing. Emotional labour is concerned with establishing and maintaining affective states: subjective feelings of comfort, security, well-being, safety and worth. Derived from a study of airline cabin staff by Hochschild (1983), this idea adds a new dimension to the analysis of the work of nursing. It is the 'how' rather than the 'what' of the activity that is highlighted. Superficially, there may seem to be little in common between an intensive care ward and a jumbo jet. But aircraft, like hospitals, are 'institutions cradled in anxiety' (Revans 1964). Throughput of patients and passengers is high. Instrumentality predominates. Danger, crisis, failure and death are potentially overwhelming for all parties in the enterprise. Space is confined and the normal range of behaviour restricted. Intimacy with total strangers is not only allowed but legitimated. Nurses and cabin staff make use of sexual allure and play on patient and passenger fantasies. Patients and passengers are dependent on others for survival. A key function of both cabin staff and nurses is to create an atmosphere of normality. Homeliness is seen as an important aspect of both environments. Making the cabin seem like your own front room or the ward like your own back bedroom is believed to reduce the fear engendered by unfamiliarity. Staff are expected to offer reassurance as well as rehydration, comfort as well as cuisine provençale, understanding as well as unguent. In each case the latter is the medium for conveying the message. The message, whether to passenger or patient, is that each is unique, important, valued and that the steward or nurse is concerned in a deeply personal way about their comfort, their anxieties and their needs. The emotional labour lies in the maintenance of states of well-being among passengers or patients. It is not window dressing or packaging though it may deteriorate into that if too great a demand is made of staff by the managers of emotional labour. It is not a byproduct or unintended consequence of physical or intellectual activities. Emotional labour is the essential element which defines and differentiates. For nursing there is, perhaps, a higher goal in that nursing involves the use of self in an intentionally therapeutic way to create and maintain a sense of well-being among patients.

Patients judge nurses on their emotional style (Smith 1989). Their competence they take for granted. That this may, in some cases, turn out to be unwarranted makes it all the more important that the technical aspects of nurses' work should be rooted in research-based practice so that we do, indeed, act in such a way that we do the patient no harm. The value patients place on emotional work alerts us to the idea that they may not respond in expected ways to nursing care, however technically excellent, unless nurses get what Hochschild calls the 'deep acting' right. They must convey information, through actions rather than solely through words, about emotional care in order to facilitate other aspects of care. A nurse cannot '*make* a patient comfortable' and she certainly cannot bring about a change through the medium of words alone. She can only recognize discomfort, attend to a patient's wishes or needs, express her concern and then, with the patient, use technical skills to solve the problem that faces them both. You only have to read Victor Zorza's account of how a nurse in a hospice struggled to make his daughter Jane comfortable to understand just how difficult this is (Zorza and Zorza 1980). Concentrating on the emotional labour of nursing does not mean that what we do at a technical level does not matter so long as we get the feeling right. The implication is that technical care, however excellent, may fall short of its therapeutic intent unless attention is paid to the emotional aspect of care.

It is a short step from the idea of well-being to that of healing. Healing is the restoration of the feeling of well-being, the replacement of comfort for discomfort, ease for disease, security for insecurity and, in the hymn writer J.S.B. Mansell's words, 'Trust for our trembling and hope for our fear' (English Hymnal No. 42).

## CATEGORIES OF THERAPEUTIC NURSING

Most nursing care is not delivered and received via a continuous didactic relationship but through serial relationships. This raises questions about the level at which the 'nurse–patient relationship' may be held to exist in practice. This, in turn, raises questions about the very possibility of therapeutic nursing particularly where this is grounded in the therapeutic use of self.

Muetzel (1988) has argued that the adoption of primary nursing is a prerequisite for the practice of therapeutic nursing. Binnie (1987) has stated bluntly that nursing structures are in the main inimical to the introduction and support of primary nursing. On this basis therapeutic nursing is likely to be practised in very few places at present though the idea is gaining currency. Wharton and Pearson (1988) write that 'The complex, therapeutic role of both primary and associate nurse, rooted in close relationships and an environment for healing and growth hinges, we believe, on the hands of the nurse being used therapeutically in giving direct care'. If this sounds more like the prayer of St Theresa than a procedure manual it is because many such assertions are at the moment tentative hypotheses or propositions which are awaiting research. Where is the research evidence, for example, that the use of night sedation has fallen notably since the initiation of massage for sleeplessness? This may well be the experience of the nurses working in that particular situation but before such practices are taken up in other areas, it is important to demonstrate the link between the two variables. The implication that it is the controlled experiment itself which destroys what it sets out to study and, therefore, fails to produce positive evidence should be strenuously resisted. At the same time, it must be recognized that in social situations any intervention of any kind may bring about observable and even measurable change. The particular intervention may not be causally linked with the observed change as, for example, with the use of placebo drug therapy. The intervention may simply offer the opportunity for an exchange between nurse and patient and the therapeutic result may stem from the quality of that exchange. Such complicated issues have to be faced if we are not to introduce new practice on an inadequate footing.

Ersser (1988) has suggested five broad categories for describing the therapeutic approach to nursing. These are the nurse–patient relationship, creating a therapeutic environment, giving information, providing comfort and holistic health practices. McMahon (1989) has added a sixth, that of tested physical interventions. While a literature search using 'therapeutic nursing' may not yield much in the way of research-based references (Hockey 1989b), exploration of the component elements may be more productive.

Bond and Bond (1982) used the Delphi technique to explore in a systematic way what nurses wanted to see researched, the rationale for this approach being that 'Utilization of research would be more likely to occur if the initial research had high social relevance'. Nearly half the items (48%) related to nursing practice. While the term 'therapeutic nursing' does not appear, communication, the management of pain and the care of the terminally ill were ranked highly in terms of their importance for both nurses and patients. Determining methods of encouraging greater utilization of research findings in nursing practice was high on the agenda but in terms of its value to nurses themselves, rather than to patients. This is an interesting perceptual difference suggesting that research is seen as having the potential to improve the practice of nurses but not as a major contribution to the welfare of patients.

It is not the purpose of this chapter to present a bibliographic review of research on therapeutic nursing. It is sufficient to demonstrate that there is an emerging literature on this topic though much of it is not research based.

The material on touch is extensive and illustrates the use of a number of research methodologies. Classic experimental work was carried out on the importance of touch to baby monkeys (Harlow and Harlow 1966). That scientific or positivist methods have to be used in proofs of practice does not imply the denial of the uniqueness of the individual patient and the individual nurse. The randomized crossover trial (Keller and Bzdek 1986) may well be the most appropriate research design for establishing the relative effectiveness of therapeutic touch in pain control while the understanding, use and value to the patient of therapeutic touch in a practice setting may best be explored through ethnographic methods. Touch, for example, may signify acceptance, inclusion and belonging. It may confirm feelings of self-worth or even bring about awareness of being in the world. These may be important benefits in their own right or may help people to be less aware or tuned in to their pain. The relationship between the objective fact of pain and the subjective experience of the patient or use of touch and the subjective meaning of touch to the individual is not clearcut. Neither pain nor touch can be measured in precisely the same way as temperature and drug dosage, though analogue scales may be very useful both in research and practice (Bondestam et al. 1987). Only each individual patient can say what constitutes for him or her tolerable and intolerable levels of pain or whether therapy, of whatever kind, has reduced the awareness of pain. As the above study demonstrated, nurses tend to underestimate the degree of pain experienced by patients and to overestimate the therapeutic effect of drugs. When we get to notions of 'unruffling the field' and 'modulation of energy' (Wright 1987) we would, perhaps, do well to submit such hypotheses to the most rigorous scientific testing. They are expressed in what appears to be a scientific format rather than in terms of patients' experiences, beliefs and understandings and must therefore expect to be investigated through experimental research.

There have been many attempts to study the environment, particularly in so far as it touches psychiatric patients, where the concern has been not simply with the physical environment but with the social milieu. The therapeutic community as an exercise in the deliberate management of patients through group living goes back at least to the late 1940s. Moos (1973) has categorized environments within the framework of human ecology in a wide-ranging typology which goes far beyond what nurses normally think of when they concern themselves with the patients' immediate ward environment. Comfort is one of the less studied aspects of therapeutic nursing. There is, for example, work on comfort and pain (Eland 1988), the comfort needs of cancer patients (Fleming *et al.* 1987) and on self-care and comfort (Richeson and Huch 1988). Cameron (1988) explored the concept with patients while they were still in hospital using informal interviews and observation. In her abstract she writes, 'Current thought appeared to relegate comfort to an inferior position of soothing rather than to a dynamic process that altered the uncomfortable state'. She uses a grounded theory approach and develops the concept of integrative balancing to describe the process by which patients attempt to redress the disequilibrium which they experience in hospital. While one might question her assertion that 'It could reasonably be said that the motive underlying almost every patient action was a striving to increase comfort', her work does suggest that comfort is a high priority for patients and that nurses may fail to recognize that patients are actively in pursuit of comfort and can be helped or hindered by the extent to which nurses share their understanding of what is involved.

Some things can be shown to 'work' without our being able to explain why in our present state of knowledge or understanding. That may be an adequate basis for adoption into practice on a temporary basis, a working hypothesis, but even if only non-invasive activities are involved questions about whether, how and why they work must continue to be asked. Some things do not even need to be proved through nursing research. Nursing research does not, for example, need to prove that institutionalization may give rise to sensory deprivation (Heron *et al.* 1956). Nursing research should concentrate, instead, on the application to nursing of such findings generated in other arenas.

## OUTCOMES FOR PATIENTS

Advanced nursing practice, therefore, is concerned with the very basics of nursing: with independent practice initiated by nurses related to the core of nursing and with emotional labour. It focuses on healing, has a deliberate therapeutic intent and relies on the nurse's use of self. Krulik, quoted by Bircumshaw (1989), has stated that 'It is very questionable if the true core of nursing . . . the caring, the interpersonal interaction, ethical judgement, priority decision making, etc. can be quantified'. The essential inability to quantify does not mean that these ideas cannot be explored through research. Not long ago doctors would have argued that diagnosis was a matter of specialized knowledge, experience and gut feeling which could not yield to research. The process whereby decisions are made can be extrapolated and used to fuel a computer-based 'expert system'. The resultant diagnostic decisions, which can take into account more information than a doctor can readily manipulate unaided, are more accurate than those based on more traditional methods. Unnecessary operative procedures are avoided and hospital costs reduced (de Dombal 1979). There is no inherent reason why some of the secrets of nursing should not be yielded up in similar ways and using similar methodologies. Nightingale (1859) herself was convinced that these things could be elucidated:

> Let people who have to observe sickness and death look back and try to register in their observation the appearances which have preceded relapse, attack, or death, and not assert that there were none, or that they were not the *right* ones.

Research does not eliminate clinical judgement. It does offer ways in which such judgement may be supported and improved.

While therapeutic nursing may have as its rationale the bringing about of beneficial outcomes for patients, the nature of such outcomes and the demonstration that they are beneficial pose problems for both practitioner and researcher. Who is the arbiter of benefit? What is the trade-off between short-term and long-term benefit? What happens when nurses and patients disagree about the value of the outcome? Only the patient knows what really works in matters of pain and comfort. But the nurse must also be aware of the objectively dangerous consequences of any attempt to avoid all pain and discomfort.

Many of the subjective outcomes for patients, though they have a value in their own right, probably depend in part for their efficacy on a treatment equivalent of the Hawthorne effect. When nurses spend more time talking to patients (McBride 1967, Tarasuk *et al.* 1965) patients' perception of well-being is increased. Many of the reports of good outcomes for alternative physical therapies may simply reflect that they all require time spent together by patient and therapist and it is the longer encounter and the occasion for communication which this affords which is the important element.

At the individual level, the process of nursing is assessing the problem, deciding on appropriate nursing intervention and evaluating the outcome. Where the same time of intervention can be shown to have similar outcomes for other patients, we have moved into researching the practice. Case comparison is a perfectly legitimate way of developing knowledge. In principle, nursing process documentation should offer a rich harvest for clinical nursing research. In practice, the information recorded is often not detailed or accurate enough to provide data for research. Computerized storage and retrieval systems at ward level could bring about a major change in the quality of available data. Information on outcomes and evaluation of the contribution of the nursing intervention to that outcome are rarely made explicit (Report of the Nursing Process Evaluation Working Group 1986). If practitioners are unable to specify the effects of what they do then it is unlikely that research into nursing outcomes for patients will get very far. There is a need not only for greater clarity in determining what is independent nursing intervention but also for work to be done in specifying outcomes which might be directly attributed to nurses and their work.

There are outcomes of varying order. There are long-term objective outcomes, such as five-year survival rates of QUALYs (quality-adjusted life years), in which the impact of nursing is assumed to be negligible and short-term subjective outcomes, such as a terminally ill patient feeling comfortable and pain free for several hours, in which it is allowed that nursing may have made a major contribution. The former may find their way into performance indicators while the latter are likely to remain at the level of an entry in the nursing record. It is nonetheless an important outcome of nursing care for that patient. The problem for nursing is how to present such small-scale outcomes in order that the value of nursing be recognized beyond the immediate situation.

In addition, many people other than the nurse are involved in the care of patients. They, too, feel that they have a unique therapeutic relationship with patients. It is not easy to see what part of the overall outcome for patients might be attributed to the input of nurses. Objective outcome measures, such as length of stay, readmission rates and survival rates, may be a useful way of approaching the overall effectiveness of a hospital, ward, service or specific therapeutic regimen, whether the latter is initiated by doctor or nurse, but have little to contribute to the understanding of the process. Nursing is a process. It is the way in which care is given which is the *independent* variable. But we have to demonstrate that the caring is in the quality and that the quality of the caring matters.

## IMPLEMENTING RESEARCH FINDINGS IN PRACTICE

It is received wisdom that the findings from nursing research do not inform practice. Brett (1989) has looked at the diffusion of research-based practices among qualified nurses in the USA and has shown that most nurses are aware of some items of validated practice, such as closed sterile drainage systems, but that relatively few know about others, such as the idea of deliberative nursing, an approach of skilled communication which allows the nurse effectively to ascertain the patient's real needs. There is, moreover, a gap between knowing about a practice and actually using it all the time. Though 94% of Brett's respondents knew about the importance of regular changing of the intravenous site, only 27% claimed always to ensure regular change was carried out in practice. Although 34% knew about deliberative nursing, only 9% claimed always to make use of the technique in assessing patients.

It could be claimed that looking at items of practice in this way merely confirms the shopping-list approach to both practice and research and that we should be looking at different ways of exploring how far research does inform work in real practice settings. The focus should not be on the individual nurse but on behaviour in the place of work.

Various explanations have been put forward for the research–practice gap. Nurses do not make use of research for a variety of reasons enumerated by Hunt (1981). Perhaps one of the additional reasons is that they do not subscribe to the view of 'nurse as scientist', a concept which Kennedy (1980) maintains has led medicine to take the wrong path. Moira Hunt (1987) sees the problem in terms of nurses' lack of ownership of information and involvement in the research process. Action research is often put forward as *the* method for nursing as it involves practitioners but does not always appear to yield results commensurate with the effort involved.

It is not that the positivist approach is never appropriate for nursing research but that not all problems to which practitioners seek solutions can be addressed in this way. Susman and Evered (1978) argue that 'Positivist science is deficient for generating knowledge for use in solving problems that members of organizations face'. Important for our concern with why research findings are not implemented in practice is their contention that positivist science leads to research being seen as an:

> ... accumulation of social facts that can be drawn on by practitioners when they are ready to apply them. This conception encourages a separation of theory from practice because published research is read more by producers of research than by practitioners.

If we are worried about the need to take on a holistic view of the patient we need also to concern ourselves with a holistic notion of nursing in which not only are research and practice not separated but also researcher and practitioner are not always different people. The creation of nursing development units and the growth in opportunities for practitioners to undertake research training courses tailored to their specific needs indicate that the inherent dangers of such a split are being recognized and action taken to bridge the chasm before it gets too wide.

The terms 'therapeutic nursing' and 'deliberative nursing' do not figure as yet in the expression of priorities for research. As our perceptions of what constitutes nursing and our understanding of the nature of the nurse–patient relationship change, so must our notions of what constitutes appropriate and worthwhile research. Not only shall we ask different 'research questions' but we shall also draw from different theoretical perspectives. It is the nature of the question posed, not the problem identified, that determines the appropriateness of theory, methodology, research design, tools and tests.

Jonathan Miller (1989), in speaking of film editors, said, 'As with any hands-on craft the editor would not be able to spell out the principles on which he works'. It is one of the tasks of nursing research to distil such principles from observation of the craft-in-practice, to articulate them in clear and unambiguous terms and to validate them against the experiential knowledge of the nurse and the patient.

## ACKNOWLEDGEMENTS

I am grateful to Philip Burnard, Sandy Kirkman and Paul Wainwright for their constructive criticism on the draft and to several other colleagues for tracking down elusive references.

## REFERENCES

Binnie, A. (1987) Primary nursing: structural changes. *Nursing Times*, **83**(39), 36–7.
Bircumshaw, D. (1989) How can we compare graduate and non-graduate nurses? A review of the literature. *Journal of Advanced Nursing*, **14**, 438–443.
Bond, J. and Bond, S. (1982) *Clinical Nursing Research Priorities: A Delphi Survey*, Health Care Research Unit, University of Newcastle upon Tyne and Northern Regional Health Authority.
Bondestam, E., Hovgren, K., Johansson, F. G. *et al.* (1987) Pain assessment by patients and nurses in the early stages of acute myocardial infarction. *Journal of Advanced Nursing*, **12**, 677–682.
Brett, J. L. (1987) Use of nursing practice research findings. *Nursing Research*, **36**(6), 344–349.
Buckledee, J. and McMahon, R. (1994) *The Research Experience in Nursing*, Chapman and Hall, London.

Cameron, B. L. (1988) The nature of comfort to hospitalized patients. Unpublished MSc thesis, University of Wales.

Department of Health and Social Security (1989) DHSS *Handbook of Research and Development 1988*, HMSO, London.

De Dombal, F. T. (1979) Computers and the surgeon. *Surgery Annual*, **11**, 33–57.

Eland, J. M. (1988) Pain management and comfort. *Journal of Gerontological Nursing*, **14**(4), 10–15.

Ersser, S. (1988) Nursing beds and nursing therapy, in *Primary Nursing*, (ed. A. Pearson), Croom Helm, Beckenham.

Fleming, C. *et al.* (1987) A study of the comfort needs of patients with advanced cancer. *Cancer Nursing*, **10**(5), 237–243.

Harlow, H. F. and Harlow, M. K. (1966) Learning to love. *American Scientist*, **54**, 244–272.

Heron, W., Doane, B. K. and Scott, T. H. (1956) Visual disturbances after prolonged perceptual isolation. *Canadian Journal of Psychology*, **10**, 13–16.

Hochschild, A. R. (1983) *The Managed Heart: Commercialisation of Human Feeling*, University of California Press, Berkeley.

Hockey, L. (1989) The birth and development of two research units: similarities and contrasts. Paper read at the RCN Conference on Research in Nursing: Retrospect and Prospect, London, September 12th.

Hunt, J. (1981) Indicators for nursing practice: the use of research findings. *Journal of Advanced Nursing*, **6**, 189–194.

Hunt, M. (1987) The process of translating research findings into practice. *Journal of Advanced Nursing*, **12**, 101–110.

Institute of Medical Ethics (1989) *Bulletin*, **49**, 6.

Jennings, B. M. and Rogers, S. (1988) Merging nursing research and practice: a case of multiple identities. *Journal of Advanced Nursing*, **13**, 752–758.

Keller, E. and Bzdek, V. M. (1986) Effects of therapeutic touch on tension headache pain. *Nursing Research*, **35**(2), 101–105.

Kennedy, I. (1980) The Reith Lectures: unmasking medicine. *The Listener*.

Lathlean, J. and Farnish, S. (1984) *The Ward Sister Training Project*, Nursing Education Research Unit, King's College, London.

Luker, K. A. (1983) An evaluation of health visitors' visits to elderly women, in *Nursing Research: Ten Studies in Patient Care*, (ed. J. Wilson-Barnett), John Wiley, Chichester.

Luker, K. A. and Kenrick, M. (1992) An exploratory study of the sources of influence on the clinical decisions of community nurses. *Journal of Advanced Nursing*, **17**, 457–466.

McBride, M. A. B. (1967) Nursing approach, pain and relief: an exploratory experiment. *Nursing Research*, **11**, 337–341.

McMahon, R. (1989) Therapeutic nursing, theory and practice. Paper read at the First National Conference on Therapeutic Nursing, Oxford, March 22nd.

Menzies, I. (1960) A case-study in the functioning of social systems as a defence against anxiety. *Human Relations*, **13**(2), 95–123.

Miller, J. (1989) *Equinox* (Channel 4).

Moos, R. (1973) Conceptualisation of human environments. *American Psychologist*, **28**, 652–665.

Muetzel, P.-A. (1988) Therapeutic nursing, in *Primary Nursing*, (ed. A. Pearson), Croom Helm, Beckenham.

Nightingale, F. (1859) *Notes on Nursing*, (republished 1980), Churchill Livingstone, Edinburgh.

Nuffield Provincial Hospitals Trust (1954) *The Work of Nurses in Hospital Wards*, (The Goddard Report), NPHT, London.

Pearson, A. (1988) Primary nursing, in *Primary Nursing*, (ed. A. Pearson), Croom Helm, London.

*Report of the Nursing Process Evaluation Working Group to the DHSS Research Liaison Group* (1986) (ed. J. Haywood), Nurse Education Research Unit, Report No. 5, King's College, London.

Revans, R. W. (1964) The morale and effectiveness of general hospitals, in *Problems and Progress in Medical Care*, (ed. G. McLachlan), Oxford University Press, Oxford.

Richeson, M. and Huch, M. (1988) Self-care and comfort: a framework for nursing practice. *New Zealand Nursing Journal*, **81**(6), 26–27.

Robinson, J., Stilwell, J., Hawley, C. and Hempstead, N. (1989) *The Role of the Support Worker in the Ward Health Care Team*, Nursing Policy Studies 6, Nursing Policies Studies Centre and Health Services Research Unit, University of Warwick.

Smith, P. (1988) The emotional labour of nursing. *Nursing Times*, **84**(44), 50–51.

Smith, P. (1989) Emotional labour, nursing work and the research process: measuring quality of life. Paper read at the Royal College of Nursing Research Society Annual Conference, University College, Swansea, April 14th–16th.

*Supporting Research and Development in the NHS (The Culyer Report)*, (1994) HMSO, London.

Susman, G. I. and Evered, R. D. (1978) An assessment of the scientific merits of action research. *Administrative Science Quarterly*, **23**, 582–603.

Tarasuk, M. B., Rhymes, J. P. and Leonard, R. C. (1965) An experimental test of the importance of communication skills for effective nursing, in *Social Interaction and Patient Care*, (eds J. K. Skinner and R. C. Leonard), Lippincott, Philadelphia.

Wharton, A. and Pearson, A. (1988) Nursing and intimate physical care – the key to therapeutic nursing, in *Primary Nursing*, (ed. A. Pearson), Croom Helm, Beckenham.

Wright, S. M. (1987) The use of therapeutic touch in the management of pain. *Nursing Clinics of North America*, **22**(3), 705–714.

Zorza, V. and Zorza, R. (1980) *A Way to Die*, Andre Deutsch, London.

# 10

# An exploration of touch and its use in nursing

Elizabeth Tutton

**INTRODUCTION**

The practice of nursing involves a high level of human contact. One of the means of providing this contact is through the use of touch. However, the use of touch is a complex and multidimensional process. Individuals experience the process of giving touch and receiving touch in a unique way. Influencing factors such as family norms, experience and culture affect the meanings ascribed to the experience of touch. Differing situations and people involved in the process will also change how touch is experienced. Touch is highly significant in the work of nurses and is worthy of serious consideration as nurses are in a powerful position to determine how people experience the touching process.

There are many obvious examples of nurses using touch in their work. Nurses hold hands with patients who are experiencing a traumatic procedure, such as having their stitches or a drain removed. They touch patients in order to lift them into more comfortable positions. Touch is also necessary when nurses facilitate the relearning of dressing or walking skills by patients. The nature of nursing work allows nurses the privilege of close bodily contact at the very beginning of a relationship with a patient. Touch often occurs at the first meeting, a light touch on the arm to reassure a patient or in the performance of admission procedures such as taking a pulse or blood pressure. Often the first contact is of a more intimate nature and involves the provision of help with toileting or cleaning the patient's body. Touch is therefore an integral part of nursing care, but how frequently do we as nurses consider its use? Do we always use touch appropriately? Are we using touch to its fullest potential in order to provide high-quality nursing care? Le May and Redfern (1987) demonstrate that in one elderly care setting the majority of touch provided by nurses was related to the performance of a procedure. This suggests that other forms of touch may be underutilized.

The use of touch in nursing is not a new topic for discussion. Estabrooks (1987) provides evidence of a well-developed use of touch in American and Canadian nursing literature in the early 19th century. Currently there is a resurgence of interest in touch and its use in nursing (Davies and Riches 1995, Heidt 1991, Le May 1986, Turton 1989). There may be several reasons for this interest. The first may be concerned with an attempt to counteract the dehumanizing effects of a patient's stay in a modern hospital. Murphy (1984) indicates the highly stressful nature of a 'high-tech' hospital environment, which can adversely affect patients' well-being. Naisbitt (1982) suggests that nurses are in an ideal position to use touch to provide a high level of personal contact in an alien hospital environment. Second, nurses are constantly reviewing the principles from which they practise. The current trend in nursing is moving away from a concept based on a medical model of practice towards practice that encompasses holistic principles (Pearson and Vaughan 1986). The principles of holistic practice, treating the person as a unified whole, underlie most forms of complementary therapy. Similarities between the goals of nursing and those of complementary therapies have led many nurses to use some of these therapies to enhance their nursing practice (Holmes, 1986, Tutton 1987, Wise 1989). For example, the use of massage as a form of touch within nursing is increasing. Its use along with other advances in nursing care has been shown significantly to increase the quality of care nurses provide (Pearson et al. 1988).

This chapter is divided into two main parts: the first explores the use of instrumental, expressive and therapeutic touch and the second considers massage as a nursing intervention. A general discussion of each form of touch is followed by a brief research critique of some of the major studies investigating these areas. At the same time it is hoped that individuals will explore their own beliefs and values about touch and how they use it in their own practice. A series of exercises is provided throughout for this purpose. The reader is also given the opportunity to experience massage in the form of an example of a foot massage. Finally, methods of evaluating the use of touch in practice are considered.

## INSTRUMENTAL, EXPRESSIVE AND THERAPEUTIC TOUCH

**Exercise 1** Write down a brief description of three different incidents where you touched a patient. What were you hoping to achieve by touching them?

Nursing research has often placed touch within a framework of communication theory, viewing it as a form of non-verbal communication (Le May and Redfern 1987, Sims 1986, Tutton 1987). Estabrooks (1987) questions this deductive approach. From a review of early nurses' writings, she suggests that touch should be viewed as an integral part of the concept of comfort. The provision of comfort in the form of touch was a key role of the nurse that appears to have been neglected in more recent literature.

According to Sims (1986a), the use of touch in nursing can be divided into four categories:

1  Instrumental touch
2  Expressive touch
3  Therapeutic touch
4  Systematic touch.

Watson (1975) defines instrumental touch as a deliberate physical contact made as part of a procedure, such as performing an aseptic technique or supporting a patient learning to walk again. Expressive touch is seen as spontaneous and affective in nature. A hug to comfort a patient who is feeling unhappy is demonstrating expressive touch. This division, though useful as a starting point, is rather simplistic as it does not consider the intentions of the person providing the touch. It also does not take into account the receiver's experience of the touching process. Empirical work has demonstrated that these categories need further exploration. The intensive care unit (ICU) nurses in Estabrook's (1989) study identified three categories of touch: caring touch, protective touch and task touch. Caring touch was seen as 'real touch' which often contained an 'emotional intent' and had a therapeutic benefit for the patient. Protective touch was used to physically protect the patient and physically and emotionally protect the nurse. Task touch was seen as the daily important work of the nurse. Each of these categories of touch could occur on their own. However, caring touch and protective touch were used separately but either of them could occur in combination with task touch.

Therapeutic touch involves the transference of energy from one person to another with the intention to heal (Krieger 1979). This form of touch normally occurs without direct skin-to-skin contact. Systematic touch could be seen as synonymous with massage, which can be defined as a purposeful manipulation of the soft tissues of the body with the intention of enhancing the receiver's well-being.

**Exercise 2** Can you identify any of these categories of touch in your three descriptions?

### Instrumental touch

Instrumental or task touch is essential for the performance of nursing tasks. Watson (1975) assumed that touch in health professionals is primarily instrumental in nature. Le May and Redfern (1987) observed 1420 touches during 318 interactions between nurse and patient. Of these, 1216 (85.63%) were instrumental and 181 (12.75%) were expressive and 23 (1.62%) indefinable. This study had a sample of 30 patients and took place on a long-stay elderly care ward. Although generalizations beyond this care setting cannot be made, this study provides evidence to support Watson's assumption.

The emphasis on the use of instrumental touch may relate to the nurses' working patterns. A system of task allocation, where nurses are given one or more tasks to perform with a large group of patients, may mean that no one person is aware of the interrelated nature of the patient's needs. The scope for appreciation of instances where other forms of touch may improve a patient's well-being could be limited. Melia (1987) suggests that student nurses are quickly socialized into the ward culture with its emphasis on getting the work finished. This ethos may also reduce the opportunities for forms of touch other than instrumental. Other factors such as the layout of the ward, ward furniture, patients' diagnosis, cultural background and personality of the nurse and patient may also conspire to limit touch to its instrumental form. Estabrooks (1989), from her study of ICU nurses, criticizes the negative connotation placed on instrumental or task touch. She suggests that this simply reflects the nature of nursing work, in this case in an ICU. The nurses in her study were able to determine if the task was 'positively or negatively experienced' by the patient. The nurses tended to mix the touch with caring or protective touch, depending on the nature of the situation. Protective touch was considered necessary to control the patient and prevent them from harm. It was also used to protect the nurse from physical and emotional harm. Touch was also used in a negative way if strategies to eliminate frustration in the nurse had not been successful.

**Exercise 3**   Identify factors in your work patterns and work environment that might make you focus on using instrumental touch.

### Expressive touch

Locsin (1984) considers that touch affects people's feelings of value and worth, their integration and ego integrity. Johnson (1965) sees touch as a behaviour that communicates comfort, love, security and warmth with implications for physical survival as well as emotional self-esteem. Barnett (1972a) indicates that people convey their inner feelings and reactions through touch to others. Locsin (1984) and Goodykoontz (1979) describe touch as a sense through which one person shares themselves with another. Goodykoontz continues that touch can communicate caring, well-being and facilitate recovery and acceptance of a diagnosis. Seaman (1982) also sees touch as beneficial as it carries messages of acceptance and caring. Touching in a caring manner is seen as therapeutic by Ernst and Shaw (1980). It also has the potential to communicate trust, according to Hollinger (1980). Click (986) has demonstrated that expressive touch has the potential to decrease, though not significantly, anxiety in patients who have had a myocardial infarction. Caring touch was considered to have two aspects, comforting touch and encouraging touch, by the nurses in Estabrooks' (1989) study. Comforting touch, such as 'holding hands, stroking a forehead', was often used with people experiencing 'grief, discomfort, or dying'. Encouraging touch was 'hopeful, future orientated, and boisterous'. These two categories were seen as fundamental to the caring role of the nurse.

Touch can also be used to convey negative emotions or to communicate distance and non-involvement. Estabrooks (1989) identifies this type of touch in relation to protective touch and task touch. Avoidance of touch may be interpreted by the patient as the nurse's dislike of them (Goodykoontz 1979). Other patients may feel uncomfortable when touched (Goodykoontz 1979, Seaman 1982).

**Exercise 4**   How do you feel when you touch other people? Write down your thoughts.

Ask someone to touch you. Discuss what you felt with them. Did what they intended you to feel match up with what you felt?

Practise using different ways of touching and explain the effects of your touch in relation to what you intended the person to feel.

**Therapeutic touch**

Therapeutic touch, or the laying on of hands, is an ancient form of healing. It involves the transference of 'energy', known as *chi* in China and *prana* in India, from the healer to the sick person. Its use in nursing was pioneered by Dolores Krieger in the 1970s. Krieger was impressed by the work of Grad and Smith, who used controlled experiments to assess the effect of the touch of Colonel Estabany, a well-known healer, on the healing of skin wounds in mice (Krieger 1975). Grad *et al.* (1961) found mice treated by Colonel Estabany healed significantly faster. The same team found a comparable effect when barley seeds were treated in the same manner. The height of the seedlings and yield of plant material was significantly higher. Krieger (1975) reports on her studies using haemoglobin as the dependent variable. In all her three studies haemoglobin values were significantly higher after treatment with therapeutic touch. Krieger then went on to test her assumption that anyone with a fairly healthy body and a strong intention to help or heal ill people could become healers. The same research study was then carried out using 32 registered nurses who had been taught healing. The results confirmed that ordinary nurses taught therapeutic touch can significantly affect haemoglobin levels in ill people.

Husband (1988) argues strongly for the use of therapeutic touch and its incorporation into nursing practice. She proposes that therapeutic touch, with its ability to produce a relaxation response and pain relief, has many possible applications in patient care. Turton (1988) believes that therapeutic touch is an 'eminently suitable therapy for nurses to incorporate into their care'.

**Exercise 5** Find yourself a quiet place and make yourself comfortable. Close your eyes. Place both your hands together as in the traditional sign of prayer. Now move your hands until they are 2 cm apart. Concentrate your mind on the space between your hands. Then slowly move your hands until they are 4 cm apart and then bring them together until they are nearly touching. Repeat this action for about three minutes.

What did you feel: Ask your friends to try this exercise and share your experiences. (For more information about this exercise read Krieger (1979), Chapter 3.)

### A review of the research studies on touch

A range of studies has considered the use of touch in nursing care. The first study, by Barnett (1972b), uses observation to identify who is being touched and where touch is occurring. From this point onwards until the late 1980s the research focuses on the effect of deliberate touch on patients' responses in a variety of sample groups. These studies have largely drawn on pre-experimental and quasiexperimental designs. More recent studies by Estabrooks (1989) and Estabrooks and Morse (1992) are more exploratory in nature. Using a qualitative perspective, they have examined how nurses learn to touch and how they perceive the process of touching.

A large study looking at where and which patients health professionals touch was undertaken by Barnett (1972b). Using observation over a four-week period on randomly selected wards and rooms, all unnecessary touch that took place was recorded. Information gathered showed that registered nurses touched patients the most, with the female nurses giving 85% more touch than the male nurses. The age of the patient was related to the amount of touch, with decreasing touch with increasing age. Most touch was given to 26–33-year-olds and 72% of touches occurred on patients who were 18–33 years old. The 6–17-year-olds and 42–49-year-olds were not touched at all. Touch levels were higher in paediatrics, labour rooms and intensive care. Barnett considered this to be related to the high stress levels in these areas. The hand received 60% of the touches and was the area that was touched most often. The amount of touch a patient received was also based on their condition, with 70% of those touched being considered to be good or fair. This study provides useful descriptive data, but it is dated and specific to that particular setting, at that specific time. It also lacks any evidence of interobserver reliability testing.

Further studies have been undertaken with pre-experimental and quasi-experimental designs, using different subject samples. Lorensen (1983) undertook a small study using post testing only, on 12 primigravida women during labour. The sample was one of convenience, with no randomization, and there was little control over the amount of touch the women in the control group received. The investigator administered a high degree of touch during labour to the experimental group. The control group received instrumental touch only. Whether this touch was perceived in a positive or negative manner is unknown. An author-designed questionnaire, for which there was no evidence of reliability or validity, was administered between 24 and 36 hours later. The results showed no significant differences. However, in answer to the question 'Who was most helpful?' four chose the nurse in the experimental group while one chose the nurse in the control group. Five subjects in the experimental group said that holding their hand was the most important thing the nurse did. Five subjects in the experimental group found massage relieved low back discomfort.

Aguilera (1967), using a quasiexperimental design with 36 psychiatric patients, investigated the use of physical contact and verbal interactions. The experimental group received simple appropriate touch with verbal commands whilst the control group received no touch. A subject attitude questionnaire was given before and after the intervention and an observation sheet was filled in. There was no evidence of reliability, validity testing of the tools or interobserver reliability and not all patient variables were considered. No statistical test of significance were used on the results. Aguilera claims that there was increased verbal interaction, rapport and approach behaviour, particularly after the eighth day, in the touch group. There was no evidence of a greater increase in verbal interaction in the evening shift. The degree of comfort of nurses was positively correlated with the degree of comfort of the subjects. There was also a higher rate of acceptance of schizophrenic subjects compared with depressive subjects by nurses. Aguilera also found a significant correlation between age and amount of touch, with younger subjects receiving higher comfort and acceptance ratings from nurses.

Taking Aguilera's study one step further, Langland and Panicucci (1982) designed a study to see if touch while giving a verbal request increased attention, verbal response and action response. They used a convenience sample of 32 elderly female patients who had been confused for six months or more. The patients were assessed using known tools and allocated randomly to each group. The experimental group received touch with a verbal request and the control group received just the verbal request. The subjects were assessed for attention using an author-designed tool which showed no evidence of reliability or validity testing. There was also no evidence of investigator or observer reliability using this tool. This subject's verbal response was tape recorded and physical action documented by the investigator and observer. Results from this study showed significantly increased attention and non-verbal response when touch was used. The subjects showed no increase in relevant verbal response or in appropriate action response.

Other authors using a case study approach have found touch increases the verbal and action response. Burnside (1973) worked with a group of six elderly regressive patients with chronic brain syndrome. Using touch as part of the therapy, she increased the amount of non-verbal and verbal communication within the group. Preston (1973) also describes a case study of touch used with a request increasing the non-verbal and action response in an elderly man with organic brain syndrome.

There are two studies on touch with critically ill patients. A well-designed study by McCorkle (1974) used 60 seriously ill patients, randomly allocating them to an experimental group, who received touch to the wrist while talking to the investigator, while the control group received the verbal interaction but no touch. The observers had interrater reliability and a tape recording made of the verbal interaction was analysed using Bale's interaction process analysis which claims to have face validity and to be reliable. There were a number of significant results. A greater number of the patients in the experimental group responded positively with facial expressions. Correspondingly, a greater number of control patients responded negatively with facial expressions. The experimental group had significantly more neutral movements and fewer negative movements. Analysis of the verbal responses showed that significantly more of the experimental group responded positively, in fact, 93.3%. In the control group, 70% of the patients responded positively. Responses to the question, 'Was the nurse interested in you?' were approximately the same for both groups: 90% of the experimental group and 87% of the control group said 'Yes'. ECG readings were also taken but proved inconclusive.

The other study performed on critically ill patients was by Knable (1981). This was based on a case study approach using hand holding when it naturally occurred and describing what happened. The author combines this with pre- and postphysiological measurements. Fifteen subjects and

12 nurses were used, with the investigator as measurer and observer. The nurses chose two periods in four hours when they would normally hold hands with the patient. The results showed that hand holding lasted up to three minutes and was used primarily to provide emotional support and to establish rapport. Of 306 non-verbal behaviours recorded during the hand-holding events, 222 were positive and 85 negative. The vital signs proved to be inconclusive.

A significant movement in our understanding of the process of touch has been facilitated by the work of Estabrooks (1989) and Estabrooks and Morse (1992). The first part of this study examined how nurses use touch and what variables influenced the process of touching. The second part considered how nurses develop a touching style and how they see the process of touching. The research approach was rigorous and qualitative in nature, utilizing indepth interviews and participant observation. The sample consisted of eight ICU nurses who identified themselves as using touch in practice and considered touch to be important. The resulting data are illuminating and raise many research questions but they only show the nurses' perspective and need to be examined within the cultural context in which the research took place. In the first part of the study, Estabrooks (1989) identified the three types of touch discussed earlier in this chapter: caring touch, protective touch, and task touch. Protective touch had not previously been found in the literature on touch and therefore is worthy of further investigation. The process of touching was seen to be extremely complex, as demonstrated in this quote: 'For any given nurse–patient dyad, on any given situation, there is an emerging pattern of touching. This pattern is dynamic and sensitive to subtle changes'.

The variables affecting the way touch was used fell into three groups: those in relation to the nurse, the daily context of the work and those in relation to the patient. Individual nurses were seen to have a touching style which evolved over time in relation to the person's life and work experiences. Daily work variables focused on the nurse as a person and on the working environment. It is interesting to note that, 'The better a nurse feels physically and emotionally, the more therapeutic the nurse's touching behaviours are likely to be'. A more positive touching style was also possible if the nurse and patient were able to relate to each other. Touch was facilitated in patients who had a greater need, those who provided a positive response and those for whom the nurse 'feels bad'. Inhibitors of touch were seen as: problems in relation to behaviour, situations where the nurse is at risk and diagnosis where the patient was responsible for their condition.

The second part of the study (Estabrooks and Morse 1992) examines how nurses learn to touch and the nature of the touching process. The nurses in this study considered that they learnt to touch through three main areas:

cultural background, nursing education and work. Cultural background encompassed the family norms in relation to touch and learning within the wider society, which included sexuality. Personal experiences such as receiving a massage themselves also influenced their beliefs. Nurse education appeared to contribute little to the nurses' development in this area. The most focused period of learning about touch in relation to nursing was the working period. Initially, nurses concentrated on learning the knowledge and skills necessary for ICU practice. Once competent in these areas, they tended to focus on individuals they wished to emulate and learn from them, including their touching style. As this intense period of learning faded the nurses became affected by the routine nature of the work and became bored. At this point it seems the nurses developed their touching style which matured as the nurse matured. The process of 'cueing' or giving and receiving verbal and non-verbal messages was the dominant process for learning more about the patient at this stage.

The touching process was described as having two phases: entering and connecting. During the entering phase the nurses perceived themselves to be 'gaining permission to enter the patient's personal space'. This was achieved by talking to the patient and gathering information about the patient's likely response. The next phase consisted of talking and touching. This then continued with the addition of touch. The nurse actively sought permission to enter more intimate areas of the patient and picked up cues concerning the patient's experience of the touch. This phase was seen as facilitating a closer nurse–patient relationship. 'The nurse has now made a commitment to interacting meaningfully with the patient and to expending the emotional energy required to connect with the patient.'

In the connecting phase the interviewees identified the feelings associated with touch: the feelings of caring for the other person and the vulnerability that is often associated with caring. 'The feelings may be those of satisfaction, reward or joy if the patient does well, or they may be the less desirable feelings of emotional pain, sorrow, anger or grief if the patient does not do well.' Within this phase is the actual touch itself but this did not appear to be seen in isolation from the feelings associated with the touch.

Estabrooks (1989) and Estabrooks and Morse (1992) have provided a rich source of new insights into the discussion on touch. They have identified that the experience of touch is more than merely physical contact and the meaning within the process of touching is of great importance. Estabrooks and Morse (1992) suggest that touch is seen as a Gestalt: 'A gestalt involving voice, affect, intent, and meaning within a context as well as tactile contact'. This provides a much wider interpretation than the traditional studies on touch. Areas for further research are clearly identified. The process of cueing, the use of protective touch and the process of learning to touch all provide a good foundation for further exploration.

The other studies exploring touch have tended to be experimental in design, with convenience samples which have been randomly allocated into experimental and control groups. There has been a lack of reliability and validity testing of tools and interobserver reliability, apart from McCorkle's (1974) study. The results indicate that most touches occur on the hand and the amount of touches decreases with age (Barnett 1972b). Hand holding enhances positive, non-verbal response in critically ill patients (Knable 1981) and is most important to mothers in labour (Lorensen 1983). A verbal request accompanied by touch can increase verbal and non-verbal responses (Aguilera 1967, Langland and Panicucci 1982, McCorkle 1974). Finally, physiological measures such as vital signs and ECGs produce inconclusive evidence. Lader and Mathews (1970) question the efficacy of using physiological indices to measure autonomic changes at low levels of arousal. They claim that patient variables, obtrusive devices and artifacts can affect the measurements.

## A review of the research studies on therapeutic touch

The study of therapeutic touch (TT) is an area of great interest. Earlier studies have utilized experimental designs and gained some interesting results, particularly in relation to its effect on anxiety. However, more recent studies are endeavouring to understand the process of therapeutic touch through the use of qualitative research methods.

Five studies have looked at the effect of therapeutic touch on anxiety states. Randolph (1984) induced anxiety in 60 health subjects with the use of a silent film. Using a quasiexperimental design, the experimental group received TT during the film while the control group received physical touch. Pre- and postmeasures of skin conductance level, muscle tension level and peripheral skin temperature were recorded. Both groups showed a physiological stress response to the film but there were no differences between the two groups. It could be that the stimulus was inappropriate for the use of TT as an intervention. Normally, it takes place in a quiet relaxed environment with minimal external stimulus for healer and recipient. There was also no evidence of the practitioner's ability to practise this art.

Heidt (1981) is a key researcher in this field and, in an early study, chose a population with known high anxiety scores, a sample of 100 patients on a cardiovascular unit. Three groups were used, one who received TT, one casual touch (pulse taking) and one no touch but with verbal interaction. Heidt recorded preintervention and postintervention anxiety scores using Spielberger's state-trait anxiety self-evaluation questionnaire. The results indicated that the TT group experienced a significant decrease in anxiety and had significantly lower scores than the casual touch and non-touch groups. The control interventions can, however, be criticized. The casual touch group could have mimicked therapeutic touch to make a truer control and the non-touch group brought a new factor, verbal communication, into the design which, as the author discusses, allowed the patients to bring up concerns that could not be dealt with in the time available. This in turn could adversely affect their anxiety scores.

To make a tighter research design, Quinn (1984) used two groups, one receiving non-contact TT and the other receiving a mimicked version of TT. Quinn trained the assistants and then filmed them and tested to see if a panel of judges could tell which ones were using TT and which ones were not. Analysis showed no correlation, hence it was proved impossible visually to tell the difference. Using Spielberger's self-evaluation questionnaire, pre- and postanxiety states were taken of 60 patients on a cardiovascular unit. Possible bias could be introduced to the study from the seven different nurses giving the treatments and there was no control for the different anxiety state levels in each group. However, the results still showed a significant decrease in post-state anxiety scores in patients treated with non-contact TT.

A replication and extension of this study was performed by Quinn (1980). The study was extended by the use of a different sample group, preop cardiac surgical patients, and a larger sample (153), a no-treatment control group and the addition of physiological measures. No significant results were obtained. Quinn (1989) identified difficulties in relation to the researcher providing the therapeutic touch and the mimicked version of the therapeutic touch. Turning off the therapeutic action was problematic. Also, restricting the intervention to five minutes before the therapist felt the intervention was complete created an artificial situation which may have affected the results. A further complication was the large number of patients on medication which was not measured as a variable in the study.

Another study by Simington and Laing (1993) attempted to combine TT with a back rub. This proved problematic as the intentions behind the two different therapies were not made explicit. A three-group, post-test design utilizing Spielberger's state-trait anxiety self-evaluation questionnaire was used. The treatment group received TT and a back rub. Control group 1 received a back rub by the same nurse who performed the TT in the treatment group, but without the energy exchange. As in the study by Quinn (1989), the researcher had an effect on the control group which raises the issue of the nature of control groups. The second control group was given a back rub by a nurse unfamiliar with TT. The results indicated a significant difference in the mean anxiety scores between the treatment group and the second control group. The study does, however, have limitations. There was no pretesting of anxiety scores and hence no baseline data for comparison. Control of the environment in which the study took place was not discussed. Three minutes is possibly too short a time for an intervention of this nature. Using different researchers to control for concepts such as 'intentionality and compassion' is not possible unless the concepts themselves are analysed as part of the study.

A fresh perspective on TT was provided by Heidt (1990) in her study of seven nurses and seven patients using grounded theory. A rigorous approach was used to discover how the process of TT is experienced from the giver's and receiver's perspective. Indepth interviewing and observation were used to collect the data. The patients' and nurses' experiences were of a similar nature and so were collated together. The experience of TT was categorized into opening intent, opening sensitivity and opening communication. A summary of the findings are shown below from Figure 1 in Heidt (1990), entitled 'Therapeutic touch: opening the flow of the universal life energy').

OPENING INTENT
**Quieting**: Stilling the mind, emotions and body to feel in harmony with the universal life energy
**Affirming**: Recognizing the unity and the wholeness of the universal life energy
**Intending**: Desiring to get the universal life energy moving again.

OPENING SENSITIVITY
**Attuning**: Listening to the quality of the flow of the universal life energy
**Planning**: Using the internal and external cues about the flow of the universal life energy to make a plan of treatment.

OPENING COMMUNICATION
**Unblocking**: Clearing out the impediments and balancing the flow of the universal life energy
**Engaging**: Directing and receiving the flow of universal life energy
**Enlivening**: Pulling in and balancing the flow of universal life energy.

The nurses and patients in this study were all experienced in the process of TT and provided positive descriptions of their experience. However, this type of sample is useful for obtaining indepth knowledge concerning the process or nature of the intervention. The nurses all had a clear sense of direction that went beyond the TT. This is demonstrated in the following quote.

Nurses 'touched' their patients by offering a therapeutic relationship that engendered hope in the patient; they provided a sense of trust, enabling patients to unblock impediments to the flow of life energy; they taught patients, giving them a sense of control in planning their own health care.

A further exploration to ascertain the experience of people who have received TT was made by Samarel (1992) using phenomenology. Open-ended interviews were undertaken with a convenience sample of 20 people who had a wide range of experience of receiving TT, from two to seven days. A follow-up interview to clarify and elaborate on the data was also undertaken. Clarity is needed regarding the length of interview time as 15 minutes seems too short a time to get at the indepth information needed for this type of research. The descriptions were analysed and fell into three categories: experiences before, during and after treatment. The subjects had a memory of 'unmet physiological, mental/emotional and spiritual needs' prior to the treatment. The experience of treatment developed a raised awareness of emotions, roles and relationships. After the treatment the subjects experienced 'spiritual and personal change leading to resonating fulfilment'. The overall experience was considered to be dynamic, multidimensional and positive in that it led to personal growth.

To summarize, the earlier studies on TT used experimental designs and attempted to measure the effects of TT on physiological indices and anxiety. An inherent difficulty with this is that the intervention itself is taken out of context. Samarel (1992) and Heidt (1990, 1991) both provide evidence that people choose TT for a wide range of reasons, not just for anxiety. The use of phenomenology has demonstrated that the experience of TT is a linear multidimensional process that directs the individual towards personal growth (Samarel 1992). One-off artificial interventions are therefore of debatable value. Understanding the process of TT has also identified areas of similarity across nursing interventions. Both Estabrooks and Morse (1992) and Heidt (1990) identify 'cueing' as an important mechanism in the process of providing touch. The experimental studies also have problems in relation to the choice of control groups and the fact that the control itself has an effect on the subject. These issues remain unresolved despite the rigorous efforts of researchers such as Quinn (1984, 1989).

## MASSAGE IN NURSING

The literature suggests that touch is a means of communicating or sending messages from person to person. Massage as a form of touch has the same effect. Auckett (1979) sees massage as an expression of love through loving, caring and touching. She feels that massage can promote mother–baby bonding and sets up a metaphysical energy flow between them. It calms unsettled, irritable and colicky babies, by giving them pleasure, awareness, gentleness, closeness and relaxation. Hefferman and Mott (1984) also believe that massage is of high value in establishing the mother–baby relationship. Debelle (1981) uses massage in a clinic for babies that are causing their parents some distress. The babies are considered to be uncuddly, irritable, poor feeders, constant criers or sleep fighters. Debelle uses massage successfully to improve the communication between the parents and babies. She claims that massage helps the parents to be:

1 More aware of the babies' needs
2 Tuned into the babies' feelings and responses
3 Able to reassure the baby by maximum skin contact that the environment is safe
4 Able to help the baby relax
5 Able to relax themselves.

Jackson (1985) considers touch to be therapeutic and suggests that it should be given in a structured manner on a regular basis. She recommends massage and says it allows verbal interaction, improvement and maintenance of emotional well-being, relief of pain and muscle tension, establishment of a unifying bond between nurse and patient and socialization through one-to-one contact. Hollinger (1980) suggests that nurses can communicate trust through back rubs and reinforce feelings of well-being and self-worth. From his experience of using massage with orthopaedic patients, Mason (1988) said that massage provided the opportunity for the patient to discuss his problems with his nurse. The nurse also uses the massage sessions to pick up cues about the patient's physical and mental state. Wharton and Pearson (1988) consider massage to facilitate the development of a close nurse–patient relationship. They provide a case study of a patient who was helped to cope with a painful procedure through the use of massage.

Massage is contraindicated, according to Joachim (1983b) where there are skin lesions, blood clots, fractures or extreme arthritic pain. Breakey (1982) also indicates that patients on bed rest should not have their legs massaged to avoid mobilization of a thrombosis or emboli formation.

Most authors consider that massage may have a relaxing effect on the subject (Breakey 1982, Jackson 1977, Joachim 1983a). By association, massage may have physiological effects. Joachim (1983a) suggests that massage increases the flexibility of muscles, increases circulation by dilating blood vessels, facilitates the removal of waste products and prevents contracture and tension. Breakey (1982) agrees with Joachim and adds that massage promotes lymphatic drainage, benefits connective tissue and increases fibre networks, presumably by improving venous return. It also decreases oedema and postoperative pooling of blood and improves gastrointestinal activity. Joachim (1983a) also claims that massage decreases the use of pain and sleeping medication.

**Exercise 6** Consider the factors (those that relate to yourself, your patient or the environment) that might influence your use of massage in your area of practice.

These factors might relate to yourself in terms of your sexuality, the clothes you wear or maybe how you perceive your role. The patient's diagnoses, their appearance or how they behave might be influencing factors. Environmental factors might be that there is too much noise or too much light.

Explore these factors and consider alternatives that might facilitate the use of massage in your area of practice.

## A review of the research studies on massage

As in the previous areas of touch, massage as a nursing intervention has not received a systematic research effort. The studies identified here use different samples and a variety of outcome measures. Unlike touch and therapeutic touch, the research process has not moved forward to explore massage within the context in which it is used or explore the meanings ascribed to the process of receiving massage. The earlier studies focus on trying to identify a physiological relaxation response. Later studies combine this with attempts to measure patients' well-being. The choice of study design tends to remain in the pre-experimental, experimental domain.

A study by Kaufmann (1964) looked at the physiological and subjective responses of 36 patients who received a back rub. Each subject acted as their own control with half receiving the back rub first and half receiving it second. The control period of rest was undertaken on another day which could lead to bias if the patients' feelings or condition had changed with time. There were also four nurses administering the massage and three nurses taking recordings, which would introduce some variations in technique. The study provided no indication of random assignment of patients to each group. The results showed no statistical significance between the physiological measurements of each group. However, 31 subjects gave strongly positive responses to their back rubs.

Using ten healthy subjects, Barr and Taslitz (1970) attempted to discover if physiological relaxation occurred with massage. Each subject undertook six consecutive sessions of alternating massage and a control rest period. The results were inconclusive and gave no indication of a relaxation response. Initially, systolic and diastolic pressure decreased during massage, yet at the end of the massage there was an increase in systolic and a small decrease in diastolic pressure. Heart rate increased during massage and body temperature decreased as a result of increased sweating. However, there were no discernible trends in skin temperature, pupil diameter or axillary sweating.

More positive results in relation to physiological measures were obtained in a more recent study by Meek (1993). A quasiexperimental design with the subjects acting as their own controls, by providing baseline physiological measurements, was used. No actual control group was implemented and the researcher carried out the intervention and undertook the physiological measurements. Thirty hospice patients each received two sessions of slow stroke back massage lasting three minutes. Measurements of diastolic and systolic blood pressure, heart rate and skin temperature were taken before, immediately after and five minutes after the intervention. Each of the measures demonstrated statistically significant changes that indicated a short-term relaxation response.

Another study using 32 healthy female subjects was undertaken by Longworth (1982). The author used an experimental pre- and postintervention test design, she did not have a control session and the intervention was a massage session. Both Spielberger state-trait anxiety self-evaluation questionnaires and measurements of heart rate, blood pressure, galvanic skin response and muscle tension were undertaken before and after the intervention. The results indicated a significant decrease in state anxiety scores and no significant changes in physiological measures.

Joachim (1983b) also considered physiological factors and found that, after massage, pulse rates decreased by 5–20 beats per minute. Blood pressure readings were inconclusive. Joachim's design, however, was a weak, pre-experimental one-group pre-post test design and so strong inferences cannot be made. The sample was 15 randomly selected patients with inflammatory bowel disease. Each patient had four sessions with 30 minutes of deep breathing exercises and 45 minutes of body massage. Before and after interviews were conducted on four aspects of well-being. The design of the study made it impossible to isolate the effect of deep breathing from that of massage. However, useful qualitative data were obtained using techniques that could be incorporated into care planning. Nine patients demonstrated an increased ability to sleep and nine patients also felt more in control of their pain. Fourteen patients said they were more aware of the difference between feeling stressed and feeling relaxed. Thirteen patients were better able to calm themselves and 14 patients said massage helped them feel more relaxed. This provides an insight into the ways in which massage may be useful to individuals that go beyond the traditional view of providing a relaxation response and reducing anxiety.

A severely limited study by Rowlands (1984) had a sample of 24 elderly patients. The design was pre-experimental post-test only, with questionnaires given to all the staff and subjects in the home at the end of the study. The subjects were put into three groups: one had therapeutic touch twice a day, one had it once a day and the third group had nothing. Therapeutic touch was not adequately defined but was 'a massage'. The subjects were not randomly allocated and because of the three-group design, there were only small numbers in each group. The nurses giving the intervention were the nurses on duty at the time so over the six-week period the intervention was not standardized. There was no reliability or validity testing of the questionnaire and all the staff knew exactly who had the intervention and how often. The results were very positive but must be considered in light of the design. The mood of the experimental subjects was lightened in the first four weeks and they had greater positive behavioural responses. Both experimental groups showed an increase in sociability towards the domestics in weeks 2–6. Of the nurses, 78.3% believed the massage benefited the residents in the study, while 64% of the residents said they had a reduction in muscle tension and 65% had assisted movement. Finally, 95% of the residents felt that massage was of value to them.

In a study on the effect of teaching mothers to massage their babies to establish if it improved infant development, Booth *et al.* (1985) assigned primiparas and their infants to three groups: a powder massage group, a non-powder massage group and a control group. Each child had pre- and post-testing using Bayley scales of infant development, nursing child assessment project teaching scales (NCAP) and post-testing of a 30-minute videotape of mother–infant free play and massage session. There was no evidence of random assignment or of observer reliability testing using the aforementioned scales. The results, however, were statistically inconclusive but there was considerable positive feedback from all the mothers in the massage group.

A thought-provoking pilot study was undertaken by Sims (1986a). The sample comprised six female patients with breast cancer undergoing radiotherapy. Each of these patients received three sessions of slow stroke back massage on three consecutive days, followed by three sessions of a control rest period on three consecutive days in the following week. The subjects were randomly allocated into two groups: group 1 received massage followed by the control periods and group 2 vice versa. Before and after measurements of symptom distress (McCorkle 1981) and an author-adapted mood adjective checklist from McNair and Lorr (1964) were taken. The results must be considered in the light of the small sample size but it is interesting that from six patients, 28 spontaneous positive comments were made. Four of the six patients also started spontaneously to talk about their personal concerns. Subjects in group 1 reported a significant percentage improvement in symptom distress following the massage intervention. However, group 2 showed no difference in percentage improvement following the massage and control interventions. Following the control intervention, the percentage improvement in symptom distress for group 2 was significantly greater than the percentage improvement for group 1. For the whole sample, a 25% improvement in total symptom distress scores following massage was reported compared with 7.7% improvement following the control intervention. Using the mood checklist, group 1 reported greater improvement on one variable, tense, whereas group 2 reported greater improvement in four variables, tranquil, tense,

vitality and tired, following the massage compared with the control intervention. The whole sample reported an overall mood improvement of
17.9% following the massage compared with 13.3% following the control
intervention.

A different area of study is explored by Weinrich and Weinrich (1990).
Their intention was to see if a ten-minute Swedish massage reduced the
level of pain, measured using a visual analogue scale, in cancer patients.
Subjects were paired in relation to the frequency of administration of
pain medication. This proved an inappropriate method for pairing as pain
medication levels did not equate with pain levels. The treatment group
demonstrated higher levels of pain than the control group. Each pair was
randomly assigned to a treatment or control group. The control group
received a visit from the researcher but the exact nature of this visit was
not made explicit. There were seven data collectors in this study but no
evidence of interrater reliability was provided. The only significant results
were that the male subjects demonstrated a significant reduction in pain
levels immediately after the massage intervention. This reduction was
not apparent in the female subjects. Gender issues in relation to pain and
massage therefore warrant further exploration.

A recent study by Fraser and Ross Kerr (1993) used an experimental
design to measure the effect of five minutes of slow stroke back massage
on anxiety levels in a group of elderly people in long-term accommodation.
Twenty-one patients were split into three groups. The treatment group
received a back massage with normal conversation. One control group
received conversation only and the other no intervention. Each subject
received their intervention on four consecutive evenings. The Spielberger
state-trait anxiety self-evaluation questionnaire and physiological measures were taken prior to the study, directly after and ten minutes
later. There were no statistically significant changes in the physiological
measures. There was, however, a 'statistically significant difference in
the mean anxiety score between the back massage group and the no-
intervention group'. However, the results need to be considered in light
of the small sample size in each of the groups and lack of control of
variables within these groups. The same researcher provided the input
for the intervention and the control groups. As in other studies, the control groups themselves were having an effect on the subjects. It is also
possible that the ten-minute rest period experienced by all the subjects
could have effects of its own. Tutton (1987) found that rest periods
had both positive and negative effects on her elderly subjects. Questions
could also be raised about the value of using the anxiety scale three times
in quick succession. Familiarity with the tool may lead to bias in the
responses. The verbal responses following the massage were all very
positive, implying that a degree of relaxation, comfort and enjoyment had
been achieved.

An attempt to gather both qualitative and quantitative data in order to get a deeper understanding of individuals' experience of massage was made by Van der Riet (1993a). The study used a convenience sample of 60 gynaecological and general surgical patients randomly allocated into treatment and control groups. The treatment group received 45 minutes of Swedish massage with some reflexology of the feet. This period more adequately represents the amount of time a therapist would spend with a client. The control group, however, received no intervention at all. The Spielberger state-trait anxiety self-evaluation questionnaire was used as the measure of anxiety and was administered directly after the massage. No statistical differences were found between the two groups. The study utilized a post-test design and the control group knew they would not be receiving a massage. The control group did show evidence of higher trait anxiety scores. Mixing general and gynaecological surgery may have implications in relation to issues of gender. Attempts in the study to link length of stay and analgesia uptake to one intervention of massage without controlling the variables are unhelpful.

The second part of this paper (Van der Riet 1993b) considers the interactions that took place during and after the massage and the field notes kept by the researcher. An unstructured interview took place with the subjects after the massage session. Evidence of the use of questions and the subsequent process of analysis was not provided. The subjects described feelings of 'acceptance, respect for the body and being cared for'. It improved their sense of 'well-being and self-worth'. Some subjects felt physically more mobile. Many subjects particularly the women, felt able to talk about their emotions, life experiences and worries. All the subjects, with the exception of one, felt the effect of the massage had been calming and relaxing. Several subjects also found the massage to be healing: 'I feel this massage will heal me'. The individuals in this study are providing evidence that the experience of massage is multifaceted and has much wider implications than the earlier studies suggest. More rigorous research studies are needed to examine this area further.

Overall, the studies indicate that physiological measurements of massage-induced relaxation are inconclusive. However, subjects' responses to well-being after massage are mainly positive in nature. Several studies (e.g. Joachim 1983b, Van der Riet 1993b) have attempted to ascertain the subjects' experience of the intervention in a systematic way. More rigorous systematic qualitative research is needed to really examine the process and meanings ascribed to the experience of giving and receiving massage. The choice of experimental design for this type of intervention is problematic. As with the studies on therapeutic touch, the intervention is short and taken out of context. The use of anxiety as a dependent measure without first understanding the nature of massage and its effect on individuals is unhelpful. The use of control groups is also difficult as the control groups themselves obviously have their own independent effect. Our understanding of this intervention would be facilitated by further research examining its use in practice, with particular emphasis on the receiver's perspective.

## Principles of giving massage

Massage can be described as the manipulation of soft body tissue by the hand for therapeutic purposes. Different authors suggest variations on the method of massage. Jackson (1977) suggests using four different strokes.

*Effleurage or superficial stroking*: A longitudinal stroke, light to moderate in pressure, which warms the tissues and calms the receiver. It is usually used on the full length of the back and a massage should start and finish with this stroke.

*Petrissage or circular or deep transverse stroking*: This is a moderate to deep stroke used to feel the muscles and other tissues to discover where tension lies.

*Kneading*: This is manipulation of underlying tissue using the thumb and fingers of the hand. It is a deep manipulation and may be used on problem areas throughout the massage.

*Friction*: This is a deep circular motion using the thumb, knuckles or ends of the fingers. The pressure is concentrated in a small area.

The speed at which a massage is performed is of great importance. A rushed massage will cause tension to build up in the receiver. The action should be slow and deliberate and carried out in a relaxed manner so that rapport is established with the subject. It is essential to establish a good rhythm of movement and breathing which should remain constant throughout the massage. Joachim (1983b) and Jackson (1977) agree on how a massage should be performed. They both indicate that a quiet warm room should be chosen, away from interruptions. Both the giver and receiver need to be in comfortable positions. The giver's hands must be washed in warm water and the oil or other medium applied directly on to the hands so that it is warm before being applied to the receiver. Jackson (1977) believes that a holistic massage energy is passed from giver to receiver. The giver should therefore be centred or focused and feel free from all negative feelings, otherwise these will be picked up by the receiver. The receiver also needs to concentrate all her energy on what she is feeling and in doing so, directs positive feelings and energy towards herself as well as the giver.

**Exercise 7 Centring** Find yourself a quiet place and make yourself comfortable. Close your eyes. Concentrate your mind on your breathing and take slow, full, deep breaths. Empty your mind of all the worrying tensions of the day and replace them with thoughts of love, peace and happiness. Practise this for a few minutes, several times. For further information about centring read Krieger (1979), Chapter 4.

In practice I have found centring a useful exercise to perform for a few seconds between caring for different patients. It provides a break after the last patient and enables me to concentrate more fully on the following patient.

The massage can last as long as both parties enjoy the exercise. However, Jackson (1977) suggests that 30 minutes is necessary for a full back massage. Breakey (1982) sees a ten-minute massage as providing the relaxation necessary to induce a full night's sleep. Joachim (1983b) also feels that ten minutes is adequate to massage one part of the body effectively.

**Exercise 8   Foot massage**   Find yourself a partner with whom you feel safe and comfortable and who is prepared to join in this exercise. Decide who is going to perform the massage first. It is important that you both experience giving and receiving massage as it is necessary to understand the feelings involved in both giving and receiving touch.

Find a warm comfortable place where you are free from interruptions. You will need some oil – grapeseed oil or almond oil are useful as they are quite light and odourless – and a towel for resting the feet upon and for wiping excess oil off your hands.

When you are ready, get into positions where you are both comfortable and the feet are accessible. The person who is giving the massage now 'centres' herself using exercise 7. Now place some oil onto your hands and rub them together to warm the oil. Firmly use your hands to smooth oil over the whole of one foot.

For the purpose of this exercise, I have planned a set of massage sequences for you to follow, mainly using petrissage (see Figures 10.1–10.5). Experienced masseuses do not always follow a set procedure but use their experience and intuition. However, by describing a procedure I hope to provide a basis for future massage experiences. Throughout this first massage collect information from the receiver about the effect your touch is having on them. Your partner may want you to press harder or more softly and she may like some areas massaged more than others. In consequent massages, the receiver may want to remain quiet and concentrate on enjoying the experience of being massaged. If you should find an area that causes pain, work around the edge of this area. All the time, the giver needs to be aware of her breathing and the speed of her strokes.

At the end of the massage repeat the procedure on the other foot, then change roles so that the giver is the receiver and vice versa. Share your

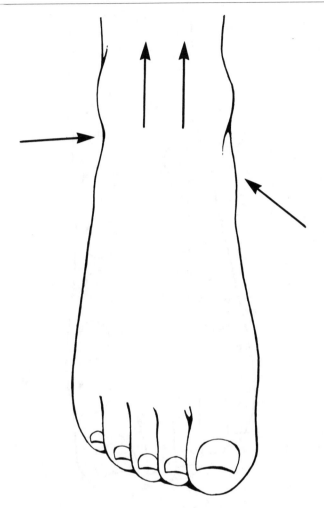

**Figure 10.1** Using alternating thumbs, stroke the area between the ankle bone in a forwards direction whilst maintaining pressure underneath the ankle bone with your fingers.

experiences with each other. In my experience foot massage has been particularly useful with elderly patients who have experienced strokes or fractured neck of femurs. At the end of a heavy day, much of it spent regaining the skills of walking, they said that foot massage made them feel relaxed, happy and cared for. I enjoyed giving the massage and felt it increased the level of rapport and facilitated disclosure between myself and my patients. Once you feel confident performing a foot massage, try massaging one of your patients.

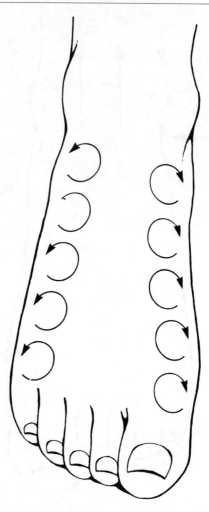

**Figure 10.2** Work with your thumbs down the side of the foot using moderate pressure and a circular movement.

### Evaluating the massage

Evaluating the effect on the patient is an important part of the massage. The information gained from the evaluation may be used as a basis for making decisions relating to the massage technique, the timing, duration or frequency of the massage or its discontinuation. The two main methods of evaluating massage are observing the effect it is having on the patient and asking the patient to provide a verbal report.

Physical observations of vital signs in patients who have received a massage have been shown to be unreliable (Barr and Taslitz 1970,

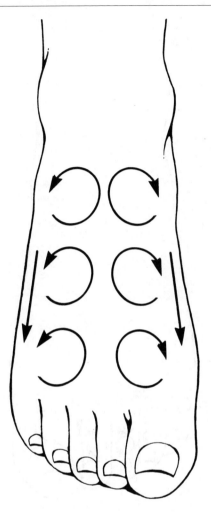

**Figure 10.3** Using the same stroke but with larger circles, work up the foot with both thumbs and then down the sides.

Kaufmann 1964). Other observable signs might be used, such as changes in the patient's appearance, depth and speed of breathing, muscle tone, posture, vocal tone or level of activity. Massage will affect people in different ways. Some of my patients fell asleep and others wanted to talk. Whatever observations are made, it is useful to have a description of the patient before and after the massage.

Asking a patient how he or she feels is a useful way of obtaining information. Tutton (1987) asked elderly patients how they felt after a back massage. They gave responses such as 'That feels comforting, soothing,

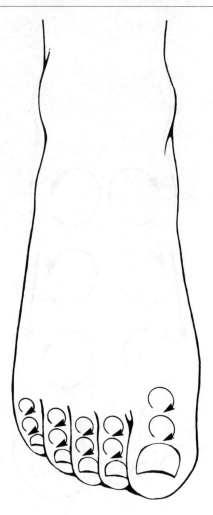

**Figure 10.4** Rest one hand underneath the foot whilst the other works on the toes. Using one hand, continue the circular action up the full length of the toe. At the end of the toe, hold firmly for a few seconds. Repeat on all five toes.

beautiful, you have a lovely touch', ' I feel relaxed, could fall asleep', 'It's not aching so much, you have eased my backache'. Alternatively, if you are using massage to relieve a specific symptom a simple scale may be used to assess the intensity of the symptom before and after the massage. For example, if a patient complains of an awful nagging ache in her left leg, a five-point scale could then be formulated using the patient's own words (Figure 10.6).

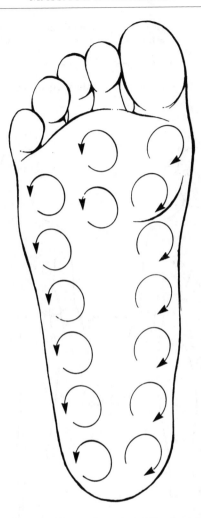

**Figure 10.5** Move hands smoothly to the sole of the foot. Work from the heel to the toes using the same circular movements. To finish, place the back of one hand against the sole of the foot and rest for one minute.

Another method used by Tutton (1987) to measure the area of discomfort is the body map (Figure 10.7). Patients mark on the body map the extent of their discomfort. The area can then be estimated using graph tracing paper and comparisons made.

| Awful nagging ache | very bad ache | a moderate ache | a slight ache | no ache |
|---|---|---|---|---|

**Figure 10.6** An example of a five-point scale used to measure symptom relief.

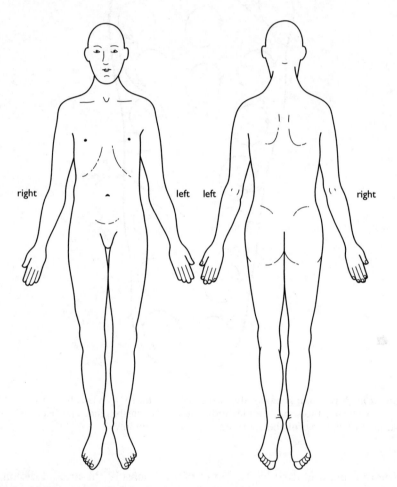

**Figure 10.7** An example of a body map that can be used to measure the area of discomfort in patients.

## CONCLUSION

Nurses, as the key providers of intimate physical care and by virtue of their continual presence, are in a prime position to use touch to its fullest potential. The selected review of the studies exploring touch have, despite flaws in the methods, revealed the possible benefits of touch to patients' well-being. Patients appreciate being touched (Kaufmann 1964, Lorensen 1983) and touch can increase attention and non-verbal responses (Langland and Panicucci 1982, McCorkle 1974) as well as verbal responses (McCorkle 1974). Therapeutic touch has been shown significantly to reduce anxiety (Heidt 1981, Quinn 1984), as has massage (Longworth 1982). Joachim (1983b) has demonstrated that massage and deep breathing can increase patients' feelings of control as well as their ability to sleep and relax. Patients' symptom distress has also been shown to decrease with massage (Sims 1986a). However, there are some interesting findings relating to who nurses touch. For instance, the amount of touch patients receive tends to decrease with age and touch often relates to the patient's condition (Aguilera 1967, Barnett 1972b). This suggests that the individual's attitude to or beliefs about the patient may affect their use of touch.

Future studies on touch need to focus on real situations where touch is used in practice and explore the experiences of the givers and receivers of touch. Research by Estabrooks (1989), Estabrooks and Morse (1992), Heidt (1990), Samarel (1992) and Van der Riet (1993b) has explored our understanding of touch by using qualitative research methods. These studies have started to provide the indepth data needed to establish the basis for further research. Finally, if touch is to be used to its full potential, nurses need to explore their own attitudes and beliefs about their patients and to analyse critically their use of touch in practice. My own positive experiences of using massage with elderly people inspired me to further exploration and I hope other nurses will feel the same.

## REFERENCES

Aguilera, D. C. (1967) Relationships between physical contact and verbal interaction between nurses and patients. *Journal of Psychiatric Nursing*, Jan–Feb, 5–21.

Auckett, A. (1979) Baby massage: an alternative to drugs. *Australian Nurses' Journal*, **9**(5) 24–27.

Barnett, K. (1972a) A theoretical contrast of the concepts of touch as they relate to nursing. *Nursing Research*, **21**(2), 102–109.

Barnett, K. (1972b) A survey of the current utilization of touch by health team personnel with hospitalised patients. *International Journal of Nursing Studies*, **9**, 195–209.

Barr, J. and Taslitz, N. (1970) The influence of back massage on autonomic functions, *Physical Therapy*, **50**(12), 1679–1691.

Booth, C. C., Johnston-Crowley, N. and Barnard, K. E. (1985) Infant massage and exercise, worth the effort? *American Journal of Maternal and Child Nursing*, **10**(3), 184–189.

Breakey, B. (1982) An overlooked therapy you can use ad lib. R.N., July, 50–54.

Burnside, I. (1973) Touching is talking. *American Journal of Nursing*, **73**(12), 2060–2063.

Click, M. (1986) Caring touch and anxiety in myocardial infarction patients in the intermediate cardiac care unit. *Intensive Care Nursing*, **2**(2), 61–66.

Davies, S. and Riches, L. (1995) Healing touch. *Nursing Times*, **91**(25), 42–43.

Debelle, B. (1981) Relaxation and baby massage. *Australian Nurses' Journal*, **1**, 16–17.

Estabrooks, C. (1987) Touch in nursing practice, an historical perspective. *Journal of Nursing History*, **2**(2), 33–49.

Estabrooks, C. (1989) Touch: a nursing strategy in ICU. *Heart and Lung*, **18**, 392–401.

Estabrooks, C. and Morse, J. (1992) Toward a theory of touch: the touching process and acquiring a touching style. *Journal of Advanced Nursing*, **17**, 448–456.

Ernst, F. and Shaw, J. (1980) Touching is not taboo. *Geriatric Nursing*, **1**(5), 193–195.

Fraser, J. and Ross Kerr, J. (1993) Psychophysiological effects of back massage on elderly institutionalized patients. *Journal of Advanced Nursing*, **18**(2), 238–245.

Goodykoontz, L. (1979) Touch: attitudes and practice. *Nursing Forum*, **18**(1), 4–17.

Grad, B., Cadoret, R. and Paul, G. (1961) An unorthodox method of treatment on wound healing in mice. *International Journal of Parapsychology*, **3**, 5–24.

Hefferman, A. and Mott, S. (1984) Baby massage – a teaching model. *Australian Nurses' Journal*, **13**(6), 36–37.

Heidt, P. (1981) Effects of therapeutic touch on anxiety level of hospitalised patients. *Nursing Research*, **31**, 32–37.

Heidt, P. (1990) Openness: a qualitative analysis of nurses' and patients' experiences of therapeutic touch. *Image: Journal of Nursing Scholarship*, **22**(3), 180–186.

Heidt, P. (1991) Helping patients to rest: clinical studies in therapeutic touch. *Holistic Nursing Practice*, **5**(4), 57–66.

Hollinger, L. (1980) Perception of touch in the elderly. *Journal of Gerontological Nursing*, **6**(12), 741–746.

Holmes, P. (1986) Fringe benefits. *Nursing Times*, **82**(20), 22.

Husband, L. (1988) Therapeutic touch: a basis for excellence, in *Recent Advances in Nursing: Excellence in Nursing*, (ed. R. Johnson), Churchill Livingstone, Edinburgh.

Jackson, R. (1977) *Massage Therapy: The Holistic Way to Physical and Mental Health*, Thorsons, Wellingborough.

Jackson, S. (1985) The touch process in rehabilitation. *Australian Nurses' Journal*, **14**(11), 43–45.

Joachim, G. (1983a) Step-by-step massage techniques. *Canadian Nurse*, **4**, 32–35.

Joachim G. (1983b) The effects of two stress management techniques on feelings of well-being in patients with inflammatory bowel disease. *Nursing Paper*, **14**(4), 5–18.

Johnson, B. (1965) The meaning of touch in nursing. *Nursing Outlook*, **13**, 59–60.

Kaufmann, M. A. (1964) Autonomic responses as related to nursing comfort measures. *Nursing Research*, **13**(1), 45–55.

Knable, J. (1981) Hand holding: one means of transcending barriers of communication. *Heart and Lung*, **10**(6), 1106–1111.

Krieger, D. (1975) The therapeutic touch: the imprimatur of nursing. *American Journal of Nursing*, **75**(5), 748–787.

Krieger, D. (1979) *The Therapeutic Touch: How to Use Your Hands to Help and Heal*, Prentice-Hall, New Jersey.

Lader, M. and Matthews, A. (1970) Comparison of methods of relaxation using physiological measures. *Behavioural Research and Therapy Journal*, **8**, 331–337.

Langland, R. M. and Panicucci, C. (1982) Effects of touch on communication with elderly confused patients. *Journal of Gerontological Nursing*, **8**, 152–155.

Le May, A. (1986) The human connection. *Nursing Times*, **82**(47), 28–30.

Le May, A. and Redfern, S. (1987) A study of non-verbal communication between nurses and elderly patients, in *Research in the Nursing Care of Elderly People*, (ed. P. Fielding), John Wiley, Chichester.

Locsin, A. (1984) The concept of touch. *Philippine Journal of Nursing*, **54**(4), 114–123.

Longworth, J. (1982) Psychophysiological effects of slow stroke back massage in normotensive females. *Advances in Nursing Science*, **4**(4), 44–61.

Lorensen, M. (1983) Effects of touch in patients during a crisis situation in hospital, in *Nursing Research: Ten Studies in Patient Care*, (ed. J. Wilson-Barnett), John Wiley, Chichester.

Mason, A. (1988) Massage, in *Complementary Health Therapies: A Guide for Nurses and the Caring Professions*, (ed. D. Rankin-Box), Croom Helm, London.

McCorkle, R. (1974) Effects of touch on seriously ill patients. *Nursing Research*, **23**, 125–132.

McCorkle, R. (1981) Non-obtrusive measures in clinical research, in *Cancer Nursing Update* (ed. R. Tiffany), Cassell Ltd., London.

McNair, D. and Lorr, M. (1964) An analysis of mood in neurotics. *Journal of Abnormal Psychology*, **69**, 620–627.

Meek, S. (1993) Effects of slow stroke back massage on relaxation in hospice clients. *Image: Journal of Nursing Scholarship*, **25**(1), 17–21.

Melia, K. (1987) *Learning and Working: the Occupational Socialisation of Nurses*, Tavistock, London.

Murphy, E. (1984) Practical management course, Module 15. High Touch techniques for managing the environment. *Nursing Management*, **15**(11), 79–81.

Naisbitt, J. (1982) *Megatrends*, Warner Brooks, New York.

Pearson, A. and Vaughan, B. (1986) *Nursing Models for Practice*, Heinemann, London.

Pearson, A., Durand, I. and Punton, S. (1988) *Therapeutic Nursing: An Evaluation of an Experimental Nursing Unit in the British NHS*, Burford and Oxford Nursing Development Units, Oxford.

Preston, T. (1973) When words fail (caring for the aged). *American Journal of Nursing*, **73**, 2064–2066.

Quinn, J. (1989) Therapeutic touch as energy exchange: replication and extension. *Nursing Science Quarterly*, **2**(2), 79–87.

Randolph, G. (1984) Therapeutic and physical touch: physiological response to stressful stimuli! *Nursing Research*, **33**(1), 33–36.

Rowlands, D. (1984) Therapeutic touch: its effects on the depressed elderly. *Australian Nurses' Journal*, **13**(11), 45–52.

Samarel, N. (1992) The experience of receiving therapeutic touch. *Journal of Advanced Nursing*, **17**, 651–657.

Seaman, L. (1982) Affective nursing touch. *Geriatric Nursing*, **3**(3), 162–164.

Simington, J. and Laing, G. (1993) Effects of therapeutic touch on anxiety in the institutionalised elderly. *Clinical Nursing Research*, **2**(4), 438–450.

Sims, S. (1986) The effects of slow-stroke back massage on the perceived well-being of female patients receiving radiotherapy for cancer. MSc thesis in Nursing, King's College, University of London.

Turton, P. (1988) *Healing Therapies: A Guide for Nurses and the Caring Professions*, Croom Helm, London.

Turton, P. (1989) Touch me, feel me, heal me. *Nursing Times*, **85**(19), 42–44.

Tutton, E. (1987) The effect of slow-stroke back massage on the perceived well-being of elderly female patients in a nursing unit. MSc thesis in Nursing, King's College, University of London.

Van der Riet, P. (1993a) Effects of therapeutic massage on pre-operative anxiety in a rural hospital: Part 1. *Australian Journal of Rural Health*, **1**(4), 11–16.

Van der Riet, P. (1993b) Effects of therapeutic massage on pre-operative anxiety in a rural hospital: Part 2. *Australian Journal of Rural Health*, **1**(4): 17–21.

Watson, W. H. (1975) The meanings of touch: geriatric nursing. *Journal of Communication*, **25**, 104–110.

Weinrich, S. and Weinrich, M. (1990) The effect of massage on pain in cancer patients. *Applied Nursing Research*, **3**(4), 140–145.

Wharton, A. and Pearson, A. (1988) Nursing and intimate physical care: the key to therapeutic nursing, in *Primary Nursing: Nursing in the Burford and Oxford Nursing Development Unit*, (ed. A Pearson), Croom Helm, London.

Wise, R. (1989) Flower power. *Nursing Times*, **85**(22), 45–47.

# 11

# An evaluation of humanism as a philosophy for nursing practice in an era of rational-scientific health care

Christine McKee and Nick Bowles

## INTRODUCTION

Humanism has been a major influence upon nurse education and nursing practice for over two decades. Regarded by some as a natural philosophy for nursing and by others as 'sugar coated and ambiguous', the basic premises and application of humanism within the postreform NHS (and other health-care systems) require a contemporary re-evaluation.

Within this chapter the drive for evidence-based practice is acknowledged and provides an opportunity to discuss the place of natural sciences as a theoretical basis for nursing. It is argued that as man and the world he occupies are unpredictable and complex, natural science is an inadequate tool to generate understanding and to guide nursing practice.

The nature of man is discussed in a review of existentialist ideas which inform humanistic theory. The key elements of humanism are critically reviewed with some contemporary responses to some of the most frequently advanced criticisms. The application of humanism to nursing practice is discussed, with reference to Paterson and Zderad's ground-breaking seminal model, Donald Schön's concept of the reflective practitioner and more recent nursing research.

This is followed with a concise examination of phenomenology, generally regarded as the research base of most relevance to humanism, and consideration of its relevance during an era which is likely to be dominated by large-scale objective research in the tradition of medical and natural science. The chapter concludes with reflection upon the relationship between nursing science and natural science and the role of humanistic nursing practice.


## THE PROMISE OF 'EVIDENCE-BASED PRACTICE'

The generation and use of knowledge is one of the major tasks currently facing health professionals. Nurses, as the largest professional group in the NHS, must come to terms with the need to be research based, to be able to demonstrate that a sound and possibly even 'proven' basis exists for that which they do to or with patients (and with 'public' money).

If the 1980's were most noteworthy as the start of the era of NHS reforms, then the mid-1990s may well be seen as the beginning of the rational, research-based NHS, in which care and treatment were increasingly informed by clinical guidelines, effectiveness literature, critical reviews, meta-analysis and evidence-based practice.

However, the road to research-based practice within nursing has been tortuous, nursing graduates are still a minority group, many nurses still do not possess research skills, are unable to critically evaluate research findings and will benefit little from published research. Those that do read widely and critically often face narrow perspectives which do not reflect the complexity of professional practice. Incomprehensible scientific or academic jargon, small-scale research and an almost complete absence of critical reviews compound their difficulties and limit generalizability to their own practice.

However, the need for clarity, for answers on what is or is not effective remains, indeed, it is imperative, as Degenberg observed: 'One of the most important goals of the NHS is to secure, through available resources, the greatest improvement in the ... health of the population' (Degenberg 1996:37).

Only two years after the major thrust of the NHS reforms, a strategy for research and development in the NHS was commissioned. Since then, centres with a specific remit on the generation and use of research-based knowledge in the NHS have been set up, including the Centre for Reviews and Dissemination, the Cochrane Database, the National Clinical Audit Information and Dissemination Centre, the UK Outcome Clearing House and the Centre for Evidence-Based Medicine in Oxford. Other centres such as the Nuffield Institute for Health are also engaged in relevant work.

At an individual level, changes are also visible. Researchers are increasingly aware of the need to promote the accessibility of their findings, by writing in a suitable manner for the readership. Some research intended for a nursing audience is exemplary in this respect – for example the freely available 'Research Highlights' series published by the English National Board for Nurses, Midwives and Health Visitors and those produced by the School of Nursing at the University of Manchester. Whilst these are undoubtedly positive developments, the research paradigm underpinning much of the 'effectiveness literature' is the so-called scientific method, which relies chiefly upon large, expensive and lengthy controlled randomized trials (RRTs), usually spanning broad sections of the population. Outcomes are determined as significant on the basis of objective, statistical evidence and are not intended to reflect the lived experience of the patients who participated in the RRT and the local variations which influenced their care, treatment and outcome. The 'gold standard' of evidence-based practice, the 'systematic review' is based upon several studies, usually RCTs, increasing sample size, reliability and ability to generalize. Weaknesses and one-off phenomena are minimized to a level of insignificance which renders them largely invisible.

The allure of certainty and the extinction of ambiguity is undeniable, as is the potential that evidence-based approaches provide for lay people (and managers!) to question so-called 'professional judgement'. Yet the suitability of this approach to knowledge creation for nurses has been questioned and the reasons for this are explored below.


## WAYS OF KNOWING

During the Dark and Middle Ages, knowledge was regarded as the preserve of a privileged minority (primarily members of religious orders) and this knowledge was derived from the Greeks. Effectively it was a static and dependent medium, which did not recognize the value of individual enquiry; for example, to learn about bees, one didn't observe bees, instead one went to the manuscripts to read what the ancients had written about them.

During the Renaissance (literally 'rebirth') this changed; indeed, the structure of whole societies shifted and many prevailing attitudes were overthrown. Pioneers like Francis Bacon taught that all knowledge had not yet been acquired, promoting an investigative fervour. Bacon's key legacy was a systematic method of acquiring knowledge, now referred to as the 'scientific method', which relies on dispassionate experimentation to discover natural laws or incontrovertible facts.

An important part of the scientific method is the notion of 'determinism', i.e. that if the same experiment is performed under the same conditions, the same outcome will be observable time after time. For centuries scientists believed that determinism itself was a law of nature and that, given an adequate understanding of the initial conditions and all the mechanisms involved, an outcome could always be predicted. Hence, man, nature and the universe were regarded as predictable.

Throughout the ensuing centuries scientific achievements have been dramatic, largely based on this method. Consequently, many disciplines, including nursing, have attempted to use its philosophies and methods to advance their own understanding. Benner and Wrubel (1989) argue that the majority of present-day nursing theories are in the tradition of classic 17th century science and as such maintain that a human being, like the universe, can be considered machine-like, orderly, predictable, observable and measurable.

However, application of the scientific method to nursing has not been as successful as in other fields. It tends to have a dehumanizing effect and encourages a fragmentation of the individual into parts and systems, the antithesis of holism. Aggleton and Chalmers (1986) suggest that nurses commonly regard nursing models as being mechanistic in their identification of human needs and consequently they dehumanize the 'process of nursing by drawing an analogy between a human being and a machine'. This is an orientation which underpins task allocation and labelling, inhibiting close or intimate nursing care.

A further problem with the scientific method is that it often doesn't work, as it is a poor predictor of outcomes in complex situations. Benner (1985) cites Merleau-Ponty (1962) in arguing that no strictly bottom-up explanation, i.e. explanation from the cellular level up to the lived experience of health and illness can adequately predict or accurately explain the particular course of an illness. Nor can it explain the maintenance of health; laboratory data frequently do not match the illness experience, nor do people live or die strictly according to biochemical or physiological accounts.

It is interesting to observe that even in the natural sciences the scientific method and determinism have not been completely successful. In the 1920s the confusing world of quantum mechanics proved what some scientists had suspected for some time: that determinism is not a law of nature. Specifically, scientists who were attempting to predict the position and motion of the electron in its orbit around the atom's nucleus found that it could not be done. They concluded that motion within the atom, the fundamental building block of the universe, is governed by probability. Later studies of photons (light particles) have proved even more perplexing, with some physicists suggesting that the act of observing photons affects their behaviour! Hence the world we live in is not totally predictable, after all.

Given that man is neither wholly determined by observable phenomena nor entirely predictable and behaves in a way which may not be understood by reductionist analysis, an alternative model for understanding and interaction is required. One such model is humanism, derived from the philosophical school of existentialism. These are discussed below.

## EXISTENTIALISM

Existentialism is a philosophy most closely associated with Jean Paul Sartre (1977). Essentially antipositivist (and therefore descendent from the European neo-Kantian tradition), existentialism is a complex philosophy which many authors have selectively described and augmented, to the point where it has been suggested that there are as many existentialisms as there are existentialist philosophers (Clemence 1966). However, few would disagree that existentialism is the study of human existence. A derivative of the Latin verb *'exsistere'*, literally to stand out from, emerge or become, existentialism concerns being, becoming and choices. Hence existence is emergence, a process of becoming, rather than a defined and static state of being (Graham 1986).

Analysis of the existentialist literature indicates the presence of several key themes.

1  Individual existence is not a state of being, rather it is a process of becoming
2  The individual makes him/herself, through the courageous and honest use of freedom in the face of situational limits such as illness, grief, anxiety and solitude (Clemence 1966)
3  With freedom come choice and personal responsibility
4  Aloneness is a fundamental condition of life, as the individual nature of lived experience traps us within our own separate realities which we are never able to comprehend or communicate completely
5  Determinism and human predictability are wholly rejected, on the grounds that one cannot predict what one cannot fully understand, i.e. another person
6  The belief that life and others are to be studied from the inside out or from the 'view of the lived life' (Gulino 1982); hence phenomenology should be used in the study of being
7  Groups, classes and categories should not be applied to individuals, whose will may transcend such classification.

In short, human beings are unique and unpredictable and may only be viewed humanistically, i.e. as a whole and with emphasis upon the individual's own perspective.

## THE RISE OF HUMANISM

In the late 1960s humanism emerged as a psychological school whose key protagonists include Carl Rogers and Abraham Maslow. Humanism grew out of European existentialism and the seeds (if not the 'flowering') of equality and democracy in 1960s North America (Brown and Pedder 1994). It represents an attractive and beneficent alternative to the existent psychological schools of psychoanalysis and neobehaviourism and has attracted supporters in psychology and mental health, education, social work and in particular nursing.

Just as humanism represents an alternative to psychological traditions, its use as the underpinning of nursing, as a 'human science' (Watson 1985), also permits differentiation from the rational, scientific tradition of medicine in which 'the individual is rarely viewed as a whole person' (Busfield 1986:26). Indeed, the adoption of humanism within nursing is regarded by Bevis (1982) as a maturational high point for the nursing profession, which espouses fundamental values of equity, respect for persons and caring (RCN 1987).

In recent years, these values have been associated with the language of choice, empowerment and partnerships between client and nurse, the emergence of individualized patient care, primary nursing and the 'new nurse' (Salvage 1990) whose use of self may be both 'therapeutic' (Travelbee 1966) and 'beneficial' (Redfern 1996).

Yet this approach and its philosophical underpinnings have been widely criticized. Mulholland (1995) argues that the fundamental idealism of humanism ignores social realities, including class and gender inequalities, which are inextricably linked with ill health and the power differential between practitioner and client. This view is also expressed by Masson (1993) in a work which is predicated on the basis that therapy diverts attention from the real causes of human misery, fosters dependency and therefore diminishes the 'dignity, autonomy and freedom' of the person who seeks help. Mulholland (1995) adds that as existentialists hold individuals responsible for their own predicament, 'victim blaming' may replace understanding. He goes on to cite Seedhouse (1986), arguing that a 'sugar coating of ambiguity' is the feature which attracts nurses to humanism, possibly as a vehicle to maintain epistemological mystique within an era of proletarianization or, more prosaically perhaps, out of intellectual laziness. Others have questioned whether patients actually want the 'new nursing'. Kadner (1994) argues, not unreasonably, that nurse–patient intimacy may not always be necessary or even welcome and may be intrusive. This is echoed by Waterworth and Luker (1990), who argue that patients do not always want to be involved in their own care, and by Salvage (1990) who, whilst an articulate and convincing exponent of the 'new nursing', warns against the use of quasi-psychotherapeutic nursing interventions.

The majority of these criticisms ignore the task-oriented legacy from which nursing has emerged, which subordinated the patient to the smooth running of the organization, and the medical illness–cure model, which subordinated the needs of the individual to the cure of their illness. If therapy diverts attention from social ills, then illness traditionally diverted attention away from the person. Humanistic nursing seeks to redress this imbalance and values the person's subjective perception of their predica-ment. If the client exercises their right to opt for a 'passive, dependent role in relation to their carers' (Redfern 1996) then this is acceptable; indeed, as Bowlby observed, to an extent it is almost an inevitable part of illness (Hunter 1990). Fiduciary nurse–client partnerships cannot be imposed!

Furthermore, attacks on the existential underpinnings of humanism as precursors to victim blaming are naive, as the authors hold the opinion that victim blaming is incompatible with an empathic understanding of the client's situation and the application of the core values articulated by the Royal College of Nursing, described above. Humanistic nursing regards the client's 'wishes, goals, needs and resources' as its starting point and draws upon an existential base in that the client's achievement of these wishes is regarded as the result of the client's own activity (Holmes 1990). In short, humanistic nursing is oriented to helping the client exercise control over his/her situation; 'it dismantles the dehumanizing' aspects of health-care provider organizations (Holmes 1990) and is congruent with the post-NHS reform reconceptualization of patient as informed consumer. Humanism is a philosophy *of* nursing and *for* nursing and fits within a consumer-oriented framework.

## APPLICATION TO NURSING CARE

Humanism is one of several modes of thought guiding nursing theory. Others include systems, developmental and symbolic interactionist theo-ries, all of which are closely linked to the scientific method and, as such, are deterministic. Systems theory seeks to place the individual at the centre of an interlocking feedback system, often no larger than the immediate family which supposedly can be understood and adjusted, quite possibly in line with the professional's view of how things should be. Symbolic interaction-ism (threads of which can be seen in most nursing models), whilst an interesting approach to the divination of meaning, can be mechanistic. As Pearson and Vaughan (1986) suggest, symbolic interactionism holds that a person's responses to a given situation can be predicted. Likewise, developmental theory centres around growth and change which occur in recognized stages and are caused by identifiable variables and move in a predictable direction (Pearson and Vaughan 1986).

In contrast, only humanism recognizes the individual's ability to construe circumstances idiosyncratically and act in a unique way (Sarvimaki 1988). Humanistic nursing regards the person as a unique and essentially unpredictable whole and emphasizes the validity of an individual's lived experience. This experience is irreducible to component parts or interpretive eclecticism.

Paterson and Zderad (1976) offer a description of humanistic nursing which, whilst the subject of some well-placed criticism (McKinnon 1991) and bearing the esoteric hallmarks of American nursing theory, remains an enabling and positive interpretation of humanism in practice. They describe the humanistic approach to nursing practice as a 'system, mode of thought or action' in which human interests, values and dignity are of primary importance. The person is regarded as a whole rather than a series of problems to be solved and the act of nursing as the nurturing response of one person to another in need. They urge the nurse to be with the patient in the fullest sense, which requires attention and communication of the nurse's therapeutic availability.

In order to be completely effective in this way, the nurse must herself approach nursing as an existential experience. Nursing is itself a lived experience, a response to a human situation which the nurse shares with another. It involves a transactional relationship which requires self-awareness, respect for the other and personal commitment. It cannot be imposed by an outside authority, any more than liking for another person can be decreed.

For those nurses wishing to apply humanistic ideas, Paterson and Zderad (1976) elucidate the principles in terms of actions within the nurse–client relationship. These they term 'meeting', 'relating', 'presence', 'call and response'; each is discussed below.

### Meeting

At the first meeting, the patient and nurse each brings their own set of goals and expectations. They both share the implicit expectation that the nurse will be helpful and that the patient needs assistance. Beyond that, each is a unique individual bringing all that they are or are not and, if the meeting is planned, each comes with feelings of anticipation, anxiety, dread, hope, fear, pleasure, impatience, hostility, dependence, responsibility. Each has a choice of openness and each may have a different view of the precise need and the kind of help required. In addition, the nurse may have prior knowledge of the patient and may bring preconceived ideas, labels or stereotypes which should be consciously processed and dropped.

### Relating

Humanistic nursing and humanistic communication is founded on the work of Buber and his 'I–Thou' paradigm, which identifies two classes (the authors prefer to think of these as ends of a continuum) to describe the quality of interpersonal communication (Duldt and Giffin 1985). One end of the continuum is referred to as 'I–It', in which one person views another as an object, ignoring their unique 'human characterization', consequently devaluing and dehumanizing the person (Duldt 1991). The other paradigm is 'I–Thou', in which the communication enables each to value the other, develops and is perceived as humanizing on both sides (although as Dudlt (1991) points out, if the nurse feels neutral but the client feels the nurse is 'coming across' as humanizing, then this is perfectly acceptable).

## Presence

Presence involves being with the patient in the fullest sense, being open and available. The nurse may be attentive but refuse to give of him or herself. Actions may not necessarily signify presence, but presence can be revealed directly and unmistakably in a glance, touch or tone of voice. This is a theme Benner (1984) develops and one which she regards as a key element of nursing expertise. Contained within genuine dialogue is a quality of unpredictability or spontaneity, which requires openness, receptivity and availability.

## Call and response

Call and response are transactional – the patient calls for help, the nurse responds. The nurse calls for the patient's participation and the patient responds. The patient's call may be non-verbal and may be indicated by posture, colour or facial expression. The nurse's response (i.e. in terms of urgency, content etc.) is influenced by her perception of the patient's independence, motivation, rehabilitation, growth and strengths.

## PLANNING CARE

Paterson and Zderad (1976) give no clear guidance concerning a goal-directed nursing care plan, perhaps due to a belief that the philosophy underpinning care plans contains an element of determinism and pre-dictability, which humanism rejects. The 'goal' is the increased well-being of the client, expressed in terms which have meaning to him. In attempting to divide the patient into a list of problems, the nurse may lose sight of the complex relationships between those problems, which are often as important as the problems themselves.

To illustrate this principle, an analogy may be drawn with a protein molecule, which is a long chain of amino acids. This chain is folded over on itself to form a compact, ball-like structure. This shape allows the protein molecule to interact with others. Any effort to string out the protein molecule in order to itemize its component amino acids 'denatures' the protein so that, having lost the shape it depended on, one can no longer understand how it functions. Likewise, an attempt to characterize the patient as a list of problems can lead to only a partial understanding of his situation.

Donald Schön (1983) has also raised concerns over the positivist problem-solving process. He suggests that practitioners inclined to a positivistic stance may respond to complex situations by selectively ignoring data which appear to confuse or disconfirm their prior understanding, i.e. to fit professional knowledge, a self-defeating mechanism well known in a clinical context to cognitive therapists. He refers to this as 'cutting the situation' to fit professional knowledge. Nurses who follow a problem-solving approach may find themselves narrowing their field of vision to take in only the problems which look as though they can be solved and stepping over those which appear insoluble. Moreover, the nurse who is orientated towards active solving may feel helpless in situations where she doesn't know what to do when simply being with, presencing and understanding are all that is needed.

Schön (1983) goes on to argue that a positivistic epistemology of practice rests upon three principles: the separation of means from ends, the separation of research from practice and the separation of knowing from doing, none of which holds in the 'real' world. As an alternative, Schön proposes his now well-known theory of 'reflection-in-action' as a description of what really happens in practice. This may be described as a conversation with the situation, during which practitioners will reflect on intuitive understandings of the phenomena which are derived from their own repertoire of familiar examples and themes. Using this approach, ideas are exchanged backwards and forwards, means and ends are framed interdependently, knowing and doing are inseparable. Therefore, the problem-solving cycle may be seen to be an inadequate vehicle for this dynamic process. The implications for nursing record keeping are discussed below.

## APPLICATION TO CLINICAL RECORD KEEPING

Humanistic nursing is potentially less limiting than problem-solving approaches because the nurse is not trying to 'solve' problems, but to draw upon the client's understanding and co-create a reality in which both can achieve a deeper understanding of the client's situation and enable the client to take control of his health situation. However, rejection of the familiar four-stage problem-solving cycle does not imply rejection of rigorous record keeping. On the contrary, Paterson and Zderad (1976) advocate a phenomenological approach, which should be as rigorous as the lived experience of being with the client.

If a humanistic nurse were to follow this guidance she would carefully record what she comes to know, that is, the knowable responses of the individual being nursed, the nurse's own observations and responses and also her experiences as a participant. The nursing record may in part take the form of a journal, but may bear little relation to standard forms of nursing or multiprofessional documentation.

In the late 1990s a number of developments are under way which will influence the manner in which nurses record their observations in clinical records and other forms of documentation. In the UK the foundations have been laid for an NHS-wide computer network which, it is expected, will enable transmission of electronic clinical records almost instantaneously. As these records will be available to health professionals in different locations, disciplines and specialisms, the possibility of differing interpretations of their content has been considered. In response, a national thesaurus of clinical terms has been compiled which will be available to clinicians at the point of data entry. This has some significance for the phenomenologists who prize the nuances of linguistics and who may reject preconceived classification systems. However, if one accepts that a mere fraction of the lived experience can be recorded, then it could also be argued that what is written into the record should have as wide a meaning as possible for the largest part of the potential readership.

It may be that the most valid container for full and vivid phenomenological records is the nurse's own professional portfolio, where the documentation of her experiences as a participant would be in keeping with the reflective nature of portfolio keeping and would also be confidential. It is not difficult to imagine that a humanistic nurse who applied the phenomenological approach to record keeping in a clinical setting may face a range of negative reactions, some born out of ignorance, perhaps, but others arising from the very real need for all members of the nursing team to have clear guidance to assist the delivery of nursing care when they are on duty. A further problem may be that the nurse's accounts of her own experience must perforce be written in such a way that they are not likely to upset or offend the client (who in the UK now has access to clinical records) and also that the nurse does not disclose so much of her self that she feels exposed or embarrassed. To draw an analogy with the author's own work, a common failing in some therapeutic encounters is that the novice worker commonly encourages high levels of personal disclosure from the client at an early stage in the relationship, with the result that clients feel embarrassed and often withdraw. It would be regrettable were this to happen to a nurse who attempted to fully document her experiences in the clinical record. It is not difficult to see how these factors may render such accounts so insipid that the phenomenological approach could not be said to be effective, and would be best undertaken in a personal reflective form.

A middle road can be taken, however, if the client is fully involved with the documentation of his care. If clinical terms are used, then an account of what this means to the client will also be documented (this has risk management benefits also). Goals should be written in the client's own words and these words should be used in nurse–client interactions. Some nurses encourage clients to describe their experience as a story which, if the client agrees, forms part of the clinical record. The authors have seen this technique used with the terminally ill, newly ostomized patients who, whilst reticent to talk, wanted to communicate, and with people recovering from anorexia nervosa. In essence, what fundamentally matters is that the client recognizes and 'owns' the documentation as relating to him; if it was a 'photo-fit', it should be recognizable! This is a challenge for all nurses, whether they subscribe to humanistic principles or not.

## PHENOMENOLOGY: THE RESEARCH BASIS OF HUMANISM

The growth of humanism reflects a move away from reductionist, determinist or mechanical explanations of human behaviour. This is a significant change and to some extent, it mirrors trends within scientific thinking, towards the recognition that predictability, causality and order are not fundamental laws of nature. A parallel may be drawn between the universe around us which, whilst not completely known to us, can be approached ever more closely and another individual, who may be understood more fully using the research method of phenomenology.

Phenomena can be defined as any object or occurrence perceived by the senses. Natural, objective science cannot accommodate subjective experience (Strawson 1974); indeed, it has been suggested that even the language of positivistic science is too impoverished to give an adequate account of the occurrences of everyday life (Benner and Wrubel 1989). Phenomenology, by contrast, is the study of individual experience and relies upon the individual's perception.

The phenomenological method of enquiry focuses upon subjective experience and refutes positivist concepts of cause and effect. It is not concerned with prediction or control, but with understanding the individual's inner life and experiences, as part of an interactive environment which affects and is affected by the person. Husserl, the founder of phenomenology, was committed to the clarification of experience (Graham 1986) and of consciousness. To this end he put forward a phenomenological method which encompasses intuition (with a focus on the phenomena of consciousness), discovery of the various constituents of such phenomena and their relationships and finally description or communication of these perceptions.

This approach has given rise to a range of ethnographic methodologies and has been a supporting element in the emergent feminist research paradigm which applies quite different values from those traditionally prized by positivist researchers. It has also invigorated the tradition of storytelling (or reflection) in a nursing context (Benner 1991, Bowles 1995, Diekelmann 1993) and the collection and archiving of oral histories and personal stories in order that the views and the very lives of individuals can be validated, shared and preserved. A striking example is the archive of Holocaust survivors which Steven Spielberg is currently developing, in a personal quest which began with the making of the film *Schindler's List*.

## APPLICATIONS TO RESEARCH

The use of humanistic nursing has rich implications for research, as virtually every nursing situation can be a research situation. A key antipositivist criticism is that the role of the clinician in developing knowledge is overlooked, a view offered by Benner and Wrubel (1989) who go on to argue that research knowledge, especially that generated elsewhere, may come to be viewed uncritically as a product to be used. The lack of ownership nurses may feel with regard to the product of others' research is discussed by Schön (1983), who argues that a positivistic basis to practice separates research from practice yet for many practitioners, practice is a kind of research, enquiry being a transaction with the situation in which knowing and doing are inseparable. In short, nurses who use a phenomenological method for everyday nursing situations are researchers.

In many ways, since the first edition of this work appeared there have been dramatic changes in the nature of clinical research. The gulf which once separated researchers from clinicians in the UK has largely disappeared; funding bodies, for instance, often specify a high level of collaboration between clinicians and academics as a criterion for funding. Joint appointments are still in vogue, as are secondments between academic and service organizations. At the level of the individual, reflection-in-action is now a concept familiar to the majority of registered nurses, who may receive academic credit for evidence of reflective practice and who, in years to come, will be required to produce similar evidence to maintain their registration with the UK Central Council.

Just as the outdated classifications of idiographic and nomothetic research are largely regarded as narrow and irrelevant, the distinction between positivist and antipositivist research is to some extent becoming more blurred. Even Watson (1985) accepts that the 'human science' of nursing and the natural science of medicine are complementary, best regarded as two ends of a continuum.

The 'action research' (Carr and Kemmis 1986) paradigm is now well accepted as an ideal vehicle to advance practice locally or in the 'real world', as Robson (1993) would have it, and whilst evidence-based practice and the accompanying guidelines industry are building up momentum, there is currently very little 'product' from this 'high-tech' approach which has any specific relevance for nursing practice.

Humanistic nursing, with its 'high touch' (Wright 1991) existential and phenomenological basis may still provide the most accessible and appropriate opportunity for the development of nursing knowledge from clinical practice, with the nurse–client relationship central to the process. Paterson and Zderad suggest that compiling and synthesizing phenomenological descriptions over time will build and make explicit a science of nursing, a view broadly supported, and indeed, used by Benner (1984) and others, for example Heinrich (1992) and Uden *et al.* (1992), and most recently in the illuminating and thought-provoking series of nursing narratives carried in both of the UK's most widely read nursing weekly's.


## CONCLUSION

Humanistic nursing is an expression of the values upon which nursing itself is founded. It regards the person as an unpredictable and unique whole, not a collection of parts or problems. It is expressly concerned with the relationship between nurse and client and gives the nurse the means to provide committed and genuine human contact in the often impersonal clinical environment. It is an approach which demands professional maturity and commitment and is wholly consistent with the individualized patient care ethos familiar to most registered nurses.

The humanistic approach (or model) offered by Paterson and Zderad described in this chapter requires careful consideration and interpretation, as it was first published two decades ago and, as even its enthusiastic supporters would admit, it contains some rarefied terms and only semi-workable concepts. With regard to documentation, for instance, rejection of currently used documentation is not an option for the vast majority of nurses and instead, a middle road must be taken. Several suggestions have been made in this work for the purposes of illustration. In a sense the nature of the documentation matters less than content and, as stated earlier, a humanistic nurse will ensure that the content reflects the unique human characteristics (Duldt 1991) of the client and humanizes care as fully as possible.

Finally, whilst growing from a phenomenological basis, nursing science is not incompatible with natural scientific approaches as each paradigm may illuminate and complement the other. But the communication of the *meaning* of human experience will always be the preserve of the phenomenological approach and its application in practice is the key function of the humanistic nurse.

## REFERENCES

Aggleton, P. and Chalmers, H. (1986) *Nursing Models and the Nursing Process*, Macmillan, London.

Benner, P. (1984). *From Novice to Expert: Power and Excellence in Clinical Practice*, Addison-Wesley, Menlo Park.

Benner, P. (1985). Quality of life: a phenomenological perspective on explanation, prediction and understanding in nursing science. *Advances in Nursing Science*, **8**(1), 1–14.

Benner, P. (1991) The role of experience, narrative and community in skilled ethical comportment. *Advances in Nursing Science*, **14**(2), 1–21.

Benner, P. and Wrubel, J. (1989) *The Primacy of Caring*, Addison-Wesley, Menlo Park.

Bevis, E. (1982) *Curriculum Building in Nursing*, Mosby, Kansas City.

Bowles, N. B. (1995) Storytelling: a search for meaning within nursing practice. *Nurse Education Today*, **15**, 365–369.

Brown, D. and Pedder, J. (1994) *Psychotherapy*, Routledge, London.

Busfield, J. (1986) *Managing Madness*, Hutchinson, London.

Carr, W. and Kemmis, S. (1986) *Becoming Critical: Knowing Through Action Research*, Deakin University Press, Geelong, Victoria.

Clemence, S. M. (1966) Existentialism: a philosophy of commitment. *American Journal of Nursing*, **66**(3), 500–505.

Degenberg, K. V. (1996) Clinical Guidelines: improving practice at local level. *Nursing Standard*, **10**(9), 37–39.

Diekelmann, N. (1993) Interpretive research and narratives of teaching. *Journal of Nurse Education*, **32**(1), 5–6.

Duldt, B. (1991) I–Thou in nursing: research supporting Duldt's theory. *Perspectives in Psychiatric Care*, **27**(3), 5–12.

Duldt, B. and Giffin, K. (1985) *Theoretical Perspectives of Nursing*, Little Brown, Boston.

Graham, H. (1986) *The Human Face of Psychology*, Open University Press, Milton Keynes.

Gulino, C. K. (1982) Entering the mysterious dimension of other: an existential approach to nursing care. *Nursing Outlook*, **30**, 352–357.

Heinrich, K. T. (1992) Create a tradition: teach nurses to share stories. *Journal of Nurse Education*, **31**(3), 141–143.

Holmes, C. (1990) Alternatives to natural science foundations for nursing. *International Journal of Nursing Studies*, **27**(3), 187–198.

Hunter, V. (1990) John Bowlby: an interview. *Psychoanalytic Review*, **78**, 159–175.

Kadner, K. (1994) Therapeutic intimacy in nursing. *Journal of Advanced Nursing*, **19**, 215–218.

Masson, J. (1993). *Against Therapy*. HarperCollins, Glasgow.

McKinnon, N. (1991) Humanistic nursing – it can't stand up to scrutiny. *Nursing and Health Care*, **12**(8), 414–446.

Merlau-Ponty, M. (1962) *Phenomenology of Perception*, Routledge and Kegan Paul, London.

Mulholland, J. (1995) Nursing, humanism and transcultural theory: the 'bracketing out' of reality. *Journal of Advanced Nursing*, **22**(3), 442–449.

Paterson, J. G. and Zderad, L. T. (1976) *Humanistic Nursing*, John Wiley, New York.

Pearson, A. and Vaughan, B. (1986) *Nursing Models for Practice*, Heinemann, Oxford.

RCN (1987) *In Pursuit of Excellence: a Position Statement on Nursing*, Royal College of Nursing, London.

Redfern, S. (1996) Individualised patient care: a framework for guidelines. *Nursing Times*, **92**(5), 33–36.

Robson, C. (1993) *Real World Research*, Blackwell, Oxford.

Salvage, J. (1990) The theory and practice of the 'new nursing'. *Nursing Times*, **86**(4), 42–45.

Sartre, J. P. (1977) *Essays in Existentialism*, Citadel Press, New Jersey.

Sarvimaki, A. (1988) Nursing as a moral, practical, communicative and creative activity. *Journal of Advanced Nursing*, **13**, 462–467.

Schön, D. (1983) *The Reflective Practitioner*, Temple Smith, London.

Seedhouse, D. (1986) *Health – the Foundations for Achievement*, John Wiley, Chichester.

Strawson, P. F. (1974) *Freedom and Resentment*, Methuen, London.

Travelbee, J. (1966) *Interpersonal Aspects of Nursing*, Davis, Philadelphia.

Uden, G., Norberg, A., Lindset, A. and Marhaug, V. (1992) Ethical reasoning in nurses' and physicians' stories about care episodes. *Journal of Advanced Nursing*, **17**, 1028–1034.

Waterworth, A. and Luker, K (1990) Reluctant collaborators: do patients want to be involved in decisions concerning care? *Journal of Advanced Nursing*, **15**(8), 971–976.

Watson, J. (1985) *Nursing: Human Science and Human Care: a Theory of Nursing*, Appleton-Century Crofts, Norwalk.

Wright, S. (1991). A search for the therapeutic dimensions of nurse-patient inter-action, in *Nursing as Therapy*. (Ed. R. McMahon). London, Chapman Hall.

# Therapeutic nursing in acute care

12

Gerald S. Bowman and David R. Thompson

## INTRODUCTION

Every practising nurse intuitively knows that nursing decision making and ensuing action can enable a patient to survive a life-threatening crisis, maintain a satisfactory life or prepare for a dignified death. Often the patient and family realize this too. These nursing interventions may vary in complexity and, in many instances, nurses will not know precisely what it is that has made an impact on the patient, thus making it difficult for them to articulate and convince others of the value of nursing. If nurses wish to persuade others of the value of nursing then they require credible evidence to support their claims, i.e. they need to demonstrate clearly that specific nursing interventions result in successful recovery or other positive outcomes for patients.

Unfortunately, the evidence attesting to such effects is scant. Generally, it is accepted that no consensus exists about how best to assess the effectiveness of nursing (Seers and Milne 1997). The issue of what constitutes evidence is also hotly debated. Currently, randomized clinical trials (RCTs) are considered the gold standard for evidence but the number of these published in nursing journals is relatively small, being around 500 in addition to 20 reviews of the effectiveness of nursing (Cullum 1997).

However, there are a number of factors that lend support to the notion that nursing can be therapeutic. These factors may be internal, such as the nurse's knowledge, experience, skills and personality, or external, such as the nature of the organization, its philosophy and the operation of authority, responsibility and accountability, the opportunity for patient contact and the patient's personality. It is such factors that will ultimately determine whether a nurse can change, in a positive and measurable way, a patient's health state.

This chapter aims to discuss: the nurse–patient relationship; assessment; organization of care; and therapeutic nursing in acute care. Many of the examples used to illustrate therapeutic nursing are selected from the field of coronary care, which is of particular interest to the authors.

## NURSE–PATIENT RELATIONSHIP

The relationship between the nurse, patient and family is the central facet of therapeutic nursing. It will determine the atmosphere in which recovery is promoted and contribute to the achievement of an optimum level of independence and quality of life. It is not uncommon for some nurse commentators to oversimplify or sentimentalize this relationship, for example, in describing caring as 'loving' (Jacono 1993). The reality is that the nurse will meet many people as patients, family members or friends and to believe that each and every nurse can cope with numerous sentimental relationships is unrealistic and unfair to both the nurse and the patient. When they meet for the first time, they do so as complete strangers and the circumstances (illness, sickness or disease) and previous experience of 'being a nurse' or 'being a patient' will dictate the type of relationship that emerges.

Patients are generally accepting and forgiving, especially when they recognize goodwill, which engenders trust. The concepts of duty and good-will are important in the nurse's relationship with the patient and family. Importantly, these concepts can be readily enacted and appreciated by the recipients with the prospect of minimal emotional forfeit on the nurse's part. As cognitive concepts, they are non-selective and can be more consistently applied than other, more intense emotional relationships sometimes described in the nursing literature. In the acute care setting, 'duty' is seen as a sense of doing that which is right or what nurses are morally obliged to do. In the therapeutic relationship, this would mean being non-judgemental towards the patient and family, avoiding stereotyping the patient or making unnecessary assumptions and conveying an appropriate degree of understanding or compassion for their predicament. Goodwill is concerned with the intention to do something that will achieve an end. To perform this intent, nurses have to make decisions or judgements as to what is the best thing to do or wisest thing to say (Mackenzie 1972). It is simply not possible for nurses to know their patients completely and mistakes will inevitably occur, but by creating trust the way is open to positive, helping relationships.

A lack of commitment to the patient may lead to a unilateral relationship, affecting trust and the nurse's ability to influence the patient's health beliefs and behaviour (Morse 1991). Acutely ill patients invariably seek or need the help of others. They are often confused by their symptoms and are unable to undertake activities that may ameliorate their problems because their ability or knowledge may be deficient. Traditionally, the health-care system assumed control over the patient's life during the stay in hospital. In the current, more egalitarian health-care system, much is said about offering patients more control but in reality many subtle pressures conspire against this and actually encourage conformity. There is some evidence that nurses, when compared to other health professionals, have more desire to control patients (Sellick 1991). Patients equate caring behaviour with competence in key areas of work where nurses 'know' how to respond effectively to a variety of practical situations, are able to make key decisions, take time to answer questions and teach patients about their illness (Cronin and Harrison 1988). In practice, nurses will find a wide range of needs among patients regarding decision making and control. Some patients will wish for others to make decisions and act on their behalf, others may desire this provided they understand the reasons for decisions made and yet others may want each and every decision and activity concerning them discussed with and agreed by them beforehand. Offering patients a level of involvement in decision making to which they have agreed gives them a degree of control in their affairs that provides reassurance and comfort. The sensitivity of the individual nurse to what the patient wants regarding personal control indicates a highly sophisticated care system which, when effective, may be therapeutic for the patient. The attitudes of the nurse will significantly influence the nurse–patient relationship. Possibly the most important attitude nurses have is their view of the relationship between themselves, the patient and the family. An unrealistic concept of this relationship can be damaging to the patient and the nurse and can be antitherapeutic.

In forming new relationships, it is not uncommon for misunderstandings to occur. Nurses may stereotype a patient, presuming they know his needs (Farrell 1991). On admission to hospital, patients and their relatives will be experiencing a variety of emotions, including relief at being admitted, anxiety about their predicament, trepidation about novel experiences and concern about coping following discharge (Bowman et al. 1992).

Some patients will choose not to engage in relationships or activities believed by nurses to be in their own best interest. This is the right of every patient and it should be respected once he has made a conscious and informed decision.

## ASSESSMENT

The quality of a relationship will depend on how well the nurse attempts to know the patient and family. Nurses should understand patients' health problems, including how they feel about them, how they cope with them and how they are likely to respond to recommended changes in health behaviour. In the acute care setting, the nurse has often only a short period of time in which to accomplish this. A systematic nursing assessment is the means by which the nurse can get to know the patient. This allows the nurse to identify and agree with the patient a range of problems and to make decisions with patients that are in their best interest. This is likely to result in reassuring them and gaining their trust as well as initiating processes that may promote comfort, relieve symptoms and facilitate adaptation.

What is important for the relationship to be therapeutic, however, is the quality of the nursing assessment, which is more likely to result in improved relationships between the patient and nurse, continuity in care and the organization of individual procedures around the patient's specific circumstances and needs.

The nurse's behaviour is most important at the stage of admission because she knows the system into which the patient and family are entering and can exert some influence within it. Molzahn and Northcott (1989) argue that factors such as cultural background, gender, socioeconomic status, experience and role will be influential in affecting the perception of both the nurse and the patient. Nurses tend to perceive patients as being more stressed than they actually are and overestimate their worries (Carr and Powers 1986). Other evidence indicates that, at a more specific level, nurses' assumptions are frequently wrong. For example, when preparing patients for a barium enema, nurses believe patients want more information than they actually need: in reality, patients are mainly interested in knowing the purpose and benefits of the procedure (Schuster and Jones 1982).

Pain is often incorrectly estimated. Nurses who have not experienced wound pain tend to overestimate the amount experienced by patients (Ketovuori 1987). Even in specialized areas of care, like coronary care, nurses frequently under- or overestimate pain (Bondestam *et al.* 1987, O'Connor 1995). Such discrepancy is likely to be due to poor assessment. O'Connor (1995) found that nurses tended to record the location and verbal statements of pain, but the quality, intensity and duration of pain were found to be inadequate. Incorrect estimate of chest pain results in patients either receiving no treatment or ineffective treatment (Bondestam *et al.* 1987). These few examples indicate how poor assessment can lead to misunderstandings and the undermining of the therapeutic relationship.

The majority of acutely ill patients will want to know what role is expected of them, be involved in some way in decisions that affect them and have some input in the direction of interpersonal and environmental components of their care (Dennis 1987). It is important to note that acutely ill patients will gain from nurses who make themselves emotionally available, modify events appropriately and give a feeling of control to the patient; this will offer patients much reassurance at a time when their lives are seriously undermined (Boyd and Munhall 1989). Medically ill patients who have little expectation of recovery and lack hope do not cope well (Feifel *et al.* 1987) and may not wish to be actively involved in the recovery process. To effect positive health-care changes, it is the nurse–patient interaction that promotes consensus, achieved through negotiation with the patient (Kasch 1985). For nurses to feel more certain about interpreting patients' behaviour and to feel more positive towards a patient, regular participation in care activities is important (Athlin and Norberg 1987).

Inappropriate knowledge and skills can militate against therapeutic nursing. Knowledge and skills should be provided within the context of a philosophy of practice which is about nursing, not about medicine. Many nurses are better able to explain medical concepts and strategies than nursing ones and this is likely to affect their priorities and practices. Nurses require a broad knowledge base in order to appreciate a problem or manipulate events for a particular patient at a precise point in time; too often, nurses subjugate their care to the hierarchy of theory offered by the medical community (Visintainer 1986).

## ORGANIZATION OF CARE

The therapeutic environment is dependent upon the organizational structures and processes. Therapeutic nursing is unlikely to flourish in an organization that is strong on ritual and routine. Rigid ward practices and routines do not allow for truly individualized patient care and the tedium that often results can produce negative views about patients (Astrom *et al.* 1987). Where limited resources and underfunding are apparent, nurses may begin to ignore patients, take up technical tasks and appear uncaring to patients (King's Fund 1994). These deficiencies strongly militate against a therapeutic environment. A quality work environment for nurses primarily includes adequate staffing, positive work relationships, reasonable material rewards and control over work (Attridge and Callahan 1990).

Present nursing structures do not allow nurses the latitude in their work to cope with these complex relationships effectively. Smith (1992) used the concept of emotional labour to understand how nurses cope with their work. Emotional labour is evident in those occupations which have contact with the public, are required to produce an emotional state in their clients and allow the employer to have control over the employees' emotional activities. Emotional labour is the suppression of personal emotion in order that others experience a sense of being cared for. In her study, Smith (1992) found that nurses who felt cared for by more senior staff felt better able to care for patients.

The way in which a registered nurse's work is designed can reduce the opportunity for contact with patients. Work steeped in the tradition of running the ward, undertaking multiple administrative or managerial responsibilities, pursuing an unreasonable volume of medical objectives and having a lack of clarity and continuity in patient assessment or personal authority and responsibility in patient care issues will discourage the development of a rational therapeutic relationship.

A lack of leadership qualities in senior nurses can also undermine the prospects of a therapeutic nursing environment and can blunt the enthusiasm and progress made by well-motivated staff. Practising nurses need to know that their operational philosophies are accepted and actively and visibly supported by their senior colleagues.

Much nursing time can be wasted on activities valued by the system but which have relatively little intrinsic worth and prevent therapeutic nursing from taking place. Perhaps one of the better examples is the volume of observations indulged in by nurses. The continuing practice of measuring and recording temperatures, pulses, respirations, blood pressures, weights and the like beyond a time when they provide useful actionable information is endemic in acute care settings. It is likely that uncritical faith in routine observations prevents a better use of nursing time (Burroughs and Hoffbrand 1990).

Current skill mix exercises could work against effective therapeutic nursing if registered nurses are sacrificed for health-care assistants. The best available information identifies registered nurses as giving the best value for money, providing better quality of care and outcomes (Carr-Hill *et al.* 1992).

Some of the most notable nursing achievements have occurred in the least desirable settings and this offers a clue as to the nature of nursing. Possibly the most significant aspect of nursing is not just meeting a patient's level of expectation, but exceeding it. Patients' expectations have been raised by legislation which confers certain fundamental rights. In order for nurses to be effective and therapeutic, some degree of economic commitment is necessary. Often this is dictated politically and tends to be targeted at achieving a particular objective, such as the reduction of waiting lists. Those who manage budgets need to appreciate that nursing care centred upon the patient and delivered by appropriate staff is likely to result in quality outcomes for the patient.

Work should be designed to give the nurse the optimum opportunity for contact with patients (Bowman and Thompson 1995). Nurses' motivation will, to some extent, depend upon the way in which their work is structured. Work that is characterized by variety is usually attractive, utilizes the individual's knowledge and skills, offers autonomy and responsibility and permits access to other individuals involved in patient care. In the health service, few people work in a truly independent way but autonomous practice within a multidisciplinary team where there is genuine interdependence is often more satisfying and motivating than working alone (Robertson and Smith 1985).

If nursing is a therapy, it must have its own unique characteristics that produce a desired therapeutic effect. There will always be an overlap of roles between nursing and medicine and the relationship between the two professions should be complementary and mutually supportive. However, in practice, nursing and medical communications are often inadequate, do not take place on neutral ground and rarely facilitate an open exchange of opinions (Wilson-Barnett 1986). Nurses are in a position to assert to medical colleagues their views on the value of nursing. Some doctors, however, take the view (probably correctly) that nurses choose to be submissive and deferential to them (Stanley 1983). It is comparatively easy for a strong, united professional group, like medicine, to split and confuse a weak, disunited, poorly led group, like nursing. This prevents the weaker group acquiring its own authority, which may be perceived as a threat. With the increasing emphasis on a shortened hospital stay for patients, the focus is sharpened upon the medical objective of 'cure' and discharge. Thus, care is only valued as a means to an end (Reed and Watson 1994).

Although emphasis has been placed on the nurse–patient relationship and the mode of organization of care as the main focus in therapeutic nursing, the provision of equipment can clearly have an important impact on the quality of patient care and outcome. Lack of choice in appropriate equipment can lead to problems for patients and be antitherapeutic. For example, poor or inappropriate choice of urinary catheters can adversely affect the quality and standard of catheter care (Mulhall *et al.* 1992).

## THERAPEUTIC NURSING IN ACUTE CARE

In a study of patients with heart failure, Jaarsma *et al.* (1997) found four composite themes of nursing care described in practice: basic nursing care; assessment and observation; symptom-relieving interventions; and patient education. In theory, at least, nurses are in a position to influence independently three important variables concerned with patient health outcomes: to provide comfort and aid healing; to offer information; and encourage independence. Success in these key areas is the cornerstone of true therapeutic nursing.

In acute nursing environments patients are frequently initially moribund. During this period there may be many interventions of a medicotechnical or nursing nature that the nurse should be familiar with in order to help and support the patient and family. The patient is often perplexed and may experience powerlessness through loss of control (Roberts and White 1990). In descriptive studies of cardiac patients (Jaarsma *et al.* 1995) and partners

(Thompson *et al.* 1995), experiences during the early stages of recovery and convalescence included expectations about advice and information, emotional reactions, changes in physical condition and deleterious effects of treatment and convalescence.

Adjustment to an acute illness that becomes chronic has importance not only for the patient and his family but for the health-care resource too. Poor adjustment to an illness that becomes chronic can incur significant financial costs (Browne *et al.* 1994).

Using a grounded theory approach to study coronary patients, Johnson and Morse (1990) examined the process of adjustment after a heart attack and found that it incorporated four stages. The first stage involves patients' attempts to defend themselves against a threatened loss of control by trivializing symptoms and distancing themselves from events that appeared unreal to them. In the second stage, patients struggle to come to terms with the heart attack. The third stage involves the use of numerous strategies to re-establish a sense of control. If this is successful, the patients progress to the final stage which includes an acceptance of limitations, a refocusing on issues other than a heart attack and a perceived sense of mastery. Some patients were unable to adjust and found it necessary to occasionally abandon the struggle to re-establish control. Nurses can help the patient and family through the process of adjustment by appropriate education and support. To do this effectively, they need to have acquired the necessary skill, knowledge, motivation and support (Noble 1991).

The nurse can play a major role in encouraging adjustment in both the patient and the family during and following this acute stage. For example, after the acute phase of a heart attack patients' and partners' beliefs about the cause of the illness influence their emotional and practical response (Maeland and Havik 1989). Educational counselling given by nurses improves knowledge and satisfaction (Raleigh and Odtohan 1987, Steele and Ruzicki 1987, Thompson 1990), reduces anxiety and depression in both the patient and partner (Raleigh and Odtohan 1987, Thompson and Meddis 1990a,b) and may correct damaging health habits (Carlsson *et al.* 1997).

Patients need to feel at ease with their nurse: there is evidence that the mere presence of a nurse can exert a negative physical influence on the patient. For example, Lynch *et al.* (1974) showed significant increases in heart rate and a doubling of the frequency of abnormal heart beats in patients when they were in contact with nurses or doctors. Comfort is a major nursing objective. Kolcaba and Kolcaba (1991) define three types of comfort: state, which is a sense of ease and peaceful contentment; relief, which is relief from discomfort; and renewal, being strengthened and invigorated through comfort. For a patient to feel 'comfort' in the way described would clearly be therapeutic. Strategies to enhance comfort and be therapeutic can be diverse. Guzzetta (1989) assigned patients in a coronary care unit at random to either a control group or a relaxation and music therapy group of three sessions over two days. The treatment group had a lower heart rate, peripheral temperature and incidence of cardiac complications.

Touch has been shown to have a therapeutic effect (Heidt 1981, Krieger 1974), but therapeutic touch has many dimensions and requires some experience and skill to develop a style that operates the cues necessary in the touching process (Estabrooks and Morse 1992). In acute care settings, where time is of the essence, touch is likely to enter into the relationship at an early stage and may influence relationships virtually from the time of admission.

There are many factors involved in a patient's receptiveness to information, the most significant being whether an issue is perceived to be important (Hinds 1990). Generally, simple and appropriate information-giving, teaching or counselling will have the greatest impact, but knowing what is appropriate demands an understanding of the patient and their needs. Vague, general advice is probably of little value; more individualized information specific to the patient is what is required (Murray 1989). For example, coronary patients who have received individual teaching are more likely to report less anxiety and to modify identified risk factors. In the early stages following a heart attack, patients and partners need specific information, which is easy to understand and delivered on a regular basis (Hanisch 1993).

In a study based on 'caring' concepts, Fridlund *et al.* (1991) placed myocardial infarction patients into either a control group, where they received information and participated in discussions concerning return to work and leisure activities, or a treatment group, where they received a rehabilitation programme in which they learnt strategies to cope with lifestyle change and life stress and received support. The treatment group showed significant improvements, including increased physical capacity, fewer reinfarctions, higher life satisfaction, better relationships with the partner and better leisure and sex life. These results were consistent at six months and one year.

Patients appreciate these types of programme. Castelein and Kerr (1995), in a study of cardiac patients' satisfaction with lifestyle, found that caring interest shown by staff in a programme designed to meet the individuals' needs were the features appreciated most by patients during recovery.

In a randomized controlled trial of men who had suffered a first heart attack and their partners, Thompson (1990) showed that a simple programme of in-hospital counselling conferred significant benefits on the couple. The treatment group received four half-hour sessions of educative-supportive counselling provided by a coronary care unit nurse at one, two, three and five days after admission. Prior to each session, a detailed 'blind' assessment took place. The control group received usual care. At five days, there were significant differences between the two groups, with reductions in anxiety and depression and improvements in satisfaction and knowledge being reported by the treatment group. These improvements were sustained at one, three and six months. These fairly dramatic effects occurred within five days and after three half-hour sessions. The results were even more impressive with the partners. This study was the first to show that a simple and early nursing intervention could have a significant impact on the outcome for cardiac patients and partners and illustrates the influence that appropriate and timely interventions by nurses can have on patient and family health outcomes.

Developing a supportive relationship between the patient and partner can be productive following the patient's discharge. In a longitudinal study of coronary patients, Riegel and Dracup (1992) found that those who had received more social support from family and friends than desired experienced less anxiety, depression, anger and confusion and more vigour and self-esteem. They concluded that overprotection on the part of family and friends may facilitate psychosocial adjustment in the early recovery period rather than leading to cardiac invalidism.

Nurse–patient contact after hospital discharge following an acute illness also brings benefits to the patient. For example, Unden et al. (1993) demonstrate that structured contact with a nurse two weeks after discharge positively affects feelings of depression, quality of life and satisfaction.

The family is the most significant link for the majority of patients and it could be argued that all nurses should practise family nursing. Certainly, therapeutic nursing demands the inclusion of each patient's partner and each family member should be treated as a client (Friedemann 1989). For example, families who become involved with the hospital care of a patient who has suffered a stroke cope better initially following discharge (Field et al. 1983). Frederickson (1989) found that family members' anxiety was reduced by talking to the nurse during routine care.

Therapeutic nursing is dependent upon knowledgeable, skilled practitioners whose work is primarily research based. Heater et al. (1988) performed a meta-analysis of 84 subject studies and 4146 individual subjects from nurse-conducted experimental research over an eight-year period. They found that research-based nursing practice can offer patients significantly better outcomes than routine, procedural nursing care. Pearson et al. (1989), using a number of assessment methods, found the quality of care delivered to patients in acute hospital care to be significantly and consistently higher when therapeutic nursing was the mode of delivery.

The commitment to high-quality therapeutic nursing demands much of the nurse, including competence in psychomotor, cognitive and affective skills and the linking of theory to skills (Fitzpatrick et al. 1992). This is illustrated in an observational study of acute medical and surgical patients

(Lundgren *et al.* 1993), which found poor care and handling of peripheral intravenous cannulae in half the cases studied, with over 60% of all patients experiencing some degree of thrombophlebitis and some patients still experiencing cannula site pain five months later.

## CONCLUSION

It is likely that the whole package of nursing care is more important than the sum of its parts in provoking a therapeutic effect. However, a belief in nursing as a therapy in its own right is not sufficient. Objective evidence needs to be accumulated that will indicate those aspects of nursing care that are proven to be effective, those that are suspected to be effective (but which await confirmation) and those that are not effective. Even if such evidence does become available, political expediency or financial considerations may dictate that there will be little or no support for therapeutic nursing.

## REFERENCES

Astrom, S., Norberg, A., Nilsson, M. and Winblad, B. (1987) Tedium among personnel working with geriatric patients. *Scandinavian Journal of Caring Science*, **1**, 125–132.

Athlin, E. and Norberg, A. (1987) Caregivers' attitudes to and interpretation of the behaviours of severely demented patients during feeding in a patient assignment care system. *International Journal of Nursing Studies*, **24**, 145–153.

Attridge, C. and Callahan, M. (1990) Nurses' perspectives of quality work environments. *Canadian Journal of Nursing Administration*, **3**, 18–24.

Bondestam, E., Hovgren, K., Gaston-Johansson, F. *et al.* (1987) Pain assessment by patients and nurses in the early phase of acute myocardial infarction. *Journal of Advanced Nursing*, **12**, 677–682.

Bowman, G. S. and Thompson, D. R. (1995) Strategies for organising care, in *Towards Advanced Nursing Practice: Key Concepts for Health Care*, (eds J. E. Schober and S. M. Hinchliffe), Edward Arnold, London, pp.222–251.

Bowman, G. S., Webster, R. A. and Thompson, D. R. (1992) The reactions of 40 patients unexpectedly admitted to hospital. *Journal of Clinical Nursing*, **1**, 335–338.

Boyd, C. O. and Munhall, P. L. (1989) A qualitative investigation of reassurance. *Holistic Nursing Practice*, **4**. 61–69.

Browne, G., Roberts, J., Weir, R. *et al.* (1994) The cost of poor adjustment to chronic illness: lessons from three studies. *Health and Social Care*, **2**, 85–93.

Burroughs, J. and Hoffbrand, B. I. (1990) A critical look at nursing observations. *Postgraduate Medical Journal*, **66**, 370–373.

Carlsson, R., Lindberg, G., Westin, L. and Israelsson, B. (1997) Influence of coronary nursing management follow up on lifestyle after acute myocardial infarction. *Heart*, **77**, 256–259.

Carr, J. A. and Powers, M. J. (1986) Stressors associated with coronary bypass surgery. *Nursing Research*, **35**, 243–246.

Carr-Hill, R., Dixon, P. and Gibbs, I. (1992) *Skill Mix and the Effectiveness of Nursing Care*, Centre for Health Economics, University of York, York.

Castelein, P. and Kerr, J. R. (1995) Satisfaction and cardiac lifestyle. *Journal of Advanced Nursing*, **21**, 498–505.

Cronin, S. N. and Harrison, B. (1988) Importance of nurse caring behaviours as perceived by patients after myocardial infarction. *Heart and Lung*, **17**, 374–380.

Cullum, N. (1997) Identification and analysis of randomised controlled trials in nursing: a preliminary study. *Quality in Health Care*, **6**, 2–6.

Dennis, K. E. (1987) Dimensions of client control. *Nursing Research*, **36**, 151–156.

Estabrooks, C. A. and Morse, J. M. (1992) Towards a theory of touch: the touching process and acquiring a touching style. *Journal of Advanced Nursing*, **17**, 448–456.

Farrell, G. A. (1991) How accurately do nurse perceive patients' needs? A comparison of general and psychiatric settings. *Journal of Advanced Nursing*, **16**, 1062–1070.

Feifel, R., Strack, S., and Nagy, V. T. (1987) Coping strategies and associated features of medically ill patients. *Psychosomatic Medicine*, **49**, 616–625.

Field, D., Cordle, C. J. and Bowman, G. S. (1983) Coping with stroke at home. *International Rehabilitation Medicine*, **5**, 96–100.

Fitzpatrick, J. M., While, A. E. and Roberts, J. D. (1992) The role of the nurse in high-quality patient care: a review of the literature. *Journal of Advanced Nursing*, **17**, 1210–1219.

Frederickson, K. (1989) Anxiety transmission in the patient with myocardial infarction. *Heart and Lung*, **18**, 617–622.

Fridlund, B., Hogstedt, B., Lidell, E. and Larsson, P. A. (1991) Recovery after myocardial infarction: effects of a caring rehabilitation programme. *Scandinavian Journal of Caring Science*, **5**, 23–31.

Friedemann, M. L. (1989) The concept of family nursing. *Journal of Advanced Nursing*, **15**, 211–216.

Guzzetta, C. E. (1989) Effects of relaxation and music therapy on patients in a coronary care unit with presumptive acute myocardial infarction. *Heart and Lung*, **18**, 609–616.

Hanisch, P. (1993) Informational needs and preferred time to receive information for phase II cardiac rehabilitation patients: what CE instructors need to know. *Journal of Continuing Education in Nursing*, **24**, 82–89.

Heater, B. S., Beeker, A. M. and Olson, R. K. (1988) Nursing interventions and patient outcomes: a meta-analysis of studies. *Nursing Research*, **37**, 303–307.

Heidt, P. (1981) Effect of therapeutic touch on anxiety level of hospitalised patients. *Nursing Research*, **30**, 32–37.

Hinds, C. (1990) Personal and contextual factors predicting patients' reported quality of life: exploring congruency with Betty Neuman's assumptions. *Journal of Advanced Nursing*, **15**, 456–462.

Jaarsma, T., Kastermans, M., Dassen, T. and Philipsen, H. (1995) Problems of cardiac patients in early recovery. *Journal of Advanced Nursing*, **21**, 21–27.

Jaarsma, T., Abu-Saad, H. H., Halfens, R. and Dracup, K. (1997) Maintaining the balance – nursing care of patients with chronic heart failure. *International Journal of Nursing Studies*, **34**, 213–221.

Jacono, B. J. (1993) Caring is loving. *Journal of Advanced Nursing*, **18**, 192–194.

Johnson, J. L. and Morse, J. M. (1990) Regaining control: the process of adjustment after myocardial infarction. *Heart and Lung*, **19**, 126–135.

Kasch, C. R. (1985) Towards a theory of nursing action: skills and competency in nurse–patient interaction. *Nursing Research*, **35**, 226–230.

Ketovuori, H. (1987) Nurses' and patients' conceptions of wound pain and the administration of analgesics. *Journal of Pain and Symptom Management*, **2**, 213–218.

King's Fund (1994) *Londoners' Views on the Future of Healthcare*, King's Fund, London.

Kolcaba, K. Y. and Kolcaba, R. J. (1991) An analysis of the concept of comfort. *Journal of Advanced Nursing*, **16**, 1301–1310.

Krieger, D. (1974) Healing by the laying-on-of-hands as a facilitator of bio-energetic change: the response of in-vivo human hemoglobin. *Psychoenergetics*, **1**, 12–15.

Lundgren, A., Jorfeldt, L. and Ek, A.-C. (1993) The care and handling of peripheral intravenous cannulae on 60 surgery and internal medicine patients: an observational study. *Journal of Advanced Nursing*, **18**, 963–971.

Lynch, J. J., Thomas, S. A., Mills, M. E., Malinow, K. and Katcher, A. H. (1974) The effects of human contact on cardiac arrhythmia in coronary care patients. *Journal of Nervous and Mental Disease*, **158**, 88–99.

Mackenzie, N. (1972) *The Professional Ethic and the Hospital Service*, English Universities Press, London.

Maeland, J. G. and Havik, O. E. (1989) After the myocardial infarction. *Scandinavian Journal of Rehabilitation Medicine*, **22**(suppl), 1–87.

Molzahn, A. E. and Northcott, H. C. (1989) The social basis of discrepancies in health/illness perceptions. *Journal of Advanced Nursing*, **14**, 132–140.

Morse, J. M. (1991) Negotiating commitment and involvement in the nurse–patient relationship. *Journal of Advanced Nursing*, **16**, 455–468.

Mulhall, A., Lee, K. and King, S. (1992) Improving nursing practice: the provision of equipment. *International Journal of Nursing Studies*, **29**, 205–211.

Murray, P. J. (1989) Rehabilitation information and health beliefs in the post-coronary patient: do we meet their informational needs? *Journal of Advanced Nursing*, **14**, 686–693.

Noble, C. (1991) Are nurses good patient educators? *Journal of Advanced Nursing*, **16**, 1185–1189.

O'Connor, L. (1995) Pain assessment by patients and nurses, and nurses' notes on it, in early acute myocardial infarction. *Intensive and Critical Care Nursing*, **11**, 183–191.

Pearson, A., Durant, I. and Punton, S. (1989) Determining quality in a unit where nursing is the primary intervention. *Journal of Advanced Nursing*, **14**, 269–273.

Raleigh, E. H. and Odtohan, B. C. (1987) The effects of cardiac teaching program on patient rehabilitation. *Heart and Lung*, **16**, 311–317.

Reed, J. and Watson, D. (1994) The impact of the medical model on nursing practice and assessment. *International Journal of Nursing Studies*, **13**, 57–66.

Riegel, B. J. and Dracup, K. A. (1992) Does overprotection cause cardiac invalidism after acute myocardial infarction? *Heart and Lung*, **21**, 529–535.

Roberts S. L. and White B. S. (1990) Powerlessness and personal control model applied to the myocardial infarction patient. *Progress in Cardiovascular Nursing*, **5**, 84–94.

Robertson, I. T. and Smith, M. (1985) *Motivation and Job Design*, Institute of Personnel Management, London.

Schuster, P. and Jones, S. (1982) Preparing the patient for a barium enema: a comparison of nurses' and patients' opinion. *Journal of Advanced Nursing*, **7**, 523–527.

Seers, K. and Milne, R. (1997) Randomised controlled trials in nursing (editorial). *Quality in Health Care*, **6**, 1.

Sellick, K. J. (1991) Nurses' interpersonal behaviours and the development of helping skills. *International Journal of Nursing Studies*, **28**, 3–11.

Smith, P. (1992) *The Emotional Labour of Nursing*, Macmillan, Basingstoke.

Stanley, I. (1983) Where do we stand with doctors? *Nursing Times*, **79**(38), 46–48.

Steele, J. M. and Ruzicki, D. (1987) An evaluation of the effectiveness of cardiac teaching during hospitalization. *Heart and Lung*, **16**, 306–317.

Thompson, D. R. (1990) *Counselling the Coronary Patient and Partner*, Scutari Press, London.

Thompson, D. R. and Meddis, R. (1990a) A prospective evaluation of in-hospital counselling for first time myocardial infarction men. *Journal of Psychosomatic Research*, **34**, 237–248.

Thompson, D. R. and Meddis, R. (1990b) Wives' responses to counselling early after myocardial infarction. *Journal of Psychosomatic Research*, **34**, 249–258.

Thompson D. R., Ersser S. J. and Webster R. A. (1995) The experiences of patients and their partners 1 month after a heart attack. *Journal of Advanced Nursing*, **22**, 707–714.

Unden, A. L., Schenck-Gustafsson Axelsson, P. O., Kaisson, I., Orth-Gomer, K. and Ydrefors, A. M. (1993) Positive effects of increased nurse support for male patients after acute myocardial infarction. *Quality of Life Research*, **2**, 121–127.

Visintainer, M. A. (1986) The nature of knowledge and theory in nursing. *Journal of Nursing Scholarship*, **18**(2), 32–38.

Wilson-Barnett, J. (1986) Ethical dilemmas in nursing. *Journal of Medical Ethics*, **12**, 123–126,135.

# The political dimension

**13**

Nigel Northcott

Our past is not our potential.                    Ferguson (1980)

Nurses are urged to look beyond the immediate frustration of not being able to give all they would wish for today's patients and to do all in their power to be sure that tomorrow's people get the nurses and nursing they deserve.                    Henderson (1987:vii)

This foreword to Trevor Clay's book *Nursing: Power and Politics* (1987) by Virginia Henderson calls upon nurses to safeguard the future of the profession, which is by no means inevitable. In the final chapter of the first edition of *Nursing as Therapy*, Alan Pearson identified the need to prepare nurses for a future that will see a new era in nursing (McMahon and Pearson 1991). The 'threatening' nature that this new era of nursing as therapy poses, he asserts, can only arise by political means (McMahon and Pearson 1991:207).

This chapter explores the political status of nursing from an historical and contemporary perspective and invites nurses to learn from our experiences and continue the struggle to assert ourselves on behalf of our patients. Nursing as therapy is a powerful political stance that seeks to place nursing on an equal footing with all other health-care professionals. In this, it seeks to assert itself as a therapy in its own right and, further, as one that should not be subject to the invidious medical gatekeeping that so often dominates health-care access.

## POLITICS AND POWER IN NURSING – A CALL TO 'ARMS'

Cormack (1990) suggests that politics is any activity concerned with the acquisition of power and is most often associated with the study of government. Ellis and Hartley (1988) confirm that politics reflects the way that people in a democratic society influence decision making and resource allocation. Political power is defined by Rogge (1987) as '. . . the ability to influence or persuade an individual holding a government office to exert the power of that office to affect a desired outcome'. Clearly if nursing as therapy is to be established in its own right, then nursing must mobilize political power to ensure change.

Politics cannot be avoided by nurses (Holmes 1991). Indeed, Salvage (1992) and Bilton *et al.* (1981) suggest that all interpersonal interactions are political as they are predicated by power. Jean Watson (1990) confirms that 'the personal is political'; thereby nurses are political and nursing is political. Nurses and nursing cannot be neutral; they either perpetuate the status quo and are conservative or they challenge it and are radical. The conservative stance in not challenging established practice serves to reinforce and validate it and thereby perpetuate it. The concept of nursing as therapy requires nurses to challenge the many established practices and beliefs about nursing and the status of nursing; to use politics and therefore power to improve the position for all people as well as the profession.

This invitation to challenge or, indeed, to continue to challenge was clearly identified by Clay (1987), who suggests that participation in the political life of the country is the alternative for individual nurses to the silent frustration of the past. Writing as he did as the head of the Royal College of Nursing in the UK, Clay confirmed that the choice was not between action or no action, but what form that action should take. Indeed, he indicates that the frustration arising from the status of nursing, if not tackled politically, might be resolved by industrial action. Reassuringly, the use of industrial action has only been taken up by a very small minority of nurses in the past. The principle of nursing as therapy is that it should do the patient no harm and should strive to protect the best interests of patients. To avoid a major contradiction in the values and principles represented in this book, nurses must choose the political option to achieving change rather than using industrial muscle. This choice appears to have been made by many nurses if Hewison's (1994) assertion that the phrase 'the politics of nursing' has become an acceptable part of the profession is true.

The rapid developments in health-care policy in the UK in the past 20 years have seen a number of radical changes in the management of health care and organizational structures that are echoed elsewhere in the developed world. These changes neither reflect the needs of specific patient groups or nursing developments, nor do they enhance the status of nursing

(Stewart 1987). It is against this background that this chapter represents a call to arms. The way in which the largest professional group of staff in the health-care industry has been and can be so marginalized and ignored is disgraceful and unacceptable in what we describe as democratic countries. If the politics of nursing has been accepted in principle, it is now timely to act upon the rhetoric and promote change and state that if you are not with us, you must be against us.

## WHERE HAS NURSING COME FROM?

The notion of nurses as the doctors' handmaidens is as deeply entrenched as is the gender identification of male doctors and female nurses. The stereotype of a nurse as an average intelligence female nurturant follower persists (Lumby and Zetler 1990). Whilst it does, nurses' aspirations to have caring recognized as being as important as curing are unlikely to be achieved. Indeed, much of the development of the nurse's role (the extended and expanded role of nursing) might be a feature of medical paternalism and dominance rather than assertion of the professional status of nursing. Lawrence Dopson (1984), writing about a symposium on nursing history, reports Fannie Storr, the Director of Nurse Education at Gloucester, showing that the 'extended role' is not new. 'In 1763, Mrs Taylor was paid 3d (<1p) for bleeding a patient. It was less than a doctor would be paid.' He further reports Miss Storr's beliefs that doctors' main criterion in deciding whether to allow nurses an expanded role was: would it save them getting up at night? Perhaps she was correct in asserting that it was only when thermometers became cheap and recordings needed to be taken regularly that nurses were 'asked' to take this on. Generally nursing work is seen to be less valuable, 'her' work less pressing and 'her' opinions less worthy. Crane, cited in Chambliss (1996), suggests that to doctors, the nurses are there to carry out the physician's orders – with nursing as a sort of 'lesser medicine'.

Chambliss develops the concept of 'the patient as object' and suggests that much health care is depersonalized; 'one becomes the object of looking and talking'. Looking that is often invasive and frequently repeated and talking that is more often 'at' or 'to', rather than 'with'. This objectification will get worse if management (financial control), education and research are allowed to dominate caring. The 'caring for people' expectations of health care may not themselves be met by such a dominated system, let alone permit any 'caring for' to occur.

Dalley (1993) makes a clear distinction between 'caring for', as the practical tasks of tending to someone who is dependent which is more in line with society's expectations of masculine roles and functions, and 'caring about', which has a distinctly affective component and is much more closely associated with female social roles. Of course, it is necessary for all health-care professionals to combine these roles regardless of their gender to ensure we treat what the patient suffers. However, it would seem that, at present, much health care is dominated by caring for and is masculine. Nursing as therapy would therefore be seen as feminine as it is also concerned with caring about.

Nursing as a whole is still predominantly seen as an extension of natural women's work; nurturing and caring in a position of limited privilege (Salvage 1985), a position that is reinforced by the paternalism of the medical profession. Chambliss (1996) suggests that paternalism gives rise to a lack of respect which leads to universal resentment for nurses. Chambliss further illustrates this point by quoting the characterization of nurses as the 'physician extender', a cost-effective substitute in areas where there are not enough physicians. In part, the blame for this may be placed at the door of the numerous nurses who, in accepting nursing as inferior to medicine, try to enhance their own prestige by a drift towards medicine. This drift is seen in the enthusiasm for emergency room work, intensive therapy and interest in the pathophysiological aspects of health care.

Nursing also has the demands of being a 24-hour service in which the nurse 'comes and stays' while other professions and administrative staff 'come and go'. Because of this difference, 'visitors' to the clinical setting (doctors, administrators, other clinical professionals and 'loved ones', etc.), legitimately or not, leave, prescribe or dictate work for the nurse. This disruption and delegation is often undertaken in a manner which confirms the 'lower' status of nursing and increases the endless nature of nursing work. The opportunity for nurses to unite politically may also be inhibited by this never-ending nature of their work that, if left, will compromise patients and thereby themselves and their values.

The inequality of power between nurses and doctors can also extend to the plight of patients. 'Doctors are often wealthy, and nurses fairly well off. Patients, in contrast are disproportionately poor . . .' (Chambliss 1996). This contrast might equally apply to other aspects of social position and status. Doctors are more often middle aged, assertive and well educated, nurses younger, submissive and educated and patients older, dominated and often poorly educated. These stratifications are clearly not precisely defined and are an overgeneralization, but they may offer a great deal in explaining the hegemony that pervades health care.

Given that 90% of nurses are women and health-care industries are generally male dominated, the view of nursing as an extension of women's work is not surprising. This position is made worse by the working patterns of women (as nurses); 9% of UK nurses work part-time (Appleby and Brewins 1992) and many combine working as a nurse with significant child-rearing and domestic duties. The average career length for nurses is 8.5 years (Hancock 1989) and many choose to focus this upon bedside work, where their influence is less, rather than move to management or leader-ship roles (Jones 1985). Nurses are often able and indeed required to exert significant operational power, but often lack the position, status and authority to influence strategy, usually having to bow to medicine, politi-cians and administrators ('men in suits'), who have the power. There are fewer female role models in senior and authoritative positions to help reshape attitudes and promote confidence in women at all levels of nursing. In 1992 an initiative by the NHS Management Executive in the UK sought to promote women into senior posts, a move that would put women (nurses) in a position to enhance equitable health and social policy for themselves and their professions. However, such initiatives take a great deal of time to make a significant impact and do little for the majority of the workforce.

## THE CURRENT SITUATION – A CROSSROADS OR TURNING POINT?

> For many years we have heard that nursing is at the crossroads. Nursing never seems to get over being at a crossroads. Indeed, nursing has been at a crossroads many times, but instead of taking a new road, leaders in the profession always choose to continue bearing the burden of continuing to live out the subservient role . . . Nursing is no longer at a crossroads. It is at a turning point. (Ashley, quoted in Chine and Wheeler 1985)

Three major issues have impacted upon nurses and nursing as they approach the end of the millennium: new nursing work, changes in nurse education and the shifting focus of health-care needs and provision. Nurses have only partly brought these changes about themselves. Other profes-sions and economic influences have been responsible for much of the change that brings nursing to the turning point for a new future.

### The shifting focus of health-care needs and provision

The resurgence of socialist or new socialist governments in the UK (New Labour), in Europe and the Antipodes signals a move away from the capitalist focus on individualism that has dominated for many years. The shift in the relationship between the community, state and individual offers both an opportunity and the expectation that nursing and nurses will realign their status and practices.

Four major eras in health care, education and social structures within societies have existed this century. In the UK before 1945, the state did little and the community provided (or in many cases did not!). Post-1945 saw the arrival of the welfare state with health care, social care and education for all. Post-1979 saw Thatcher's celebration of the individual as a means to cut escalating costs and unwieldy bureaucracies. Her major health-care reforms came at a time when, in her own words, society ceased to exist. The final era arising in the mid-1990s came as more people realized there are more losers than winners in most competitions. The new era is epitomized in the work of Amitai Etzioni who first used the term 'communitarianism' (Etzioni 1995). His work reasserts the values of collective function and an awareness of interdependence and mutuality. This shift towards a less competitive society comes at a time when demands for health care are at unprecedented levels. This is a result of flourishing technological advances, ever-expanding health-care expectations from the public and unprecedented levels of health-care spending.

Ferguson (1980) uses the metaphor of Humpty Dumpty to suggest how change might arise. 'All the king's horses and all the king's men could not put Humpty together again – so why didn't they ask the queen?' It must be time for new solutions if all the old ones have failed. It would be profound folly merely to do more of the same if that is not working! Changes in health-care provision and delivery will be essential to meet the changes in society and health-care need.

Alain Enthoven, the Stanford University professor who inspired Margaret Thatcher to reform the NHS, is now suggesting that Britain could manage on a quarter of its current number of hospital beds. O'Sullivan (1996) reports that much of the work undertaken by doctors could be undertaken by nurses and he further notes that by the year 2000, the US could reduce by 25% its number of doctors (150,000) if best practice were followed. In New Zealand reforms designed to curb public spending 'excesses' have led to highly innovative measures to ensure that health-care spending is focused on effective practice. This clearly brings under the spotlight the friction that seems to be inevitable between doctors, administrators, politicians and all other health-care professions if health-care industries are to turn their attention truly to the needs of their customers. The centre of health care is still strongly dominated by medicine although many initiatives have tried to put politicians or administrators in its place. Nursing must try to resist the temptation of merely substituting one hegemony for another and instead 'take sides' with the consumers of health care.

Nurses have recognized the inadequacy of the medical diagnosis as the primary directive of nursing need (Tierney 1984) and the tradition of the recent past to focus nursing on disease and task rather than the patient. It is now timely to apply this principle more widely and build on such initiatives as community psychiatric nurses, midwifery-led maternity care and 'hospital at home', all approaches to care that illustrate new nursing work, a concept discussed later in this chapter.

Steiner and Vaughan (1996), in their ground-breaking work on 'intermediate care', promote a new term but not a new concept. Intermediate care focuses upon support, nurturing and education of people (often the domain of nursing) and not primarily upon medical needs. Their model of care is holistic and emphasizes home care for a large number of individuals as well as an in-between service. However, such initiatives, which will inevitably promote nursing as therapy, will only succeed if much of the current health-care politics is overturned, in particular, the domination by medical precedence of much health-care activity and its gate-keeping role. These initiatives may also offer a creative solution to the difficulties of the 'bed-blocking' patients that Ham (1996) identifies, as well as providing the primary point of health care for many patients. Intermediate care would offer the nurse a role as an equally important member of a multidisciplinary team that focuses on people's needs.

### New nursing work

... the nurse's primary responsibility is to those people who require nursing care. (ICN 1973)

However, here lies a major problem; what is nurses' work? Certainly, any return to the days when medicine delegated to nurses aspects of its own role that it no longer wished to retain, must be resisted if the central tenet of the ICN is to be preserved. In the UK, the creativity of the UKCC in both its Code of Conduct (UKCC 1992a) and Scope of Practice documents (UKCC 1992b) offers nurses the widest possible remit for practice, the only proviso being that the practice should serve the patient's best interests and that appropriate training has been received. The notion of 'new nursing work', to replace the somewhat confusing and unhelpful terms of 'extended' and 'expanded' roles of the nurse, has led to a number of initiatives that clearly represent political as well as professional statements.

Nurse prescribing, albeit limited at this time to pilot sites of community nurses or within the confines of local protocols, is clearly an indicator of a major shift in professional power. The emergence of clinical nurse specialists and nurse practitioners has not happened without a struggle and there is still much to done given the major policy change they represent. Nursing beds and nurse-led services are still few in numbers but are evidence of a shift in power that offers an excellent opportunity for nursing to establish itself as a therapy. Griffiths and Evans (1995) offer a valuable insight into the provision of a nurse-led inpatient service in the UK. Their summary of the evaluations of the early moves towards this type of service suggests that they have great promise with regard to care outcomes and nursing as therapy. It is however, interesting to note that no explanation is given as to why Beeson ward in Oxford is now closed as a nurse-led service. Might we speculate that it was before its time and was too much of a political threat to medicine to be allowed to continue? Or perhaps when it started to succeed rather than fail, it had to be closed for fear of the revolution spreading?

Midwives have used their position of autonomy in the management of maternity care as a lever for independence from nursing. However, this status of autonomy is now increasingly adopted by community nurses, clinical nurse specialists and individual practitioners who all demonstrate a shift in power towards nursing self-determination as opposed to being a subset of medicine.

### Changes in nurse education

Changes in nurse education, in terms of both education processes and products, help to explain the political power basis of nursing as well as the changes that have occurred to that position. The level and type of educational attainment is one of the determinants in increasing the confidence with which nurses participate in policy determination (Albarran 1995).

The Wood Report into nurse education was the first to propose the separation of education from service (Clay 1987), but its visionary views were accepted by neither the government or the profession (or at least its leaders). Up to this point nurse-training programmes were essentially low-cost, low-profile enterprises that produced nurses whose most important skill was obedience. This preparation may well have played a major role in hindering the development and changes that nursing required to enable it to assert itself politically. The control of schools of nurse 'training' by the matrons and directors of nursing service persisted until 1969 when the new syllabus moved to a more educational process that required some independence from service needs. Of particular note, it was not until 1970 in the UK that the first part-time course for mature students was introduced. Prior to this, the intake had been predominantly of young single women.

It was not until the Nurses Act (1979) that the door opened on wide-scale reform of nurse education in the UK with the mandate '... to establish and improve the standards of training and professional conduct for nurses, midwives and health visitors'. Execpt for a number of pilot schemes and individual innovations, over 40 years of debate about nurse training culminated in the emergence of Project 2000 (UKCC 1986). This was seen very much as a dilution of the complete separation into higher education that Dr Harry Judge had recommended (Judge 1985). However, it did allow the emergence of the concept of the knowledgeable doer, the nurse charged with developing a questioning attitude. It also promoted educational methods that conferred learner status on all involved in education, the students and tutorial staff all adopting a lifelong learning, enquiring mind, a fundamentally different political stance. These educational changes challenged the status quo to such an extent that the energy to further knowledge by systematic investigation (research) became a feature of nursing's professional behaviour. Furthermore, the UK has also adopted the mandatory ongoing education of all practitioners that is a feature of most of the nurses in the developed world (UKCC 1990).

My own nurse training led to a state registration in nursing which was portrayed as a lifelong passport to the world of nursing. Against today's educational programmes, this training might not even get academic credit for the first year of a baccalaureate or Project 2000 higher education diploma. My training was also a manifestation of nursing as a suppressed 'profession': we stood when doctors entered the lecture room, most of the learning was memory based (and assessed) and respectful obedience was the main vehicle to success.

The move into higher education is now completed in the UK, but this has brought with it additional political pressures. The educational establishments themselves, whilst welcoming the numbers of students that nursing has brought to a capitation-based system, have also sought to influence the education of nurses. The power within the senior hierarchy of the university sector must not be underestimated, especially as in a number of them, medicine ('the old adversary') is a powerfully established force. The new academic authority must also avoid the distinct risk of pushing nursing into academic excellence without ensuring practice excellence. Equally, pressure on nurse education arising from the system of negotiating contracts between the purchaser (service side) and providers via a consortium could once again place it at the mercy of powerful clinicians and directors of nursing ('matrons').

## NURSES AS POWERMONGERS!

On of the stereotypical images of the nurse as a battleaxe (Salvage 1985) portrays the side of nursing where the politics and power are not of the oppressed but of the oppressor. This oppression manifests itself in behaviour and attitudes that demean patients and fellow nurses and may of course be a backlash to the systematic oppression of the profession. However, this does not condone it.

Lancely (1985) identifies the use of controlling language by nurses, which may not be deliberate but remains a profound political stance of either domination or suppression. The use of terms such as 'dear', 'love' and 'old boy' exemplifies an overt political statement of power as does the automatic use of first names. This form of control was also widespread amongst nurses themselves. In my own nurse training (1971–1974), I was always addressed by trained nurses as 'student nurse' emphasizing my inferior status, a status confirmed by a uniform that clearly indicated my position in the hierarchy. The use of a belt buckle is an interesting external signal of authority from trained nurses that perhaps the whole wearing of a uniform represents. It is significant that in a number of the nurse-led services – health visiting, community psychiatric nursing, paediatric hospital at home and clinical nurse specialists – the wearing of uniforms has been abandoned.

Equally, the use of certain interpersonal behaviours is a manifestation of political control. Closed questions are a very efficient way of accumulating information but they also have the effect of asserting authority and preventing the patient articulating their real concerns. Keeping dialogue functional safeguards the nurse from identifying demanding emotional needs and, indeed, from using nursing as therapy.

In my own experiences as student nurse, I was subject to the distinct oppression of hierarchical working. Student nurses did not speak to ward sisters without first being spoken to and all work was prescribed by the 'workbook'. Even the provision of meal breaks was more of an order than an invitation. It was very much the sister's ward and you made beds, served meals and practised as she dictated, not according to any commonly agreed reasoning. This considerable power within nursing ward hierarchies has been the subject of much debate (Ogier 1982) and certainly the past ten years have seen remarkable flattening and more appropriate use of power. The ability of hierarchies to produce institutional control over patients' lives was first described by Goffman (1961) and controlling patients to a greater or lesser extent is often still a feature of nursing practice. This control manifests itself in a number of ways, from totally planning the patient's day to restricting visitors and excluding carers from providing or helping to provide patient care. I am sure that many of these organizational policies arise from ignorance or through unquestioning acceptance, rather than from malice. However, it remains the case that developed management systems that delegate authority and reject oppression, such as magnet hospitals (McCivre 1983) and primary nursing (Manthey 1980), are not fully established. Such, perhaps, is the power of the status quo.

## THE FUTURE – MASTER (*SIC*) OF OUR OWN DESTINY?

Trevor Clay (1987) dedicates his book on the power and politics of nursing '. . . to all those nurses who fought so many battles for the profession, and for those who will'. Such battles are the hallmark of the political struggle of individual nurses and the profession at large. He concludes his book by noting the pessimism about the possibilities of achieving change that is abroad in nursing. 'Too many nurses are willing to give up the fight, whether for education, pay or an extended role for nursing even before it has started'. In 1996, as the the downfall of 17 years of Conservative rule in the United Kingdom became more obvious, Niall Dickson (1996) predicted an opportunity for nursing, midwifery and health visiting to create a more equitable distribution of power between professions and to develop new models of care. He went as far as to suggest that changes in the NHS could lead to nurses setting up in practice and employing salaried doctors!

Nursing as therapy is not about domination of patients any more than it requires domination of other professional groups to secure it. It is about equity and effectiveness, about ensuring that all parties have an equal say and that the best care is provided because it is efficacious, not because its practitioners dominate. In the process of becoming familiar with how power and politics are interlinked, nurses have the potential to demonstrate how the caring nature of nursing can also make the whole political process less combative.

So when Dr Mahler (1985), the Director General of the WHO, states: 'If millions of nurses in a thousand different places articulate the same ideas and convictions . . . and come together as one force then they could act as a power house for change', he throws out a remarkable challenge and a curt reminder. Power can corrupt and strength can come from unity. Nursing must rise to the challenges and become politically active individually and collectively and unite under common banners, both nationally and internationally. In doing so, it can demonstrate not conflict but collaboration in health care, that manifests itself in educational contracting, policy decisions, service delivery and interpersonal skills. How this unity should be achieved has already been the subject of debate (Albarran 1995). Whether it is professional or trade union unity matters little, it is unity that is needed, locally, nationally and internationally. Until our internal divisions are set aside and a common philosophy on the role of nursing in health-care policy is agreed, nursing may continue to be a political lightweight that, in the face of the overwhelming power of medicine, administration (government) and now education, will not only fail to meet its own aspirations but ultimately those of its patients.

Jo Anne Ashley (1978) points out that nursing has long been an industry that experiences the industrial alienation and economic domination that creates the dehumanization and disintegration of health-care systems. Her views echo the rhetoric of revolution and, for example, her identification of nursing consultants as the petit bourgeois clearly indicates her Marxist affiliation. This is not to say the solution lies in radical politics but it is noteworthy that Tom Peters (1994) says, 'Eradicate change from your vocabulary . . . substitute revolution'. Traditionally, political action by nurses was considered inappropriate, partly as a result of its trade union basis (Salvage 1985). The view that political agitation is incongruent with caring and the development of nursing as an aspiring profession (Jolley 1989) now has to be challenged if the future is to be secured. The adoption of the neo-Marxist ideology of Habermas (1985) arises elsewhere in this book (Chapter 2) and also, for example, in the curricula at the Deakin School of Nursing in Australia. Habermas is unequivocal in striving for a society where social differences and capitalism do not dominate. Nursing as therapy strives for a situation where the only domination is the needs of the customers and this will necessitate a call not to arms but to political awareness and struggle. In doing so, a win-win, collaborative solution to conflict may represent a novel solution but is a realistic goal.

This rise to power will occur in a world where health-care provision is inevitably rationed (Ham 1996). It is likely that national committees to advise governments on priority setting, such as now exists in New Zealand will emerge in other countries and it is vital that nursing is seen as a key player in this debate in its own right and not as an appendage of another profession (medicine). Only then can the full potential and aspirations of nursing as therapy be realized, to the benefit of economists, the profession and most importantly our customers.

## REFERENCES

Albarrran, J. (1995) Should nurses be politically aware? *British Journal of Nursing*, **4** (8), 461–465.

Appleby, J. and Brewins, L. (1992) Profile of a profession. *Nursing Times*, **88** (4), 24–27.

Ashley, J. A. (1978) Foundations for scholarship: historical research in nursing. *Advances in Nursing Science*, **1** (1), 25–36.

Bilton, T., Bennett, K., Jones, P., Sheard, K. and Stanworthy, M. (1981) *Introductory Sociology*, Macmillan, London.

Chambliss, D. (1996) *Beyond Caring*, University of Chicago Press, Chicago.

Chine, P. and Wheeler, C. (1985) Feminism and nursing. *Nursing Outlook*, **33** (2), 74–77.

Clay, T. (1987) *Nurses: Power and Politics*, Heinemann Nursing, London.

Cormack, D. (1990) Collective assertiveness, in *Developing Your Nursing Career*, (ed. D. Cormack), Chapman and Hall, London, pp. 270–281.

Dalley, G. (1993) The ideological foundations of informal care, in *Nursing Art and Science*, (ed. A. Kitson), Chapman and Hall, London.

Dickson, N. (1996) Paper prospects. *Nursing Times*, **92** (44), 56.

Dopson, L. (1984) The cut-throat world of nursing politics – 19th century style. *Nursing Times*, **80**, 19–20.

Ellis, J. and Hartley, C. (1988) *Nursing in Today's World*, Lippincott, Philadelphia.

Etzioni, A. (1995) *The Spirit of Community*, Fontana, London.

Ferguson, M. (1980) *The Aquarian Conspiracy*, Tarcher, Los Angeles.

Goffman, E. (1961) *Asylums*, Penguin, Harmondsworth.

Griffiths, P. and Evans, A. (1995) *Evaluation of a Nursing-Led In-patient Service: An Interim Report*, King's Fund Centre, London.

Habermas, J. (1985) Civil disobedience: litmus test for the democratic constitutional state. *Berkeley Journal of Sociology*, **30** (95), 116.

Ham, C. (1996) *Public, Private or Community: What Next for the NHS?* Demos, London.

Hancock, C. (1989) Women, power and public life. *Nursing Standard*, **4** (18), 9.

Henderson V. (1987) Foreword in, *Nurses: Power and Politics* (T. Clay), Heinemann Nursing, London.

Hewison, A. (1994) The politics of nursing: a framework for analysis. *Journal of Advanced Nursing*, **20**, 1170–1175.

Holmes, C. (1991) Theory: where are we going and what have we missed along the way? in *Towards a Discipline of Nursing* (eds G. Gray and R. Pratt), Churchill Livingstone, Melbourne.

ICN (1973) *International Code of Nursing Ethics*, International Congress of Nurses, Geneva.

Jolley, M. (1989) The professionalization of nursing: the uncertain path, in *Current Issues in Nursing* (eds M. Jolley and P. Allen), Chapman and Hall, London, pp. 1–22.

Jones, M. (1985) Too political. *Nursing Mirror*, **160** (20), 16.

Judge, H. (1985) *Commission on Nurse Education: The Judge Report*, RCN, London.

Lancely, A. (1985) Use of controlling language in the rehabilitation of the elderly. *Journal of Advanced Nursing*, **10**(2), 125–135.

Lumby, J. and Zetler, J. (1990) *The Image of the Nurse – 1890s or 1990s?* RCN Australia, Sydney.

Mahler, H. (1985) *WHO Features*, WHO, Geneva.

Manthey, M. (1980) *The Practice of Primary Nursing*, Blackwell, London.

McCivre, M. (1983) *Magnet Hospital! Attraction and Retention of Professional Nurses*, American Academy of Nurses, Kansas City.

McMahon, R. and Pearson, A. (1991) *Nursing as Therapy*, Chapman and Hall, London.

Ogier, P. (1982) *An Ideal Sister*, RCN, London.

O'Sullivan, J. (1996) Is the NHS safe under Dr Blair's team? *The Independent*, October 30th, p16.

Pearson, A. (1991) Taking up the challenge: the future for therapeutic nursing, in *Nursing as Therapy* (eds R. McMahon and A. Pearson), Chapman and Hall, London, pp. 192–210.

Peters, T. (1994) *The Tom Peters Seminar*, Macmillan, London.

Rogge, M. 1987 Nursing and politics: a forgotten legacy. *Nursing Research*, **361**, 26–30.

Salvage, J. (1985) *The Politics of Nursing*. Heinemann Nursing, Oxford.

Salvage, J. (1992) A European perspective. *Nursing*, **5** (6), 14–16.

Steiner, A. and Vaughan, B. (1996) *Intermediate Care*, a discussion paper arising from the King's Fund Seminar, 30th October, King's Fund, London.

Stewart, N. (1987) How to raise your political awareness. *Occupational Health*, **39** (1), 10–14.

Tierney, A. (1984) A response to Professor Mitchell's, 'A simple guide to the nursing process'. *British Medical Journal*, **288**, 835–838.

UKCC (1986) *Project 2000: A New Preparation for Practice*, United Kingdom Central Council, London.

UKCC (1990) *The Post-Registration Education and Practice Project*, United Kingdom Central Council, London.

UKCC (1992a) *Code of Professional Conduct*, United Kingdom Central Council, London.

UKCC (1992b) *Scope of Professional Practice*, United Kingdom Central Council, London.

Watson, J. (1990) The moral failure of the patriarchy. *Nursing Outlook*, **38** (2), 62–66.

# Taking up the challenge: the future for therapeutic nursing

# 14

Alan Pearson

## INTRODUCTION

The preceding chapters all, in some way, define, explore and develop the concept of therapeutic nursing and describe its performance in action. The purpose of this final chapter is somehow to bring all of this together and to outline some pointers for the future. The task is both daunting and exciting, for the future is something about which we dream, but not something which we can accurately predict.

Since the publication of the first edition of *Nursing as Therapy* in 1991, enormous changes have occurred in health-care delivery in Western countries and a 'market' orientation has developed a strong hold on those who have power over health services. The resulting 'commodification' of health care – where health care has become a product to package, promote and sell – seems at odds with the view that values the human, subjective component of nursing. Although therapeutic nursing remains very much a feature of only British and European nursing (it has not achieved much of a profile in North America, Asia or Australasia), it is interesting to observe that the concepts it embodies continue to be valued and to be highly visible in contemporary publications in most countries. In spite of the growing commercialization of health systems and the technologizing of health-care interventions, the focus of nursing on what it means to be human seems to still hold a position of central importance in an increasingly materialistic, scientific world. This chapter will set out some of the basic assumptions inherent in therapeutic nursing; historically review the evolution of nursing as therapy; outline arguments which suggest that the therapeutic potential of nursing has been devalued; and offer suggestions for the development of nursing as a therapeutic activity for the future.

## THERAPEUTIC NURSING: BASIC ASSUMPTIONS

The use of the term 'therapeutic nursing' evolved from the work of Alfano (1969), Hall (1966) and Tiffany (1977). All three were cited by Pearson (1983) and their ideas were extensively developed in the establishment of Britain's first nursing development unit at Burford Community Hospital (Pearson 1985, 1988, 1992) and the subsequent setting up of the Oxford Nursing Development Unit (Pearson 1992). These ideas were developed further by Ersser (1988), McMahon (1988) and Muetzel (1988). The Burford initiative focused on Tiffany's notion of creating an environment where the nurse is the 'chief therapist', rather than the maintainer of order which enables other health workers to apply their therapies, and on Alfano's assertion that the nurse who acts therapeutically '... sees her role not as an intervener or interpreter, but as a caring person and teacher'. Hall (1966) posited that nurses alone engage in intensely intimate activity in their professional role and that this gives rise to opportunities for human closeness which can be used to therapeutic effect. Through concentrating on the notion that nursing as caring is a therapy in its own right, the Burford participants began to think and talk about therapy as a skilled, professional activity which has a positive effect on people in as much as it leads to the achievement of health or healing. This early thinking stemmed from Alfano's (1971) distinction between professional-orientated nursing (or therapeutic nursing) and task-orientated nursing.

The writings of early civilizations refer to nursing and throughout the ages there appears to have always been a group of people engaged in nursing, although they were not always referred to as nurses. In the Middle Ages, nursing took on the cloak of altruism and many of its practitioners (either religious men and women or knights) were the highly educated of society. Nineteenth century reforms in nursing developed an opening for middle-class and working-class women to enter a workforce which was respectable and which held out romanticized opportunities. In the 20th century, nursing has espoused the new religion of science and taken on the trappings of functionalism and objectivity.

## NURSING AS CARING

Throughout all of this, however, nurses and the communities they served have been cognizant, to a greater or lesser degree, of the core of nursing – the provision of care or nurturance.

Whilst nurses can never claim to be the only health professionals who care, they can claim to be the only group whose central concern is that of human caring *per se*. Care and caring are complex concepts which beg for further exploration, yet are frequently seen as ordinary, simple and easy to put into practice.

Dunlop (1986), in her article 'Is a science of caring possible?', suggests that care can be interpreted as a deep involvement and engagement in the world which is central and necessary to any human activity. Care is seen as a global, human concept in which the care for things (concern) and caring for others (solicitude) make human existence meaningful. Care has the same root as the word 'compassion', both deriving from the Celtic word *cari* meaning 'to cry out with, to enter into the suffering'. The words 'care' and 'compassion', then, are exactly the same. Commenting on this common meaning of care and compassion, Nouwen (1980) asserts that nurses should see care as their central mission and says that, 'Out of care, cure can be born ... Care broadens your vision; care makes you see around you; care makes you aware of possibilities'.

True caring is based on an attitude of nurturing, of helping another to grow. For the purposes of this chapter, then, in referring to care or caring, I am talking about this broad, global, human concept of investing oneself in the experience of another so as to become a participant in that person's experience. This concept of caring absolutely demands an involved stance and does not, according to Benner (1985):

> ... seek to control or master but to facilitate and uncover the possi-
> bilities inherent in the situation and the person. Caring provides
> empowerment [not control. Indeed] technological self understanding
> causes a devaluation and misunderstanding of caring.

The need to place caring as a central concept in nursing has never been greater yet the caring components of nursing have become devalued and are seen as the least sophisticated and subordinate to the therapeutic interventions of doctors and paramedical therapists.

## THE DEVALUING OF NURSING AS CARING

### Nursing and caring as women's work

Throughout its history, nursing has fundamentally been concerned with human caring. Caring itself is also at the root of human history.

Because of the overwhelming dominance of a masculine, objective world view in this century, human caring has been associated with womanhood and has been persistently and consistently both publicly devalued yet privately desired. Colliere (1986) argues that, because of this, care is publicly invisible and that those who occupy themselves with it within the workforce are socially unconsidered, powerless and marginalized in terms of their perceived usefulness to society. Reverby (1987) explores this even further. In her exposé of nursing and caring as women's work, she highlights the dilemma of altruism (which is believed by the world to be the basis of nursing and caring) on the one hand and autonomy (believed by the world to be the basis of rights and thus the possession of legitimate power) on the other.

Colliere (1986) asserts that '. . . care remains invisible, priceless in health institutions as well as at home', whilst Reverby argues that caring is universally acknowledged as good and necessary, but that it is overly associated with altruism and in direct opposition to any notions of autonomy. She suggests that nurses need to 'create a new political understanding for the basis of caring and find ways to gain the power to implement it . . .', that nurses need '. . . power to practice altruism with autonomy'.

The development of nursing has been affected by the emergence of the women's movement and its political position today is closely linked with the status of women and the dominance of a masculine world view. Ashley (1976) argues that nursing has been unable to occupy the strong power base in health care that it should have because of two interrelated factors.

1  Contemporary nursing is seen as a female occupation and as legitimately 'women's work'
2  The health-care system in itself is paternalistic and this has suppressed the development of nursing.

Whilst the status of the individual and groups relates to a number of factors, gender is frequently cited as a significant issue in nursing's current and potential power base. As Vance *et al.* (1985) say:

> Feminist women and nurses have frequently experienced an uneasy relationship. Much of the energy in the women's movement has been directed toward moving into nontraditional fields of study and work. Nursing has been seen, therefore, as one of the ultimate female ghettos from which women should be encouraged to escape.

There has been and still is a tendency for nursing, despite the rise in feminist thinking and activity, to espouse masculine values and to attempt to masculinize its practice and structures in order to gain power. Espousing masculine ideology appears to have been the strategy for development in the latter half of this century.

In the UK, Nuttal (1983) reports that although in 1983 only 20% of registered nurses were male, 43.8% of district nursing officers and 50.5% of directors of nursing education were men. This may partly be a result of the limitations imposed on women by the community in terms of its prerequisites for promotion – unbroken records of employment, full-time commitment and putting work before all else. But it may also be partly due to a rejection by nurses – both male and female – of feminine, subjective thinking and rationale. Has nursing quite deliberately pursued a masculine, objective identity in order to achieve power in a scientific world? Clay (1987) suggests that: 'The opposite view, of course, is that rather than imbuing a female profession with male values, we should be working to assert, develop and generate confidence in nursing's "femaleness"'.

The apparent distance maintained between women nurses and the women's movement is therefore difficult to understand. This is especially so when one considers Mason and McCarthy's (1985) discussion on the politics of patient care. Power in nursing, like power in general, is thus exercised from a position of legitimacy, authority, professionalism and social unity.

## Traditional notions of power and gender

Colliere (1986) suggests that because of the underestimation and devaluation of women, and therefore of care provided largely by women, nursing is part of a dominator-dominated system, where largely women nurses are dominated by largely male doctors and administrators. The powerlessness and subservience of nurses is seen therefore as directly attributable to sex or gender.

Game and Pringle (1983), in their description of the sexual division of labour in health care, argue that the symbolism of doctor/father, nurse/mother is the norm and that these lead to highly sexualized power relationships. They point out that women as the majority of health-care providers (74.96%) are dominated by a male minority and that health care is characterized by obvious and ruthless sexism.

Because care is associated with women (which, in turn, denies the presence and status of large numbers of men who engage in caring activities in the home and at work) and women hold less power in society, it is devalued and has not until now been recognized as a subtle and powerful therapeutic force in health and healing.

## Re-examining gender, power and nursing

Throughout history people have been nursed by both women and men; the caring practices of those whom we would now call nurses have been highly valued by communities and nursing has been seen to be extraordinarily effective. The historical role of committed, wholehearted caring (read nursing) on the battlefield, in the sickroom and the hospital is one which cannot be dismissed.

The rendering of nursing and human caring as invisible is probably a relatively recent phenomenon. It is also not something which emerged overnight, but is probably more a product of the evolving history of Western social order. I and my colleagues Professor Bev Taylor and Cathy Coleborne were interested in exploring how nursing's history has shaped the status and nature of nursing work in Australia in the 1990s. We were not wholly surprised to find that the ambiguity which surrounds nursing appears to make it possible to both value it highly as 'goodly, kindly purist' and to see it as something which is common-sensical, unclever and an ambiguous role in health care. Furthermore, the ambiguous nature of contemporary nursing work bears a striking resemblance to nursing's state in Victoria, Australia, (and, we suspect, elsewhere) 140 years ago.

## The historical development of contemporary nursing in colonial Victoria

The primary focus of our historical study (Pearson *et al.* 1997, Pearson and Taylor 1996) was the nature of nursing and non-nursing work in Victorian hospitals from settlement to the last quarter of the 19th century. For the purposes of the study, activity which is grounded in the giving of direct, comprehensive care incorporating the meeting of physical, emotional and medically related needs of hospital patients was regarded as legitimate nursing work.

The role of the nurse in health care has been the subject of a debate which engages with the ambiguity about the role of the nurse, the boundaries of nursing work and the question of the status of women and men within the profession. A historical perspective was required in the study in order to understand how the nursing role evolved and was socially constructed in early Australia. Because Australia was essentially an outpost of the United Kingdom at that time, with strong links to continental Europe, it was also thought that this study could throw some light on how contemporary nursing has been shaped historically in both Britain and Australia. A significant absence of accounts of nurses between 1840 and 1870 and a lack of comparative analysis of male and female roles in nursing care in this period led us to an examination which reveals some of the social, political and economic influences on the delineation of nursing work and the relevance of these factors to the current status of nursing.

Contemporary historical analyses of nursing in the 19th century fail to address a number of important issues concerning the development of the nursing role. The study addressed a number of these previously unexplored areas. It involved the collation of the scattered references to the origin and development of the role and function of the nurse in this early period. The scattered information available about the roles, duties and functions of female and male nursing staff in this period reflects an ambiguous relationship between the roles and functions of the respective caregivers and demands clarification.

It also examined the portrayal of nursing in hospital histories, in annual reports and in contemporary literature. In addition, nursing, medical and public health journals, government policy documents and literary writings of or about the period were surveyed.

The study was conducted from a sociocultural and historical perspective using an interpretive methodology of textual analysis and this gave rise to a number of additional questions as the study progressed.

- How are nurses and how is nursing represented in accounts of the hospital, in Australian history and in women's history?
- How are these representations limited?
- How accurate are these accounts? (There is some evidence, for instance, that claims about the 'dissolute' character of nurses can be substantiated, but what about the other aspects of nursing activity not examined by historians?)

To envisage and write a new nursing history of the years before 1870 was to examine a particular historical view of the nurse and a 19th-century stereotype. By employing the critical categories of gender, class and work it was possible to reassess the assumptions about the nurse in history. This meant examining the historically specific social constructions of work for women and men and thus an examination of labour history was important. It was significant that histories in Australia, from hospital histories to women's history and histories of work, had neglected the nurse before 1900.

The introduction of female nurses following a Royal Commission established to consider this very move in the early 1860s and early moves to professionalize and train nurses before the popularity of Florence Nightingale emerged as a significant issue for 19th-century hospitals. We selected this as the central problem for consideration. Related to it were the decline of the male nurse and the emerging model of caring, linked to a stereotype of femininity which conceptualized caring for the sick as a female duty, role and special skill.

Current historical analyses of nursing in the 19th century failed to address a number of important issues concerning the development of the nursing role in Australia in general and in Victoria in particular. The study addressed a number of these previously unexplored areas. The study sought, then, to identify what nursing work was like in the period studied in order to understand the evolution of the nursing role in Victoria. It was hoped that this would lead to the development of some insight into the evolution of the social construction of nursing. By understanding the way in which perceptions of the nurse's role and the nature of nursing work were created through sociocultural forces, insights can be gained into the similar norms that pervade current debate.

**Setting the scene – nursing in Victoria in the mid 1800s**

An analysis of the early literature on nursing revealed ambiguities in relation to what was and what was not legitimate nursing work and which workers did and did not nurse patients. Durdin (1991), in her book *They Became Nurses,* describes the 'nursing' role and functions of the wardsman Charles Owers and his wife at the Naracoorte Hospital in South Australia.

**Mr Owers**: At 6 a.m. I go and look at my patients. Sometimes I have to give an aperient and test their water. Assist bedridden patients to wash, sometimes make their beds. Breakfast 7.30. Take tray of special diets to patients. Make up beds for bedridden patients. Sometimes dress very large wounds before the doctor comes. He comes from 10.30 to 11.30. Attend the doctor and take his instructions. Before the doctor comes I sweep passage and surgery. Dinner at 12 noon. After dinner follow doctor's instructions mixing medicine, attending to outdoor patients. I scrub the big ward, passage, surgery and bathroom once a week, sometimes oftener. Clean all the windows once a week, sometimes oftener. After dinner occupy time rolling up bandages, making lotions, ointments.

**Mrs Owers**: Commence work at 5.30–6. If female patients, go into their ward to see how they passed the night. If medicine wanted, give it to them. The night nurse sleeps in the ward. Never leave a bad patient until 10 or 11 p.m. Make my own bed and the Secretary's. (The Secretary lives at the hospital.) Make female patients' beds. Breakfast at 7.30. Clean out my own rooms. Make all the hospital linen. Cover all mattresses that require covering. Instruct the girl what to get for meals. Take all stores from the tradesman and check them. Dinner at 12 noon. Do all sewing and mending. Tea 5 p.m. In any cases which the doctor may have ordered give cocoa or milk at 9 p.m. Receive visitors and take them through the ward, sometimes a good many. I receive instructions from the doctor regarding visitors to patients. I attend the doctor when visiting female patients. I find my own sewing machine. I am chiefly employed at sewing between dinner and tea. I look after my fowls. I assist in the washing while the cook is getting breakfast. The hospital has a washing machine and wringer. Change the patients' beds once a week, sheets and pillow cases. In special cases every day. All patients are supposed to be in bed at 9.

Because this account clearly shows that in some duties there is an overlap of the nursing roles between male and female staff, it supports one of the dominant issues which emerged from the study: that nursing work was not the exclusive domain of those workers titled 'nurse' who were at that time largely female. Moreover, in other aspects it also reveals that though specific nursing duties were allocated to male and female staff, males tended to focus on nursing work as it is construed currently and females were involved in nursing work and sewing, laundry and kitchen duties.

Whittaker (1972), in her book *A Hospital in Wangaratta*, provides an account of the role of the matron as well as revealing that the head wardsman attended female patients. Whittaker draws attention to the significant point that the wardsmen were charged with observing and reporting to the surgeon the condition of patients and changes in their symptoms. In examining the duties of the wardsmen and the nurses, it seems that both engaged in nursing work and that there were no distinctions to be drawn about their respective caregiving to male and female patients. Such examples as illustrated in the books of Whittaker and Lang led us to query the exclusiveness of the image of 'female' nursing as angelic and nurturing. The origins of such an image do not appear to stem from the reality of an emerging Australian nursing profession and are more likely to be related to the work of reformers in Britain, particularly Florence Nightingale.

Florence Nightingale occupies a particular and special place in the historical discourse of nursing in Australia. When she is treated critically, she is still a figure of importance precisely because she represents the shift in nursing practices around the late 19th century. Nightingale is an icon, a symbol invoked when the discussion turns – as it inevitably does – to the training of nurses in hospitals. Undoubtedly, her work influenced change in hospitals. But when she is used by historians as a symbol of the transition from untrained nurses to more efficient nursing practices, the implication is that she caused the change to occur. Australia, however, has a different history. Certainly, some of Nightingale's work, through Lucy Osburn, had an impact in the colonies. Yet there is evidence that change was occurring prior to this in some hospitals and certainly that the ideal of efficient nursing was prominent before it became widespread. The historical space of nursing before Nightingale is filled only by stereotypes of the 'dissolute nurse' and no investigation of nursing practices, good and bad, is conducted.

Common in the general histories of nursing is a prototypical account of nursing the sick from the 'ancient world' to the 19th century. The 19th century is championed as the age of scientific discovery, reform and training. However, the history of nursing is as patchy and inadequate as many histories which are perceived to be part of the enterprise first described as 'women's history' and which are now part of a wider project to investigate gender. Australian histories of women and histories of labour raise the important questions of professionalization, the status of women's work and the problem of class. Yet these histories also neglect the early history of nursing and mostly make sweeping assessments of the hospital nurse, all claiming that she or he was merely a domestic servant and an incompetent carer of the sick. It is more through the neglect by historians to reflect upon the actual work, experience and practice of the hospital nurse than any solid belief in this view that these statements are made.

It appeared to us, then, that what was required was some investigation of the critical analysis of writing nursing history and, together with this, a thorough look at early nursing practices. Game and Pringle (1983) have married sociological theories with historical perspectives. Their text *Gender at Work* is useful (even though it has been superseded by a new generation of feminist historical inquiry) precisely because it concentrates in part on the issue of nursing. Their perspective is also politically engaged; the model of 'conflict and resistance' leads them to conclude that the main problem for women health-care workers is that female nurses are still seen as 'hand-maidens' and their struggle is still over divisions of work/labour and the hospital hierarchy, together with the space of the ward. Certainly, they get this right but elsewhere their work carries its own gendered bias:

> Nursing is a traditional women's occupation. We situate changes in nursing work in relation to the broader division of labour in the health industry ... there is a significant movement of men into the area, though not yet a masculinization of equivalent proportions. We consider the significance of the professionalization of nursing, that is, the various attempts to raise its status. One aspect of this has been the replacement of 'female' power structures (the dragon matron) with more 'masculine' notions of bureaucratic control.

Examination of the literature available led us to conclude that nursing in colonial Victorian hospitals prior to 1870 was conducted largely by male staff until some hospitals decided to increase the numbers of female staff. It was at this time that 'female power structures' (the metaphor of the family: doctor and matron set up as father and mother of a household) were introduced, usually in response to domestic crisis and disarray in hospital organization.

Further, we came to the view that this was not a 'female power structure' but a gendered model of organization which derives from patriarchal or masculinist power structures. (Game and Pringle do acknowledge this, but their use of gender as a concept is often ambiguous.)

The second major problem introduced by Game and Pringle is the question of what constitutes nursing work and this was the second dominant issue which emerged from the study. Florence Nightingale believed that nurses should not engage in 'non-nursing' tasks – 'to scour is a waste of power' – but how is this difference really defined? Certainly, when examining the primary source material this emerges as a significant problem. Dingwall *et al.* (1988) and others have suggested that it is important to recognize this difficult boundary and to 'find a way of differentiating between 'nursing work' and 'work done by nurses'". They point to kinds of nursing and the use of sources such as the regulations of infirmaries which can indicate to historians how work was imagined and idealized in the early hospital.

The study offered some illumination of nursing's current invisible position within the dominant discourses of contemporary health care. Briefly, it seems to us that the current devaluing of nursing and human caring as important components of health care arise, at least in part, out of a history which gendered nursing and caring and which created and perpetuated ambiguity in nursing work.

## Gender

Nursing work became gendered in the 1860s in Australia. Prior to that and contrary to current rhetoric on the origins and history of Australian nursing, nursing and caring were human work rather than women's work. (Which is hardly surprising given the preponderance of males in the population in these times.) The differentiation between nurses and wardsmen was clear only in respect of gender, except in cases in which workers were designated as 'male nurses'. The documented roles, responsibilities and behaviours of the female nurses and the wardsmen merged at times with the washerwomen, cooks and general hospital custodians. Accountability for actions was not clearly defined by managements and not uniformly enforced by doctors, in relation to what might be considered to be a part of nursing work. The blurring of roles and responsibilities led to conflicts, some of which were of a grave nature. The history of nursing work, therefore, as it is depicted in these accounts gives little support to the notion of female-dominated nursing or of a Nightingale model of nursing care in those early years in Victorian hospitals.

## The ambiguity of nursing work

There seems to be minimal differentiation between nursing and non-nursing work; however, some of the literature attempted to clarify what work nurses should not do, because of its connections to domestic work. The most frequent term used for non-nursing duties was 'scrubbing'. The term seems to refer to heavy domestic duties and it is used frequently in the report of the Royal Commission on Charitable Institutions, which argued for the elimination of scrubbing duties from the role of the nurse. This is typically expressed in the following exchange:

> You said you thought it was undesirable that any of the nurses should be called upon to do domestic work?
> Not scrubbing; not the heavy male nurses' work. I think you want to conserve the delicacy of touch of the woman and keep her in a position different from a servant.

This does not, however, exclude duties which may now be seen as domestic or non-nursing duties, as one respondent explained:

> I think a nurse should know how a room is to be kept clean and how to clean it, to make the patients' beds and attend to them generally; but I do not think they should do the menial work, such as using heavy scrubbers for the floor, and work of similar description.

It is clear that scrubbing floors, cleaning bathroom and lavatories were considered to be non-nursing work and that suitable work consisted of making beds, cleaning medicine glasses and giving food.

It can be seen from the literature that what constituted nursing and non-nursing work varied between institutions and within levels of nurses. Even though there was some discrimination in domestic tasks, such as scrubbing, the highest paid nurse, the matron, was given domestic duties of a supervisory nature which divorced her effectively from the direct care of patients and validated at the highest level the inherent domestic nature of nursing work.

These two issues were constantly identified throughout the study and are reflected still in the current discourse on nursing. The genderization of nursing and the ambiguity which surrounded the nursing role in the mid-1800s made it possible to decentralize nursing and caring in the health-care enterprise and we conclude that that continues to be so today.

Given this, it is intriguing to consider nursing's ancient lineage, its powerful role of generic human caring prior to the 19th century reforms in nursing and to compare this with the past 140 years. This makes me question whether nursing is merely babysitting clients while the real therapists (physicians, physiotherapists, etc.) practise their magic or whether nursing and human caring possess inherent healing potential. Are they merely supportive of medical and paramedical therapies or are they therapeutic in themselves? Furthermore, is nursing human work which draws on our understandings of each other as human beings or is it essentially women's work which is grounded in women's experience? These questions, amongst others, underpin the development of therapeutic nursing and our pursuit of them will lay the foundations on which to build a future.

## THE FUTURE

### A new era

A new era of nursing is now, I believe, in its beginnings. There have been gradual changes in world views held by society and nursing is beginning to demonstrate a shift away from its allegiance to a technical and task-orientated view towards the adoption of new values. Nursing has espoused, or so contemporary rhetoric suggests, a broader view of the person than that adopted by the biomedical model and a robust defence of the core values of therapeutic nursing. Though today's nurses are well versed in the use of biomedical technology, the basic premises of outcomes management, total quality management and other terms spawned by the purveyors of management-speak and the pursuit of customers out there in the 'marketplace', they are also firmly grounded in a view which sees practical, sensitive, intelligent caring as central to the healing enterprise.

Like nursing in the past, contemporary nursing is being influenced by and is responding to emerging world views and the perceived needs of the consumers which these views generate. High-quality health care is becoming valued in society as a whole and there is an upsurge of interest in holistic health care and complementary therapies. Within nursing, corresponding efforts to promote patient autonomy and the right to make informed choices are becoming evident and partnership between nurses and clients (as opposed to being directive) is beginning to be seen as legitimate and valued. Nurses and others are now also beginning to realize that such an orientation actually 'makes a difference' to recovery rates and healing for clients ... that nursing is a therapy as tangible and as effective as medical and paramedical therapies.

The rigorous pursuit of gendering of nursing, though rightly still a subject of interest and research, has been replaced by a view that nursing is a knowledge base and repertoire of skills which can be acquired by anyone – female or male – with the appropriate values and beliefs, through quality education.

## Towards the future

The promotion of therapeutic nursing is dependent upon developing knowledge and new understandings about nursing and generating changes in practice which these new understandings demand, preparing future nurses to view people as the owners of their own potential and utilizing political strategies to create a valuing of therapeutic nursing.

## Developing new knowledge and changing practice

Nursing needs to invest more in its research into the therapeutic effects of its practice and to use this research in a way which changes practice in reality. For the future, two major issues need to be pursued.

First, nursing units devoted to the provision of nursing as the primary therapy are now being established widely throughout the United Kingdom. Such units need to be established even more widely within different countries and cultures. Whilst the establishment of 'subacute care units' in North America and Australasia may well serve the purposes of the economic rationalists who control health systems, they systematically deny that the crucial component of such units is nursing. The establishment of nursing units serves a number of purposes. It:

- Asserts that nursing is indeed a therapy in its own right
- Creates an environment in which the unit can develop knowledge through its actions
- Provides a milieu for research and development.

Such activity will enhance the ability of nursing to build up its own substantive base and to move practice in all settings towards a therapeutic orientation.

Second, research itself needs to be a much greater feature of initiatives which foster therapeutic nursing. Politically, hard, quantifiable data are needed to demonstrate that nursing does make a difference in terms of outcomes. More importantly, however, much of nursing is too sophisticated and complex to be studied from a stance which holds that the truth can only be exposed through the statistical analysis of quantifiable data. Other stances which see subjective and qualitative approaches to research as legitimate paths in seeking knowledge are closer to nursing's orientation and may well uncover much more than politically acceptable 'scientific' studies. Such approaches, like nursing and caring, conflict with the hard, objective masculine view of the world. In developing new understandings and knowledge of nursing and in instituting desirable practice change, the setting up of nursing units and the pursuit of research utilizing a range of methodological approaches are essential to the future of therapeutic nursing.

### The preparation of future nurses

Education can play a pivotal role in supporting this new era of nursing. In terms of preparing future nurses, changes in nursing education offer considerable potential for empowering the new generation of nurses to meet future health needs. Higher education for nurses will not inevitably lead to positive development in itself, but the potential is most certainly there. The crucial variable lies in the design and offering of programmes which can best equip students with the categories of knowledge fundamental to the kind of nursing practice needed for the future.

Whilst the hospital schools of the past may have been accused of an overemphasis on practice and nursing service and an underemphasis on theoretical preparation, higher education may be accused in the future of an overemphasis on theory and an underemphasis on practice. In the drive to enhance nursing's theoretical underpinning, practice may be dismissed as non-theoretical and the fact that it is indeed a sophisticated intellectual pursuit which incorporates a variety of patterns of knowledge may be neglected. Education has both the capacity and responsibility to empower future nurses to draw on nursing's inheritance and to move forward into the emerging era of nursing by enabling students to acquire relevant categories of knowledge.

Building on nursing's past inheritance, contemporary nursing is, I believe, in an enviable position and is on the verge of what may be referred to as the liberating era of nursing. This era encompasses the context of a changing social relevance for nursing and changing world views and nursing education carries an awesome responsibility in supporting this era. I believe that a commitment to being involved in practice and health issues will help us to empower nursing graduates to meet future health needs of the population and help to further needed reforms in nursing service.

## CONCLUSION

This final chapter has attempted to overview the concept of therapeutic nursing; its evolution; the difficulties associated with developing its legitimacy in society; and the historical background to the current invisible position of nursing as a therapeutic force in health care. The future is truly a challenge. Challenge implies both exciting possibilities and obstacles and difficulties to be overcome. Guaranteeing a future for therapeutic nursing involves both of these. Bertrand Russell said in his autobiography: 'I experienced the delight of believing that the sensible world is real. Bit by bit, chiefly under the influence of physics, this delight has faded'. Maybe we need to be more sceptical about the view that the world is sensible and predictable and more hopeful, assertive and confident in our ability to show others that this is so.

## REFERENCES

Alfano, G. J. (1969) A professional approach to nursing practice. *Nursing Clinics of North America*, **4**(3), 487.

Alfano, G. J. (1971) Healing or caretaking – which will it be? *Nursing Clinics of North America*, **6**, 273.

Ashley, J. A. (1976) *Hospitals, Paternalism, and the Role of the Nurse*, Teachers' College Press, New York.

Benner, P. (1985) *From Novice to Expert*, Addison-Wesley, Menlo Park.

Clay, T. (1987) *Nurses, Power and Politics*, Heinemann, Oxford.

Colliere, M. F. (1986) Invisible care and invisible women as health care providers. *International Journal of Nursing Studies*, **23**(2), 95–112.

Dingwall, R., Rafferty, A. M. and Webster, C. (1988) *An Introduction to the Social History of Nursing*, Routledge, London.

Dunlop, M. (1986) Is a science of caring possible? *Journal of Advanced Nursing*, **2**, 661–700.

Durdin, J. (1991) *They Became Nurses: A History of Nursing in South Australia 1836–1980*, Sydney.

Ersser, S. (1988) Nursing beds and nursing therapy, in *Primary Nursing. Nursing in the Burford and Oxford Nursing Development Units*, (ed. A. Pearson), Croom Helm, London.

Game, A. and Pringle, R. (1983) *Gender at Work*, Allen and Unwin, Sydney.

Hall, L. E. (1966) Another view of nursing care and quality, in *Continuity of Patient Care: The Role of Nurses*, (eds M. Straub and K. Parker), Catholic University of America Press, Washington DC.

Mason, D. J. and McCarthy, A. M. (1985) The politics of patient care, in *Political Action Handbook for Nurses*, (eds D. J. Mason and S. W. Talbott), Addison-Wesley, Menlo Park.

McMahon, R. (1988) Primary nursing in practice, in *Primary Nursing. Nursing in the Burford and Oxford Nursing Development Units*, (ed. A. Pearson), Croom Helm, London.

Muetzel, P. A. (1988) Therapeutic nursing, in *Primary Nursing. Nursing in the Burford and Oxford Nursing Development Units*, (ed. A. Pearson), Croom Helm, London.

Nouwen, H. J. M. (1980) Reflections on compassion. Keynote address, Catholic Health Association of Canada.

Nuttal, P. (1983) Male takeover or female giveaway? . . . all the top jobs are going to men. *Nursing Times*, **79**(2), 10–11.

Pearson, A. (1983) *The Clinical Nursing Unit*, Heinemann, Oxford.

Pearson, A. (1985) Introducing new norms in a nursing unit and an analysis of the process of change. Unpublished PhD thesis, Department of Social Science and Administration, University of London, Goldsmith's College.

Pearson, A. (1988) *Primary Nursing: Nursing in the Burford and Oxford Nursing Development Units*, Croom Helm, London.

Pearson, A. (1992) *Nursing at Burford: a Story of Change*, Scutari Press, London.

Pearson, A. and Taylor, B. (1996) Gender and nursing in colonial Victoria. *International History of Nursing Journal* 2:1, 25–45.

Pearson, A., Taylor, B. and Coleborne, C. (1997) *The Nature of Nursing Work in Colonial Victoria, 1840–1870*, Deakin University Press, Geelong.

Reverby, S. (1987) A caring dilemma. Womanhood and nursing: an historical perspective. *Nursing Research*, **36**(1), 5–11.

Tiffany, D. H. (1977) Nursing organisational structure and the real goals of hospitals. Unpublished PhD thesis, Indiana University.

Vance, C. N., Talbott, S. W., McBride, A. B. and Mason, D. J. (1985) Coming of age: the women's movement and nursing, in *Political Action Handbook for Nurses*, (eds D. J. Mason and S. W. Talbott), Addison-Wesley, Menlo Park.

Whittaker, D. M. (1972) *A hospital in Wangaratta*, Committee of Management, Wangaratta District Hospital, Wangaratta, Victoria, Australia.

# Index

Page numbers printed in **bold** type refer to figures; those in *italic* to tables